A Foundation for Neonatal Care
A multi-disciplinary guide

A Foundation for Neonatal Care
A multi-disciplinary guide

Edited by

Michael Hall
Consultant Neonatal Paediatrician
University of Southampton

Alan Noble
Visiting Senior Lecturer in Physiology
University of Southampton

and

Susan Smith
Lecturer/Practitioner
School of Health Sciences
University of Southampton

Foreword by

Andrew R Wilkinson
Professor of Paediatrics & Perinatal Medicine
University of Oxford

Radcliffe Publishing
Oxford • New York

Radcliffe Publishing Ltd
18 Marcham Road
Abingdon
Oxon OX14 1AA
United Kingdom

www.radcliffe-oxford.com
Electronic catalogue and worldwide online ordering facility.

British Library Cataloguing in Publication Data

A catalogue record for this book is available from the British Library.

ISBN-13: 978 184619 148 0

Typeset by Pindar New Zealand, Auckland, New Zealand
Printed and bound by Cadmus Communications, USA

Contents

Foreword

This book will be invaluable to the wide range of professionals who have important responsibilities in the care of sick newborn babies.

The three editors have extensive experience gained from conceiving, and successfully delivering, the first university programme to train Advanced Neonatal Nurse Practitioners in the UK. Building on their success, they take an innovative approach to making the scientific background accessible to other disciplines by presenting readable descriptions about this complex and ever expanding specialty.

The transition from early interest in diseases of the newborn to the wide ranging fundamental understanding which we now have has been extraordinarily rapid. The application of this knowledge to improving clinical care and outcome has been outstandingly successful. Progress continues to be made with the introduction of therapies after vigorous trials based on detailed experimental investigation.

All this wealth of evidence can be daunting and as standards are raised neonatal care becomes more challenging. Much can be learned in the classroom and from traditional texts but often more questions are asked. Neonatology, unlike 'organ'-based specialties, encompasses almost every other discipline and to be successful requires the expertise of a wide range of professionals. Integrating their skills on a foundation of mutual understanding of the basic principles, which this book presents, will lead to further improvements.

I have no doubt that it will be of great value to all who need to understand more about the range of human developmental pathophysiology both before and after birth.

Andrew R Wilkinson
Professor of Paediatrics & Perinatal Medicine
University of Oxford
Department of Paediatrics
Neonatal Unit, Women's Centre
John Radcliffe Hospital, Oxford
May 2009

Preface

Over the past decade there have been a number of fundamental changes to newborn care provision, not least with regard to staffing of neonatal units. For medical staff there has been a reduction in the permissible working hours of doctors in training, a move to shift working patterns and a requirement for targeted education and training programmes. Over the same period there has also been increasing recognition that the provision of high-quality neonatal care is best achieved by making full use of the talents, capabilities and aspirations of all of those committed to the care of the newborn, irrespective of their professional origins. Key roles are now played by senior nurses, clinical nurse specialists, pharmacists, advanced neonatal nurse practitioners, nurse consultants, midwives, dieticians, physiotherapists and speech therapists as well as medical staff. These professions inevitably have diverse educational and training cultures and curricula, often being generic, rather than primarily focused on the neonate. In addition to these staffing issues the last decade has seen the emergence of an important new allied specialty – that of fetal medicine.

There are many neonatal textbooks, guidelines and online sources of information currently available to guide clinical practice and these are important in helping care providers safely to decide what to do and how to do it. However, it is the ability to answer the 'why' questions which often imparts to practitioners confidence in their own clinical judgement, particularly in situations where there may be competing priorities or no established guidelines.

The purpose of this book is primarily to help all of those involved in the provision of neonatal care in their understanding of some of the genetic, physiological and biochemical mechanisms which have either led to or are associated with the clinical conditions affecting their patients. Where important therapeutic principles are involved, or where there may be uncertainty about the management of rare conditions, 'key points for practice' have been highlighted, but the book is not intended to be a source of guidelines for clinical interventions. Limitations of time and space have imposed constraints on the range of topics covered and we are aware that there are important gaps; in particular, the neurological system has sparse coverage and there is no detailed discussion of immunological or inflammatory processes.

We have included a fairly comprehensive chapter relating to fetal medicine which gives an overview of the specialty and we hope that this will facilitate an understanding of the continuum of developmental physiology and pathology which is now required of neonatal care providers. Finally, the concept of how we come to make clinical decisions may be one to which many of us have given little thought but which perhaps deserves a higher priority in our considerations, and an introductory chapter relating to this emerging discipline has also been included.

Michael Hall
Alan Noble
Susan Smith
May 2009

About the editors

Michael Hall is a Consultant Neonatal Paediatrician based in Southampton with a specific interest in postgraduate education in paediatrics and neonatology. He has been medical co-ordinator of the Advanced Neonatal Nurse Practitioner training course in Southampton for the past 15 years and has led a number of postgraduate online education programmes for doctors training in neonatology, both within the UK and in Europe. He is also involved nationally in the planning and development of postgraduate examinations in paediatrics.

Alan Noble graduated with a BSc and subsequently PhD in Physiology and Biochemistry from the University of Southampton. He was appointed as Lecturer in Physiology in 1968 and was much involved in the development of the then new Southampton Medical School. He is the author of more than 50 research papers on aspects of renal and cardiovascular physiology. He is the lead author for *The Cardiovascular System* published in 2005 by Elsevier in their Systems of the Body series. Throughout his career, he has been involved in the development and delivery of numerous courses for medical, science, nursing and other allied paramedical science students. These include the Southampton course for neonatal nurse practitioners. He retired in 2008 as Senior Lecturer in Physiology but continues to have a role in some teaching programmes.

Susan Smith is a Lecturer/Practitioner based in the School of Health Sciences, University of Southampton. Susan was one of the multi-disciplinary team responsible for establishing the first training programme for Advanced Neonatal Nurse Practitioners in the UK and since then she has been one of the nursing co-ordinators for the programme. Her research interests include neonatal education and the professional development of Advanced Neonatal Nurse Practitioners.

List of contributors

Dr Mark Anthony BSc PhD MB ChB MRCPCH
Consultant Neonatologist, Oxford
Mark obtained a degree in Medical Microbiology in 1986 and graduated in Medicine in 1989, both at Bristol University. His medical student elective was in the JALMA Institute for Leprosy, India, and since then infectious disease has been an important aspect of his career. He commenced Paediatric training in 1990, was involved in vaccine trials in the Oxford Vaccine Group in 1995, had an MRC Clinical Research Training Fellowship to study in the Molecular Infectious Diseases Group at the Weatherall Institute for Molecular Medicine between 1996 and 1999, gained a PhD in the field of Molecular Pathogenesis in 2002, and worked as an Oxford University Clinical Lecturer in Neonatal Medicine from 2000–2005. He was a Locum Consultant in Neonatal Medicine in Southampton until 2006, a Consultant at Birmingham Women's Hospital until 2008, and a Consultant Neonatologist at Oxford from 2009. His main clinical and research interest is infection in newborn babies.

Sally Boxall MSc BSc (Hons) RM RGN
Consultant Nurse in Prenatal Diagnosis and Family Support
Wessex Fetal Medicine Unit
Sally trained as a nurse and midwife after graduating from Liverpool University. After qualifying in 1984 she worked as a specialist nurse in genetics, where her interest lay chiefly in working with families who were undergoing prenatal testing. Since 1996 she has worked within the field of fetal medicine, latterly as a consultant nurse in a regional fetal medicine unit.

Dr Bruce Castle MB ChB MRCOG FRANZCOG MD DDU HGSA(Genetics) LLB
Consultant in Clinical Genetics
Wessex Clinical Genetics Service
Bruce trained in obstetrics and gynaecology and was a Fetal Medicine specialist for 10 years prior to retraining in clinical genetics. His main interests are prenatal genetics, the genetics of retarded growth, and law and medicine.

Dr Max Chipulu PhD
Senior Fellow (Management Sciences)
School of Management, University of Southampton
Max has been teaching at the School of Management since 2002. His subject specialties are statistics, decision analysis and simulation; with research interests in performance measurement, multi-variate modelling and simulation. Prior to an academic career, Max worked as a mechanical engineer maintaining underground copper mining equipment.

Dr Elizabeth Cluett PhD MSc RM RGN PGCEA
Senior Lecturer
University of Southampton
Elizabeth qualified as a nurse in 1981 and a midwife in 1982. After practising as a midwife for many years, and having taken time out to have a family, Elizabeth came into Midwifery Education and achieved her MSc, PhD and PGCEA. Currently Elizabeth works as a Senior Lecturer in the School of Heath Sciences, University of Southampton, a role which includes teaching midwives and a wide range of health and social care professionals, from BSc through to PhD level. Elizabeth maintains her midwifery clinical practice as a member of a team that provides maternity care to women with complex health needs. She also has a great interest in water immersion during labour and birth as a strategy for normalising birth, and has undertaken a randomised controlled trial in the area, as well as being lead reviewer for the Cochrane Review on the topic. Her publications include the research text, *Principle and Practice of Research in Midwifery* as well as several chapters and research papers, predominantly linked to midwifery practice and/or research processes.

Dr James William Gray MB ChB MRCP FRCPath
Consultant Microbiologist
Birmingham Children's and Women's Hospitals
James has been Consultant Microbiologist at Birmingham Children's and Women's Hospitals for 14 years, where he has had a significant role in the development of specialist paediatric and neonatal microbiology and infection control services. His research interests include *Staphylococcus aureus* (including MRSA) infections, group B streptococci, infection surveillance, point-of-care microbiology testing and test accuracy studies. He has published over 60 papers, authored several book chapters and one book, and has been an Expert Advisor for the *British National Formulary for Children* (*BNF-C*) since its inception. He is an editor of three microbiology-related scientific journals.

Dr Keith Hillier BSc PhD DSc
Visiting Senior Lecturer
School of Medicine, University of Southampton
Keith's previous positions were in the Clinical Pharmacology and Education Groups in the University of Southampton (a position he held for 30 years), Makerere University in Uganda and the Nuffield Department of Obstetrics and Gynaecology in Oxford. Dr Hillier has published more than 100 refereed publications including co-authoring seminal works on the use of prostaglandins for the induction of labour and abortion. He is co-author of the textbook *Medical Pharmacology and Therapeutics* which is currently in its third edition.

Dr Rashid Kazmi MRCP FRCPath
Consultant Haematologist
Southampton General Hospital
Rashid graduated from Bahauddin Zakariya University, Pakistan in 1987. He came to the UK in 1989 and did his further medical training at the Edinburgh Royal Infirmary. In 1992 he completed the MRCP and began his training in haematology at Royal Infirmary Leicester. Later he was appointed as a specialist registrar in haematology in Liverpool where he finished his training in 1998. For the subsequent four years he worked at Oxford Haemophilia Centre, Oxford in the field of haemostasis and thrombosis. He then moved to Southampton General Hospital where he is still working as a consultant haematologist. He is the lead clinician in haemostasis and thrombosis. His main areas of interest include genetics of thrombophilias and platelet function disorders.

Dr Bashir A Lwaleed BSc PhD FRCPath
Research Fellow
University of Southampton and Southampton University Hospitals NHS Trust
Bashir graduated in Libya in 1986. He came to the UK in 1992 to undertake post-graduate studies. He was awarded his PhD from the Faculty of Medicine, University of Southampton in 1998 and became a Fellow of the Royal College of Pathologists in 2008. He has 22 years experience in clinical and experimental haematology. Bashir's main research interest is thrombosis and haemostasis. His first indexed publication appeared in 1997. In the subsequent 12 years he has published 58 peer-reviewed articles and reviews. He acts as a referee for international journals and major funding bodies as well as publishing textbook reviews. He serves on the editorial boards of a number of peer-reviewed journals.

Debra McGonigle RSCN PGDip
Advanced Neonatal Nurse Practitioner
Gloucestershire Hospitals NHS Foundation Trust
Debra has been a neonatal nurse for more than 20 years, working largely in the southwest of England, but also in Australia and the Middle East. In 1984 she completed her RSCN training at the Royal Hospital for Sick Children, Glasgow. She has just completed her Advanced Neonatal Nurse Practitioner (ANNP) training at Southampton University and is currently employed as an ANNP by Gloucestershire Hospitals NHS Foundation Trust.

Dr Magi Sque PhD
Senior Lecturer
School of Health Sciences, University of Southampton
Magi studied nursing at Guy's Hospital, London and specialised in oncological nursing. Supported by a British Department of Health Nursing Research Studentship, she completed a PhD at the University of Southampton in 1996. Her current research explores issues that concern decision making at the end of life: in bereavement, and organ and tissue donation, retention and transplantation. She leads a postgraduate module on clinical decision making.

Dr Valerie Walker MD ChB FRCPath FRCPCH
Consultant Chemical Pathologist
University of Southampton
Valerie qualified in Liverpool, where she then trained in chemical pathology and metabolism. She went on to Great Ormond Street Hospital for Children, London, as a lecturer. Here she acquired a broad experience in paediatric biochemistry and inherited biochemical disorders and a lasting enthusiasm for these fields. She has maintained an active clinical and research interest in paediatric and neonatal biochemistry at Southampton, first as Senior Lecturer and, since 1990, as Consultant Chemical Pathologist.

Dr Intan Faizura Yeop BM (Southampton) MRCPH
Specialist Registrar in Gastroenterology
The Children's Hospital for Wales, Cardiff
Intan won a scholarship to study medicine in the UK and graduated from Southampton University Medical School in 2000. She proceeded to train in paediatrics and is currently a specialist registrar in gastroenterology in the Children's Hospital for Wales, Cardiff. Her interest in clinical nutrition began in the early years of training, developed through conducting audits and writing feeding guidelines, and led to the Diploma in Child Nutrition. She also gained experience in clinical nutrition from training posts in neonatology and hepatology in Southampton and Birmingham Children's Hospital.

CHAPTER 1

Fetal medicine

Sally Boxall and Elizabeth Cluett

CONTENTS

INTRODUCTION

This chapter considers the underpinning physiology relating to fetal assessment and therapeutic interventions relating to the fetus. The key conditions within maternal and fetal medicine – including placental implantation, hypertensive disorders of pregnancy, diabetes, multiple pregnancy, infections, haemolytic disease of the new-born and intrahepatic cholestasis of pregnancy – are discussed. An understanding of these conditions is important to appreciate the interdependency between maternal and fetal well-being, especially in the presence of specific conditions. In addition, assessment techniques such as ultrasound and cardiotocography, as well as newer fetal therapies, are considered.

THE PLACENTA AND IMPLANTATION

Understanding of the placenta has come a long way since the mid-eighteenth century when the Hunter brothers showed that maternal spiral arteries carried blood to the placenta but that the maternal and fetal circulations were not mixed in the placenta.[1] The placenta is arguably the most important human organ, providing for gaseous exchange, nutrition, excretion, endocrine functions and more during the fetal period, thus determining fetal, neonatal and adult health.[2] Successful function of the placenta is dependent on complete and correct implantation. However, understanding of the processes involved in implantation remains incomplete, not least because of the challenges of gaining appropriate human specimens for study. Therefore much of the current knowledge is derived from animal studies. The following section provides an overview of the processes of placental implantation and development, as it is currently understood. This is necessary to understand a variety of maternal and fetal conditions that become evident when the process of implantation is abnormal, such as intra-uterine growth restriction (IUGR) and pre-eclampsia.

Implantation of the placenta

The process of implantation is set within the context of the uterine structures and hormonal regulation. The vascular supply to the uterine endometrium is via uterine and ovarian arteries, from which arise the arcuate arteries which run along the anterior and posterior walls of the myometrium. Radial arteries then transverse the myometrium and give rise to 100–50 spiral arteries,[3] so called because of their appearance. The normal hormonal changes associated with the ovarian cycle and early pregnancy trigger changes within the circulation. These include systematic changes, such as increased blood volume and cardiac output, and local changes within the spiral arteries, such as alteration of the endothelium.[4] These occur throughout the uterus, and can be considered as precursors to implantation. After fertilisation, the development of the blastocyst and the differentiation of the trophoblast – the outermost layer of the blastocyst – is well documented.[5] The following section focuses on the activities of the trophoblast, but simultaneously the inner cell mass would be undergoing major changes leading to embryonic development. Figure 1.1 shows a simplified diagram of the uterine structures and the blastocyst pre-implantation.

The trophoblast can broadly be considered as, first, the main trophoblast shell, which will develop into the multiple villi of the placenta bed, and, secondly, extravillous trophoblasts, which are mobile cells that proliferate and migrate into the uterine endometrium (called the decidua in pregnancy). These invasive cells adhere to the extracellular matrix of the decidua, altering the matrix to facilitate progression through it.[6] It is believed that the invasive trophoblast penetrates the spiral arteries and initially acts as a plug, restricting blood flow and hence oxygenation and

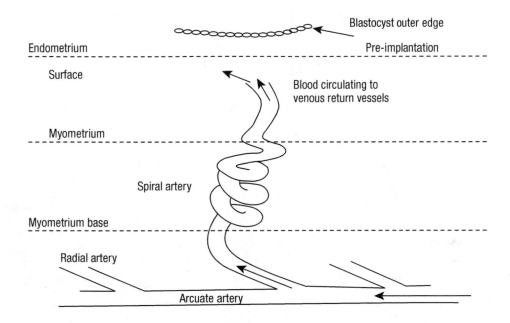

FIGURE 1.1 A simplified diagram of the uterine structures and the blastocyst prior to implantation

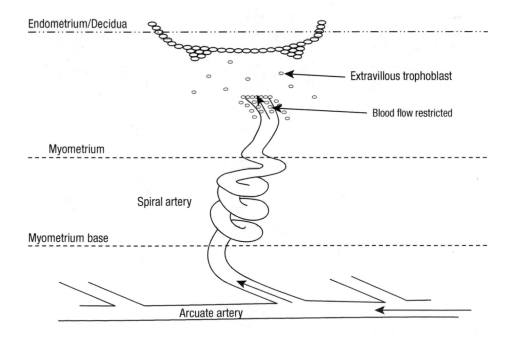

FIGURE 1.2 A diagrammatic representation of invasive extravillous trophoblast along both inner and outer surfaces of the spiral arteries

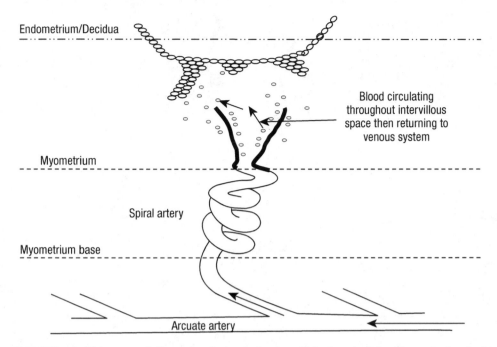

FIGURE 1.3 This remodelling of spiral arteries is within the decidual layer in the first trimester

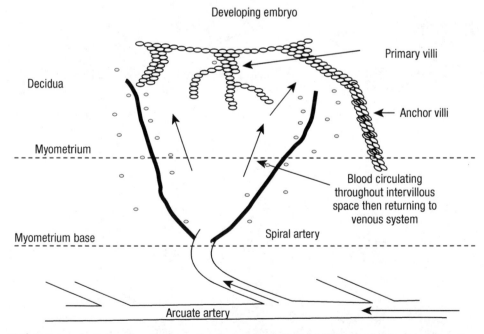

FIGURE 1.4 In the second trimester the remodelling of the spiral arteries extends well into the myometrial layer of the uterus, thus increasing the blood flow around the extensive villous placental bed

nutrition to the developing placenta/embryonic structures. This period of relative hypoxia is thought to be important in controlling the milieu in which the biochemical signalling occurs, which facilitates rapid proliferation of cells, and cell differentiation. Figure 1.2 is a diagrammatic representation of invasive extravillous trophoblast along both inner and outer surfaces of the spiral arteries.[7] It is thought that there is some 'communication' between these internal and external cells that enable the remodelling of the spiral artery walls to occur. This involves the replacement of the normal musculature of the arteries with a fibrinoid matrix[6] thus preventing the normal constriction ability of normal arteries. This ensures a low-pressure system and a free flow of blood to fill the lacunae (pools) or intervillous spaces from which nutrients can cross into the developing placenta villi. At first this remodelling of spiral arteries is within the decidual layer (Figure 1.3), but as the second trimester progresses, this extends well into the myometrial layer of the uterus, thus increasing the blood flow around the extensive villous placental bed (Figure 1.4).

The conversion of the spiral arteries starts around the centre of the placenta bed, and spreads out to the peripheral area. As the pregnancy reaches term, an additional layer of cells develops over the fibrinoid matrix, which is believed to be part of the maternal repair process postpartum.[1]

A normal, mature placenta consists of a villous tree, with villi of varying sizes including anchor villi which are embedded deeply; mesenchymal villi (the most immature villi); stem villi; intermediate villi, and terminal villi. In normal implantation, anchoring villi do not extend past the Nitabuch's layer or stria, which is an acellular fibrinoid layer that forms between maternal subepithelial connective tissue and myometrium to prevent placental implantation to deeper uterine layers. Placenta accreta occurs when implantation goes through the Nitabuch's layer, and rarely into the uterine serosa or even maternal bladder.[8] The incidence of accreta increases with the number of previous caesarean sections but is rare, occurring in 1 in 2500.[9]

Intra-uterine growth restriction

There are a variety of factors contributing to intra-uterine growth restriction (IUGR). For example, a reduction or absence of intermediate or terminal villi is associated with a significant reduction in the total surface area available for nutrient exchange, and hence is linked to IUGR. Cardiovascular adaptations by the fetus enable it to survive deficiency in nutrients by reducing blood flow to the liver, in order to prioritise the brain and other key organs. This is 'brain sparing', a consequence of which is adapted metabolic processes, which predisposes to adult disease, in particular cardiovascular disease and diabetes.[10]

Smoking is a key contributor to IUGR and its effects result, at least in part, from endothelial dysfunction. Normal placental vascular endothelium produces nitric oxide (NO), which promotes vasodilatation. Where there is reduced dilation and reduced NO there is endothelial dysfunction. Quinton et al.[11] in a small study (n = 41) using ultrasound measured flow-mediated dilation, showed women who smoked had endothelial dysfunction compared with non-smokers, and had a significantly greater incidence of neonatal birth weights below the 10th centile. Godfrey et al.[12] showed that infants of women who smoke had on average an 11% lower bone mineral content and density than infants of women who did not smoke. The reasons for this can only be theorised to be related to abnormal placental calcium absorption and transfer of these minerals secondary to maternal smoking. These examples highlight that while placental implantation is important, placental function is dependent on maternal well-being, and not just the absence of disease. Jansson and Powell[13] argued that the placenta is a sensor of maternal health and nutritional status, that can 'up or down' regulate nutritional transport to the fetus, contributing to the growth of the fetus, and thus fetal and subsequent neonatal well-being.

HYPERTENSIVE DISORDERS OF PREGNANCY

Hypertensive disorders of pregnancy are currently classified together, they are:
- pregnancy induced hypertension (also called gestational hypertension)
- pre-eclampsia
- eclampsia
- HELLP syndrome.

Although considered together, these conditions could be separate entities.

Pre-eclampsia and eclampsia

Pre-eclampsia and eclampsia are the second most common cause of maternal death within the UK with a mortality rate of 0.85 per 100 000 maternities. Pre-eclampsia is also the most common disorder associated with pregnancy, affecting approximately 10–15% of all pregnancies.[14] There is some suggestion that the incidence of pre-eclampsia and pregnancy induced hypertension is rising,[15] although the rate of eclampsia is not.[16] This is presumed to be due to better management of the condition with early use of magnesium sulphate; however, it can also be attributed to the advancements with neonatal care, which means pregnancies can be ended earlier, in reasonable anticipation of a healthy neonate. Despite improved outcomes and better understanding of the pathophysiology of the conditions, actual progress in preventing or 'curing' the condition remains elusive.

It has long been recognised that the placenta is key in the development of pre-eclampsia, and in particular placental implantation. Failure of the remodelling of the spiral arteries described above, is the pathological event.[6] Pijnenborg *et al.*[4] found that while 96% of spiral arteries undergo full remodelling in healthy uteri, this can be as low as 10% in placentae of women with pre-eclampsia. Instead of the spiral arteries being altered deep into the myometrial portion of the placenta bed, the remodelling is limited to the decidua portion, as demonstrated in Figure 1.3 rather than in Figure 1.4. This predisposes to placenta insufficiency leading to IUGR and fetal hypoxia.

However, failure of spiral artery changes alone does not seem to be the trigger for pre-eclampsia, as women without eclampsia who have IUGR fetuses also have this feature. This has led to a range of theories as to the nature of pre-eclampsia. A genetic predisposition has been mooted.[17] Other theories have included placenta debris,[18] in a two-stage process where factors, possibly due to increased apoptosis (programmed cell death), are released by the abnormal placenta and trigger endothelial cell damage in the maternal vasculature, leading to pre-eclampsia. Oxidative stress is now thought to be marker of the condition rather than a contributing factor. The current theory is that pre-eclampsia is an excessive inflammatory response to pregnancy[18] which encompasses many of the features within other theories.

The immune system is a complex but vital protective system, consisting of innate and adaptive mechanisms, both of which undergo alteration during pregnancy.[5] Indeed, without this alteration pregnancy could not succeed. An adaptive inflammatory response is part of pregnancy modifications, enabling the 'acceptance' of the invading trophoblastic cells. Redman and Sargent[19] describe normal pregnancy as a 'state of systemic inflammation' where the innate mechanism changes facilitate pregnancy, and can be seen in altered leucocytosis, complement activation, platelet and coagulation activity. Pre-eclampsia may be an extreme extension of the same immune responses, resulting in pathological changes. Impaired implantation results in placenta ischaemia, triggering local then systemic inflammatory responses. In addition to the local placenta bed ischaemia causing IUGR, there are changes to the endothelial lining of the maternal blood vessels, including enlarged cells and release of factors such as prostacyclins, NO and a variety of tissue and coagulation factors.[20] The damaged blood vessels become prone to abnormal circulating patterns, increased fibrin deposits, and further damage.

The end result of this complex multi-system condition is hypertension, and systematic capillary bed abnormalities. Although the order in which organs become affected is variable, which makes early identification based on specific symptoms challenging, the most common sign is that of hypertension followed by proteinuria, subsequent renal damage, and potentially acute renal failure. The damaged blood vessels leak fluid from the cardiovascular system into the extracellular compartments, leading to generalised oedema. The high blood pressure can trigger cerebral haemorrhage, while cerebral oedema predisposes to headaches, visual disturbances due to pressure on the optic nerve, and seizures. These are typically full tonic–clonic seizures that define the occurrence of eclampsia.

Damage to the endothelial cells of capillary beds within the lungs leads to pulmonary oedema, and potentially adult respiratory distress syndrome and, untreated, respiratory failure. Similar damage within the liver leads to altered liver function, and also liver tissue oedema, with the potential for massive haemorrhage due to liver capsule rupture. Figure 1.5 summarises the systematic features of pre-eclampsia/eclampsia.

The management of pre-eclampsia revolves around early diagnosis and currently the majority of antenatal care is focused on this. In the event that pre-eclampsia is diagnosed, the management aims to limit maternal adverse effects by controlling hypertension, using medications, for example labetalol, nifedipine or methyldopa. Magnesium sulphate is the recommended management for the prevention of imminent or actual eclamptic seizures, whilst monitoring fluid balance and maternal health stabilisation and negotiating the most appropriate point for delivery of the fetus. This is a balancing act between the needs of the fetus, monitored through ultrasound assessment of growth and well-being, and cardiotocograph (CTG) assessment, and the health of the mother. More information about the management of the hypertensive disorders of pregnancy can be found in most midwifery and obstetric texts, including Samangaya et al.[14] and Walfish et al.[21]

Systems affected in pre-eclampsia/eclampsia

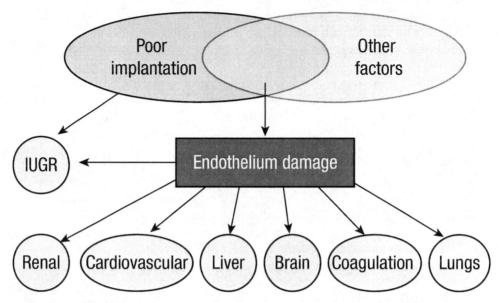

FIGURE 1.5 The body systems affected by pre-eclampsia/eclampsia

HELLP syndrome

Abnormal liver function (elevated liver enzymes) and coagulation problems (low platelets) are associated with pre-eclampsia but also the condition known as HELLP. HELLP refers to the symptoms of the condition, namely:

▶ **H**aemolysis breakdown of haemoglobin to haem and globin
▶ **E**levated **L**iver enzymes
  — aspartate aminotransferase
  — alanine aminotransferase
▶ **L**ow **P**latelets
  — less than 100 000 mm^3 – moderate
  — less than 50 000 mm^3 – severe.

While traditionally HELLP has been seen as an extension or variation of pre-eclampsia, it has been suggested that it is a separate condition based on the identification of different molecular profiles.[22]

Coagulation disruption can trigger disseminating intravascular coagulation, which can be the major factor in any associated maternal mortality. However, there is a huge range of severity, ranging from an early onset, severe disorder necessitating life-saving intervention, to – more commonly – mild pre-eclampsia or even hypertension only. Indeed, it may be that the pregnancy-induced hypertension, where the only symptom is uncomplicated hypertension, may actually be (at least in some women) a separate condition, more akin to essential hypertension.

MATERNAL DISORDERS AFFECTING THE FETUS
Diabetes

The most common medical disorder seen in maternity care is diabetes mellitus, affecting 2–5% of all pregnancies,[23] a figure that is increasing. This reflects a global trend, where the incidence of diabetes in the non-pregnant population is estimated at 2.5% and is expected to rise to 4.5 % by 2030,[24] driven mainly by a sharp increase in type II diabetes. Diabetes is a disorder resulting in abnormal carbohydrate metabolism that can be life threatening if not proactively managed. Diabetes in pregnancy increases the health risks to both the woman and her fetus/neonate. To understand the reasons for this, some understanding of glucose metabolism and the changes in pregnancy is required, as normal pregnancy can be considered a diabetogenic state.

There are key changes to glucose metabolism and insulin function to meet the needs of the developing fetal placenta unit. Figure 1.6 summaries the normal action of insulin on cells. From early pregnancy and rising steadily throughout pregnancy there is an increased maternal metabolic rate which increases maternal demands for glucose. At the same time human placental lactogen (hPL), progesterone and cortisol are secreted into the maternal system, increasing cellular insulin resistance and altering glucagon secretion[5] (*see* Box 1.1 for a summary of the glucose metabolic cycle). This means that a greater amount of maternal insulin has to be produced before glucose can be utilised by the maternal cells. This provides a period of high serum blood glucose during which the glucose is readily available for transfer to the placenta and hence to the fetus. As a result of glucose transfer to the fetus/placenta the woman's blood glucose may fall to 10–20% lower than when she is not pregnant; this results in greater swings in glucose and hormone levels, particularly at night. The gastrointestinal tract absorbs more nutrients so glucose levels are higher. Protein/ amino acid and fat metabolism are also altered; for example, serum protein and

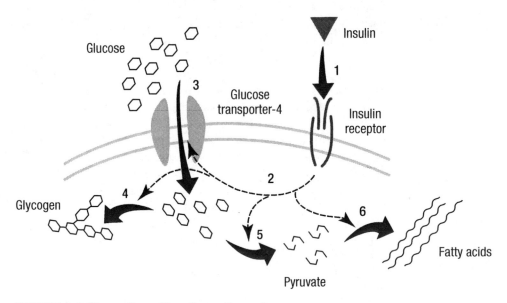

FIGURE 1.6 The action of insulin on the cell

amino acids levels are lower, due to placental uptake for use and storage. As pregnancy progress, the woman increasingly utilises her fat stores for her energy needs, leaving the glucose for transfer to the fetus.

BOX 1.1 SIMPLIFIED SUMMARY OF GLUCOSE METABOLIC CYCLE

- High serum glucose
- Insulin released from beta cells of Islets of Langerhan in pancreas
- Receptor cells activated enabling transfer of glucose into cells
- Serum glucose falls
- Insulin production stopped, glucose continues to fall
- Glucagon secreted from alpha cells of Islets of Langerhan in pancreas
- Glycolysis (breakdown of glycogen from storage) stimulated
- Glucose release into the circulation
- Serum blood glucose maintained/raised

To overcome the insulin resistance and maintain maternal homeostasis, insulin production is repeatedly increased. By the third trimester insulin production is doubled or even tripled, to have the same effect.

If a previously healthy woman is unable to increase her insulin production to this extent, gestational diabetes occurs. Women at increased risk of this are usually obese, with levels of pre-pregnancy insulin utilisation that cannot physiologically be increased enough in pregnancy. Other women who are at increased risk of gestational diabetes include those of Asian, or Afro-Caribbean origin. The ethnic increased risk is probably due to increased carbohydrate-rich diets in populations who traditionally are used to a low carbohydrate intake.

Fetal macrosomia is a recognised consequence of diabetes and occurs not only because of high maternal glucose availability resulting in increased glucose transfer to the fetus, where it is stored as fat, but also because the fetus produces more insulin to process the glucose and insulin is a growth hormone. Thus the fetus is structurally bigger with a larger bone structure, predisposing to cephalopelvic disproportion (fetal head too large to transverse maternal pelvis) and shoulder dystocia (when the diameter of the fetal shoulders is greater that it should be and hence the shoulder becomes impacted on the brim of the maternal pelvis). Both these conditions are associated with maternal trauma due to operative deliveries and with fetal hypoxia and bone fractures.

Post-natally the neonate, having been used to a high-glucose environment, is prone to severe hypoglycaemia as it has high insulin production levels, but suddenly a low glucose supply. Women who have degenerative changes due to diabetes such as hypertension or vascular impairments may have poor placenta perfusion leading to IUGR.

There is also an increased incidence of congenital abnormalities in neonates of diabetic mothers (*see* Box 1.2 for most common abnormalities found).

Early embryonic development is a complex process of cell division, differentiation, migration, organisation (organogenesis) and apoptosis (cell death) which is dependent on multiple, synchronised, biochemical signalling. Even relatively mild hyperglycaemia around the time of these processes can cause abnormalities.[25] Therefore it is vital that women with pre-existing diabetes are identified pre-pregnancy and receive preconception education and care including high-dose folic acid. Good control of the diabetes reduces the risk of abnormalities, but does not eradicate them completely.

BOX 1.2 MOST COMMON CONGENITAL ABNORMALITIES IN NEONATES OF DIABETIC WOMEN

- Transposition of great vessels
- Ventricular septal defect
- Atrial septal defect
- Hypoplastic left ventricle
- Anomalies of aorta
- Microcephaly, encephalocoele, anencephaly, holoprosencephaly
- Skeletal – caudal regression syndrome
- Spina bifida
- Tracheo-oesophageal fistula
- Imperforate anus
- Bowel atresia
- Genitourinary
- Absent kidney
- Polycystic kidneys

Another major risk for pregnancy complicated by diabetes is stillbirth. CEMACH[23] reported a stillbirth rate of 26.8/1000 births compared with 5.7/1000 in the non-diabetic population and a perinatal death rate of 31.8/1000 compared with 8.5/1000. There is now an extensive NICE clinical guideline for the management of diabetes from preconception to post-natal care.[26] The key elements of the guideline include preconception care and earlier referral for obstetric and interprofessional care for known diabetics. Screening is important for the identification of gestational diabetes. Although routine urinalysis of glucosuria has been a long-established and continuing part of antenatal care, it has both a low sensitivity and specificity, and for this reason is no longer recommended for screening.[26] The oral glucose tolerance test, undertaken at 28 weeks' gestation is now recommended for the identification of diabetes in women at increased risk.

Intrahepatic cholestasis of pregnancy

Intrahepatic cholestasis of pregnancy (ICP) may present from 30 weeks' gestation until term and is associated with preterm labour and fetal distress, including meconium aspiration and stillbirth. The incidence in the UK is 0.5–1% although it is higher in Sweden at 2%, with the highest incidence being in Chile at 22% in the Aravcania Indian population.[27] This may indicate a genetic link and a specific gene mutation has been identified in this group. There is also a higher incidence in winter which may be due to an environmental or infective/viral link although this remains unclear. Other possible causes include hormonal triggers such as raised oestrogen levels, which seems consistent with the fact that ICP is more likely in multiple pregnancies; or a link with progesterone levels.[28] Dietary factors are also possible triggers, as is a combination of these.

In pregnancy bile acids increase related to oestrogen and progesterone activity, but in ICP bile excretion is restricted. This causes an accumulation of bile acids, resulting in a rise in plasma bile acid levels. This affects nerve endings in subcuticular fat, causing pruritus. The raised circulating bile acids mean that the fetus is unable to excrete its bile via the placenta to the mother.

These fetuses may have increased amounts of meconium contributing to an increased incidence of meconium-stained liquor and possible aspiration, which may also occur at earlier gestations. The raised bile acid levels may also affect the placenta, contributing to IUGR, fetal distress, hypoxia, abnormal CTG readings and intra-uterine death (double the risk of normal population), particularly around term. For this reason delivery at 37 weeks is often advocated,[28,29] or earlier if indicated by the maternal and /or fetal condition.

The constant irritation causes lack of sleep, leading to fatigue, depression, and even suicidal behaviour. Some women experience a general malaise, and loss of appetite; this may be due to the reduction in bile entering the gastrointestinal system where it would normally have a key role in fat metabolism and absorption. There is, therefore, the potential for nutritional impairment, particularly of fat and fat-soluble vitamins, including vitamin K, and these women have a 10–22% increased risk of haemorrhage.[30] It is therefore vital that these neonates receive vitamin K following birth, and that the women are closely monitored. The altered bile acids levels also affect the prostaglandin levels that are associated with the onset of labour, and 20% of these women go into preterm labour.

Optimal management of the condition is by early diagnosis, including consideration of family history, occurrence in previous pregnancy, and previous unexplained stillbirth. Once diagnosed, disease progress can be monitored by serial measurement of bile acids, although even relatively moderate rises can be associated with adverse perinatal outcomes. Fetal monitoring using ultrasound and repeat antenatal CTG, as well as continuous CTG monitoring during labour are essential. Drug therapy options include ursodeoxycholic acid, which relieves itching and lowers serum bile salts, but there is little evidence it improves fetal outcomes. Other treatment options include cholestyramine, and S-adensyl-L-methione, but the evidence for these is inconsistent.[31] Dexamethasone may also reduce maternal symptoms.

Subsequent care includes education for life as women who have had ICP may have an excessive response to hormonal contraception/menopausal therapies and cholesterol gallstones are more likely. In subsequent pregnancies ICP is likely to recur and should be monitored for in advance of symptoms, although this can be problematic as symptoms can sometimes precede biochemical changes.

FETAL INVESTIGATIONS AND THEIR INTERPRETATION

Ultrasound scans

Non-invasive ultrasound scans (USS) can be used for screening, diagnostic and monitoring purposes. The technology may be used to exclude or confirm certain fetal abnormalities or to assess the risk of chromosomal anomalies. Ultrasound measurements are used for fetal biometry to assess growth and fetal well-being and for placental localisation. Ultrasound is a valuable tool, but its limits must be understood by those clinicians requesting the scan, and also by women accepting the offer of a scan. Optimal ultrasound images rely on the fetus being in a favourable position, with sufficient liquor to act as an acoustic medium. Images may be less clear in women with a high BMI, as the ultrasound waves have a greater distance to travel and become scattered. Women should be given verbal and written information about the local detection rates of various abnormalities, and the likelihood of detecting certain conditions.[32]

Assessment of fetal gestation is performed by taking measurements of fetal biometry: the crown rump length (CRL) before 14 weeks, and head circumference between 14 and 24 weeks. Assessment of gestational age by ultrasound is less accurate after 24 weeks as there is a wider variation in fetal size.

Fetal abnormalities such as spina bifida, gastroschisis, diaphragmatic hernia, major cardiac lesions and cleft lip are likely to be detected on a detailed anomaly scan, ideally performed around 19–21 weeks. With the advent of routine early pregnancy scanning, often performed in conjunction with ultrasound and maternal serum assessment of the risk of aneuploidy (*see* Chapter 2), certain structural abnormalities may be detected as early as 12 weeks. Some abnormalities, however, such as achondroplasia or duodenal atresia may not become apparent until later in pregnancy. Diagnosis of fetal abnormalities allows for counselling of the parents and discussion of available options including preparation for the birth in an appropriate location or consideration of termination of pregnancy.

TABLE 1.1 The 12-week ultrasound scan

Purpose	How measured
Confirmation of viability	Presence of fetal heart beat
Confirmation of gestational age	Crown rump length (CRL)
Multiplicity and assessment of chorionicity	Counting the fetuses and looking at placenta and membranes
Aneuploidy risk assessment	Nuchal translucency measurement combined with maternal serum screen
Detection of some major abnormalities	May be possible to detect anencephaly or abdominal wall defects

Ultrasound assessment of placental localisation is undertaken at the 20-week-scan stage, with further evaluation in later pregnancy if the placenta is shown to be covering the os.

The assessment of liquor volume may act as an alert to fetal anomalies: conditions such as bladder outflow obstructions or renal agenesis may present with oligohydramnios or anhydramnios. Polyhydramnios may be present in conditions where fetal swallowing is impaired such as neuromuscular conditions, or where there is obstruction within the gastrointestinal tract, such as duodenal atresia. Polyhydramnios may also be a feature of pregnancy in diabetic women due to changes in osmolarity.

TABLE 1.2 The 19–21-week anomaly scan

Purpose	How measured
Confirmation of viability (if not done before)	Presence of fetal heart beat
Confirmation of gestational age (if not done before)	Head circumference (HC)
Multiplicity and assessment of chorionicity (if not done before)	Counting the fetuses and looking at placenta and membranes
Fetal biometry	HC, biparietal diameter, cerebellar diameter, abdominal circumference, femur length compared to normal ranges
Fetal anatomical survey	Detailed examination of fetal structures
Assessment of liquor volume	Measurement of deepest pools of liquor
Placental localisation	Determination of placental position relative to internal os

Ultrasound scans later in pregnancy may be used to assess fetal growth, enabling estimation of fetal weight, and to assess fetal well-being in conjunction with liquor volume, and colour flow Doppler ultrasound to assess blood flow. Doppler ultrasound allows the operator to measure the velocity of blood flow within fetal and maternal blood vessels and hence assess utero-placental resistance or redistribution of blood flow within a fetus.

TABLE 1.3 Later pregnancy scans

Purpose	How measured
Assessment of fetal growth	Standard biometry measurements plotted on standardised or individualised growth charts
Assessment of fetal well-being	Doppler assessment of vascular waveforms Liquor volume assessment Fetal movements
Placental localisation	Determination of placental position relative to internal os

Invasive diagnostic techniques

These are used for the detection of fetal chromosomal or DNA abnormalities, particularly in women who have an increased risk of a fetus with chromosomal anomalies. Amniocentesis or chorionic villus sampling (CVS) are the most common diagnostic tests, and fetal blood sampling is available in specialist centres. Invasive diagnostic tests take samples from the pregnancy itself (amniocytes in the case of amniocentesis and placental chorionic villi in the case of CVS) so the chromosomal profile of the fetus can be determined. In certain circumstances the invasive diagnostic tests can be used for prenatal diagnosis of genetic conditions such as cystic fibrosis. DNA analysis in the majority of cases relies on prior identification of a gene mutation within the family.

Invasive diagnostic tests are not without their risks and so are often only used if there is a significant chance that a fetus has the condition being tested for, such as in a woman who has a positive result from Down's syndrome screening or where there

TABLE 1.4 Comparison of amniocentesis and CVS

	Amniocentesis	CVS
When performed	From 15+ weeks	From 11+ weeks
What is involved	Taking 15–20 mL amniotic fluid using a 20–2 g needle inserted into the uterus under ultrasound guidance	Taking a small sample of placental tissue using an 18 g needle inserted into the uterus under ultrasound guidance
Risk of procedure	1% risk of miscarriage	2% risk of miscarriage
Suitable for karyotyping	Yes	Yes
Suitable for DNA analysis for certain conditions	Yes, usually but may take longer to get results	Yes
Suitable for infection screen	Yes	No
Method of TOP if abnormality detected	Usually medically induced miscarriage	May be able to have evacuation of uterus under general anaesthesia

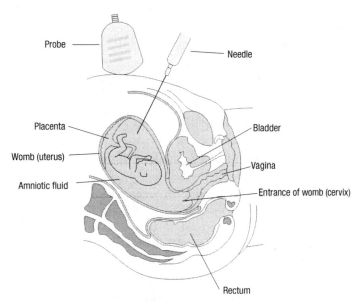

Probe

Needle

Placenta

Bladder

Womb (uterus)

Vagina

Amniotic fluid

Entrance of womb (cervix)

Rectum

FIGURE 1.7 Diagram of amniocentesis

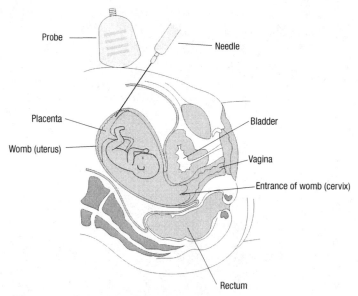

FIGURE 1.8 Diagram of chorionic villi sampling

is a family history of the condition. Risks from amniocentesis or CVS include miscarriage, preterm pre-labour rupture of membranes, or bleeding, and in the case of CVS there is a chance of confined placental mosaicism that can make interpretation of the findings more complex.

Assessment of the fetal heart rate
Fetal well-being assessment is now an important part of antenatal and intrapartum care. This assessment can utilise a variety of methods, encompassing assessment of fetal growth, position, activity, liquor volume and consistency and heart rate (HR). This section considers the latter.

The fetal heart is controlled by the cardioregulatory centre of the medulla oblongata, which in turn is controlled by the autonomic nervous system, this responds to many influences. Stimulation of the sympathetic nervous system (SNS) will increase HR, while the parasympathetic nervous system (PNS) reduces HR. The constant interaction between these systems is triggered by changes in blood pressure, oxygen and carbon dioxide tension (and the associated changed in pH) measured by baroreceptors and chemo-receptors within the aortic arch, the carotids and other large arteries, and results in fetal heart rate variability. The development of the sympathetic nervous system occurs earlier in fetal life than the parasympathetic, giving the characteristic rapid heart rate early in pregnancy and decreasing towards term (normal baseline rate at 15 weeks approximately 180 bpm, at 30 weeks approximately 150 bpm). Circulating catecholamines, i.e. adrenaline from adrenal glands, increase fetal HR. There is interdependence between the various fetal systems; for example, effective cardiac function requires oxygen and carbon dioxide transport, but equally oxygenation needs an appropriate cardiac output. The assessment of fetal heart rate (FHR) activity provides a measure of the integrity of the underlying physiological systems. There are a variety of methods to assess FHR.

Assessment methods
PINARD
The Pinard is a traditional fetal stethoscope, and the primary tool of the midwife. It enables the direct counting of the HR, giving an indication of rhythm as well as rate. It is useful antenatally and as an adjunct to abdominal palpation to aid determination of fetal position (for example breech), or for direct comparison of fetal heart and maternal pulse by one practitioner. The Pinard is also used in normal labour, when it is recommended that the FHR be recorded every 15 minutes by counting for a full minute, during the first stage of labour, and at least every 5 minutes in the second stage.[33] However, it can only be used during the uterine resting phase, and its use can be problematic in larger women, or where the woman is mobile and adopting a variety of positions during labour. In these situations a handheld Doppler for intermittent auscultation is an excellent alternative. An additional advantage of this is that the parents can hear the FHR themselves, which most find reassuring.

CARDIOTOCOGRAPHY (CTG) AND ELECTRONIC FETAL MONITORING
The development of the CTG revolutionised the assessment of FHR, enabling continuous electronic fetal monitoring (EFM) together with recording of uterine contractions, the graphic recording providing a permanent document. Doppler principles are used to measure fetal heart activity and hence measure the interval between beats. The monitoring is normally achieved via an external transducer appropriately located on the woman's abdomen, but can also be via a fetal scalp electrode (FSE). Continuous EFM is invasive, reduces maternal mobility and alters the dynamics of labour and should only be used in pregnancies where there is an increased risk of fetal compromise. This is because EFM is known to increase obstetric intervention, with the associated risks of intervention, with no evidence of benefit to the fetus/neonate in women at low risk of complication.[34]

The CTG only provides information on the FHR activity, and cannot be used in isolation as a measure of fetal well-being; it is vital that the wider maternal and fetal clinical context is always considered when interpreting a CTG and using it within clinical practice. Table 1.5 provides a list of some factors that should be considered but is not exhaustive.

TABLE 1.5 Factors that affect fetal heart rate

Maternal	Fetal	Labour related
Maternal position	Prematurity	Induction (Prostin/
Maternal disease	Growth	syntocinon)
Maternal medications	Normal fetal structures and enervation	Augmentation
Dehydration	Meconium liquor	Analgesia use
Maternal infection	Oligohydramnios and cord compression	Pethidine /epidural
pyrexia		
tachycardia		
Antepartum		
haemorrhage		
Pre-eclampsia/HELLP		

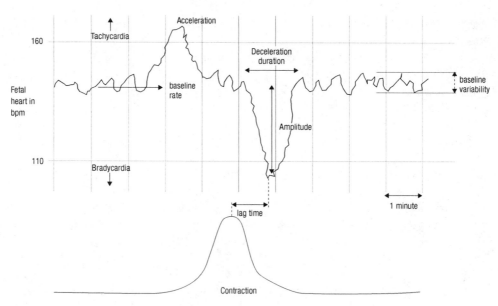

FIGURE 1.9 Elements of a CTG

TABLE 1.6 The key features of the CTG

CTG feature in term pregnancy	Explanation (bpm = beats per minute)
Baseline heart rate	Normal at term is between 110 bpm to 160 bpm This should be measured over at least 5–10 minutes
Baseline variability	This is due to the normal pattern of the autonomic nerve system activity. It is a measure of the variations in the heart rate that occur about 2–6 times per minute. Variability is normally in the range of 10–25 bpm NB this is NOT beat-to-beat variability which can only be measured on an electrocardiogram (see below)
Baseline variability in fetal sleep cycle	The healthy fetus has periods of sleep during which the baseline variability is reduced. This should never exceed 20 minutes.
Accelerations	Periods of an increase in heart rate, of 15 bpm or more, lasting at least 15 seconds. These may occur in response to fetal movements and/or uterine contractions and occur at a rate of 2 or more per 30 minutes.

The aim of EFM is the early identification of fetal pathology, in particular fetal hypoxia, to enable intervention prior to any adverse events/damage. However, a variation or perceived abnormality in one of the above features is not necessarily indicative of fetal compromise. For example, administration of analgesia, such as opioids, during labour may reduce the base rate and variability, and while this does affect fetal physiology it is not indicative of compromise or the need to expedite birth. Therefore it is normal for a CTG to be continued for at least 20–30 minutes, a duration that should enable the demonstration of a healthy fetus and all the features above, even in presence of sleep cycle. During labour where there is known to be increased risk factors, continuous monitoring is recommended, although the evidence of benefit from this is limited. However, due to ethical reasons it would now be hard to withdraw such monitoring in pregnancies perceived to be at increased risk. The most common reasons for EFM are listed below (Table 1.7).

TABLE 1.7 Indications for EFM

Maternal reasons for continuous EFM	Fetal reasons for continuous EFM
Previous caesarean section	Poor fetal growth
Pre-eclampsia	Prematurity
Post-term pregnancy	Oligohydramnios
Prolonged ruptured membranes	Abnormal Dopplers
Induction of labour	Meconium-stained liquor
Antepartum haemorrhage	Multiple pregnancy
Diabetes	Breech presentation
Other maternal disease	Other fetal abnormalities

The FHR pattern should be analysed against other key features, in particular uterine activity. Therefore a CTG should always record uterine activity in parallel with the FHR. It is good practice to also record maternal pulse and temperature and any labour features either on the recording or in the records. However, accurate interpretation of CTGs is notoriously challenging and to help recognition of key features, recording and interpretation can be helped using a mnemonic such as Dr MCQ Bravado, as shown in Box 1.3.

BOX 1.3 THE MNEMONIC DR MCQ BRAVADO USED TO AID RECORDING OF CTG FINDINGS

DR	Determine Risk
M	Fetal Movements
C	Contractions
Q	Quality
B RA	Base Rate
V	Variability
A	Accelerations
D	Decelerations
O	Overall assessment

Appropriate interpretation of the CTG is vital, and to aid this there are now agreed definitions for concluding whether a CTG is normal, suspicious or pathological.

These are clearly documented by the National Institute for Health and Clinical Excellence (NICE)[33] and are cited below (*see* Tables 1.8 and 1.9).

TABLE 1.8 Definition of normal, suspicious and pathological FHR traces[33]

Category	Definition
Normal	An FHR trace in which all four features are classified as reassuring
Suspicious	An FHR trace with one feature classified as non-reassuring and the remaining features classified as reassuring
Pathological	An FHR trace with two or more features classified as non-reassuring or one or more classified as abnormal

TABLE 1.9 Classification of FHR trace features[33]

Feature	Baseline (bpm)	Variability (bpm)	Decelerations	Accelerations
Reassuring	110–60	≥5	None	Present
Non-reassuring	100–9 161–80	<5 for 40–90 minutes	Typical variable decelerations with over 50% of contractions, occurring for more than 90 minutes Single prolonged deceleration for up to 3 minutes	The absence of accelerations with otherwise normal trace is of uncertain significance
Abnormal	<100 >180 Sinusoidal pattern ≥10 minutes	<5 for 90 minutes	Either atypical variable decelerations with over 50% of contractions or late decelerations, both for over 30 minutes Single prolonged deceleration for more than 3 minutes	

ABNORMAL CTG FEATURES

One of the common abnormal features of a CTG is a deceleration. This can be related to physiological changes in the fetus. Decelerations associated with contractions are mostly commonly associated with cord compression. These can be benign, but close monitoring for any additional signs of compromise is essential. The physiological process associated with the deceleration can be described in a series of steps (*see* Table 1.10). These decelerations are usually referred as 'early' decelerations, as they are concurrent with a contraction (*see* Figure 1.8).

TABLE 1.10 Physiology of CTG changes during cord compression associated with a uterine contraction in healthy fetus

Time point in relation to uterine contraction	Physiological state in healthy fetus	CTG reading (FHR = Fetal heart rate)
Before contraction	Umbilical vein and arteries fully patent and blood flow normal	Normal fetal heart rate baseline and variability
Start of contraction	Umbilical vein partially compressed, restricting blood flow, causing fetal blood pressure to lower, triggering response in sympathetic nervous system leading to initial increase in fetal rate	Baseline FHR increases, (often 5–10 bpm) sometimes called shouldering due to 'lifting shoulder' appearance
Peak of contraction	The umbilical vein becomes occluded and the umbilical arteries become compressed. The fetal response is via the parasympathetic nervous system leading to rapid decrease in heart rate	FHR falls, the depth of the decrease depending on the degree of arterial compression. This deceleration is concurrent with the contraction
Decreasing contraction	The umbilical arteries become patent and blood circulation returns, the vein becomes patent as contraction concludes, decreasing and discontinuing the stimulus to the cardiovascular system	The FHR increases resulting in a V-shaped deceleration that mirrors the contraction wave
Post-contraction	There is a short compensation period where FHR increases and normal physiology resumes	There is brief increase in FHR giving another 'shoulder' before return to normal FHR baseline and variability

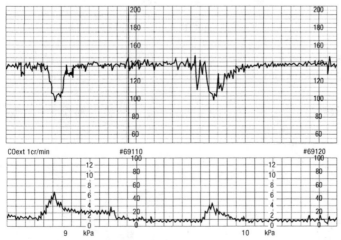

FIGURE 1.10 A CTG showing decelerations concurrent with contractions

Decelerations and a variety of other CTG abnormalities can be associated with a range of fetal conditions. The main ones are listed in Table 1.11.

TABLE 1.11 Relationship between CTG abnormality and specific fetal condition

CTG abnormality	Associated fetal state/condition
Tachycardia Generally >160 bpm but may be relative to previous baseline rate	Preterm infection/pyrexia Maternal hyperthyroidism Drugs, e.g. atropine, ritodrine Fetal cardiac anomalies Developing hypoxia Maternal anxiety/pain/dehydration Fetal activity Infection/pyrexia Maternal hyperthyroidism Drugs, i.e. atropine, ritodrine Fetal cardiac anomalies
Bradycardia Generally <110 bpm but may be relative to previous baseline rate	Hypoxia Drugs, i.e. anaesthetics, analgesics, oxytocin Maternal hypotension Cord prolapse Fetal cardiac anomalies
Decreased variability	Fetal sleep cycle Hypoxia/acidosis Prematurity Drugs, e.g. benzodiazepines, opiates, betablockers, atropine Maternal conditions, e.g. thyrotoxicosis myxodema Variety of congenital abnormalities of FHR
Early deceleration Uniform, repetitive, periodic slowing of FHR with onset early in the contraction and return to baseline at the end of the contraction. Transient episodes of slowing FHR below the baseline of more than 15 bpm and lasting 15 seconds or more	Cord compression Fetal head compression
Late decelerations Uniform, repetitive, periodic slowing of FHR with onset mid-contraction to end of the contraction which continues 20 seconds after the peak of the contraction and ends after the contraction.	Fetal distress/hypoxia

(continued)

CTG abnormality	Associated fetal state/condition
Variable decelerations – as name suggests, have variable relation with contraction, being a mixture of early and mostly late decelerations, with variable characteristics including: • Variation in amplitude (often 40 bpm or more) • Shouldering may be absent • Slower heart rate (~ 60–70 bpm) • Loss of variability during deceleration • Biphasic deceleration • Secondary rise in baseline rate • Slow return to baseline	Fetal distress/hypoxia

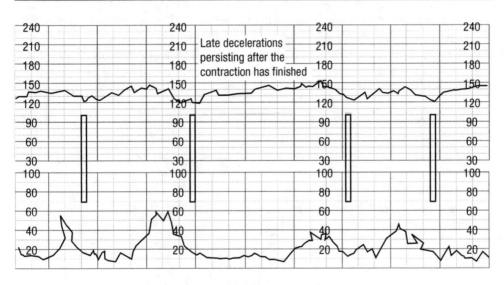

www.fetal.freeserve.co.uk

FIGURE 1.11 A CTG showing late decelerations

Fetal blood gas analysis

The use of CTG is associated with an increase in maternal inventions including operative delivery. Therefore as an adjunct to CTG, fetal blood gas analysis is recommended and has been shown to result in less intervention, in particular caesarean section, than CTG alone when compared with intermittent fetal monitoring.[34]

Fetal electrocardiograms

As technology has advanced it is now possible to record a fetal electrocardiogram (ECG). This is currently an invasive procedure that can only be acquired using a fetal scalp electrode and specialist equipment. The fetal ECG contains the same features as an adult ECG. Changes in the ST waveform, alongside comparison of the fetal CTG have been shown to have potentially more precision in the identification of fetal compromise than CTG alone.[35] However, this technology is still developing, education on its use and interpretation is required, and it is not yet part of clinical guidelines or routine practice.

Conclusion

There are various forms of fetal monitoring that provide an adjunct to the complete case scenario, and their use should be clearly documented. There are complete books on cardiography and there are computer packages that provide online instruction in CTG interpretation and the associated physiology.

MULTIPLE PREGNANCIES

Multiple pregnancy rates have risen dramatically over the last 20 years in the developed world, largely as a result of assisted reproductive techniques (ART). Not only is this a result of transfer of multiple embryos, but the techniques used in ART may also increase the chance of embryo splitting and hence an increase in monochorionic twinning as well. Newer restrictions on the number of embryos that can be transferred in the UK in IVF treatment have now limited the rise in higher-order multiple pregnancies (triplets and above) and there is increasing call for IVF single-embryo transfer for women with the best chance of achieving a pregnancy. In 2006 there were 9992 sets of twins born in England and Wales with 138 sets of triplets, and 7 quadruplet births.[36]

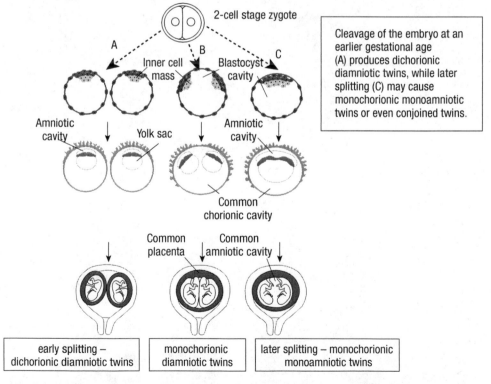

FIGURE 1.12 A diagram of the effects of timing of embryo splitting in monozygous twin pregnancies

Higher-order multiple pregnancies carry significantly increased risks of prematurity, with the potential for serious neonatal morbidity or even mortality, and multi-fetal pregnancy reduction (MFPR) may be offered to parents with three or more viable fetuses. This is best performed between 9 and 12 weeks of pregnancy, with an ultrasound-guided injection of potassium chloride (KCl). Reduction to a twin pregnancy should be discussed with the parents within the context of a discussion about the possible complications of a higher-order multiple pregnancy.

TABLE 1.12 Risks of a triplet pregnancy compared with a triplet reduced to twin pregnancy[37]

	Triplet pregnancy reduced to twins	Triplet pregnancy
Percentage of planned babies born and taken home	93%	79%
Premature birth before 32 weeks	10%	20%
Premature birth before 28 weeks	3%	8.5%
Miscarriage before 24 weeks	5%	11.5%
One or more fetal deaths during pregnancy	27/1000	92/1000

Invasive diagnosis by means of amniocentesis or CVS is possible for multiple pregnancies, but it may be challenging to ensure that both fetuses are sampled. The method chosen will depend on chorionicity.[38] There have been case reports of apparently monozygous pregnancies that are discordant for karyotypic abnormalities.[39]

Multiple pregnancies are usually identified by ultrasound, increasingly in the first trimester. Diagnosis of chorionicity is important in considering how to manage the pregnancy, and relies largely on the appearance of the placenta and membranes as shown in Figure 1.13.

All multiple pregnancies have an increased chance of maternal complications such as pre-eclampsia and exaggeration of pregnancy symptoms such as nausea and tiredness, but also an increased risk of perinatal morbidity, largely due to prematurity and growth restriction. The risks are increased in monochorionic (MC) twins compared with dichorionic (DC), due to an increased miscarriage rate, higher incidence of structural abnormalities, growth discordance and potential development of twin-to-twin transfusion syndrome (TTTS). MC pregnancies require greater surveillance with regular ultrasound scans, and planned earlier delivery than DC twins.

Twin-to-twin transfusion syndrome

TTTS affects 15–20% of MC twin pregnancies, and classically presents in the second trimester. It occurs as a consequence of intertwin transfusion through vascular anastomoses within the placenta. One twin (donor) transfuses blood to its co-twin (recipient), causing poor growth, anaemia and reduced urine production in the donor and consequent polycythaemia, and over-production of urine in the recipient. This leads to oligohydramnios and growth retardation in the donor, and corresponding polyhydramnios and high-output cardiac failure in the recipient twin. Either twin

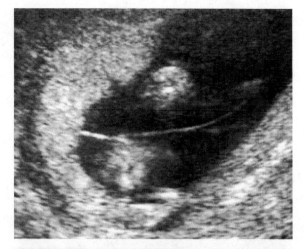

Insertion of thin membrane onto placenta (T sign) indicative of MC

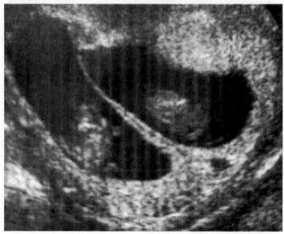

Insertion of thick membrane onto placenta (Lambda sign) indicative of DC

FIGURE 1.13 Multiple pregnancy, diagnosis of chorionicity by ultrasound scan

may die as a result of this. Severe TTTS occurring before 26 weeks is associated with high risk of fetal loss, perinatal death or long-term morbidity in survivors.[40] TTTS is graded by severity[41] and treatment options depend on the severity and gestational age.

There remains controversy about the best treatment options.[42,43] Currently two main treatments are available: *serial amnioreduction*, which attempts to reduce the risk of preterm labour secondary to polyhydramnios and may improve the haemodynamics in the placenta by reducing intra-uterine pressure and increasing the use of *fetoscopic laser ablation of the vascular anastomoses* in the placenta. Overall survival using either treatment modality in the treatment of severe disease is of the order of: 33% both twins survive, 33% one survives and 33% neither survives. However, Senat *et al.*[42] suggests that there are potentially lower neurological sequelae with laser ablation.

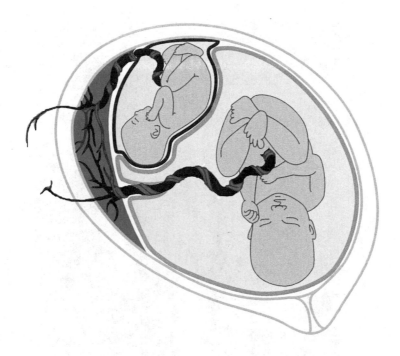

FIGURE 1.14 Diagram showing twin–twin transfusion syndrome

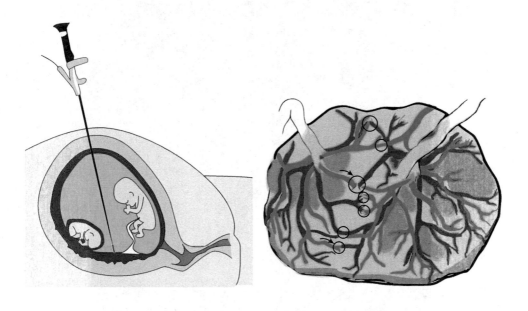

FIGURE 1.15 Diagram of fetoscopic laser ablation of placental anastomoses in twin–twin transfusion syndrome

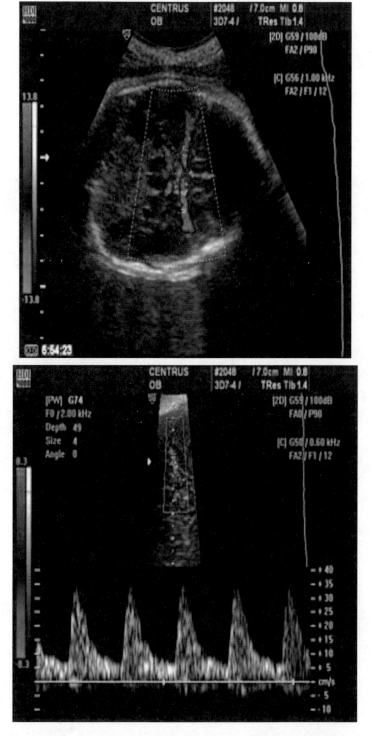

FIGURE 1.16 Ultrasound images of middle cerebral artery and Doppler waveform of measurement of maximum velocity

TABLE 1.13 TTTS staging

Stage	Liquor volume	Donor bladder	Doppler	Hydrops	Fetal demise
1	Discrepant (polyhydramnios with max vertical pocket of liquor >8 cm and oligohydramnios <2 cm)	Visible	Normal	No	No
2	Discrepant	Not visible	Not critically abnormal	No	No
3	Discrepant	Not visible	Critically abnormal (i.e. absent or reversed EDF in umbilical artery, reverse flow in the ductus venosus, or pulsatile flow in the umbilical vein)	No	No
4	Discrepant	Not visible	Critically abnormal	Yes	No
5	Discrepant	Not visible	Critically abnormal	Yes	One or both twins are dead

Monoamniotic pregnancies

These occur as a result of cleavage of a single zygote between day 9 and day 12 after conception, and results in two fetuses within the same amniotic cavity and with a single placenta. Mortality associated with this sort of twinning is up to 30% and is largely associated with fetal malformations, prematurity, complications from cord entanglement and acute TTTS, which may be difficult to recognise. Management includes US surveillance for TTTS, consideration of treatment with sulindac (a non-steroidal anti-inflammatory drug) which reduces fetal urine output and hence amniotic fluid volumes and also restricts fetal movement (which may increase cord compression) and planned early delivery by caesarean section.[44]

Fetal death of one twin

Spontaneous or iatrogenic death of one of a set of twins will have implications depending on chorionicity and gestational age. DC twins have discrete separate placentas, and so, although fetal death of one twin may cause spontaneous labour, the risk of death or morbidity to the second twin is low.

However, MC twins, because of their shared placental connections, are at significant risk of death or neurological handicap. In the event of the death of one twin the second twin is at risk because there can be an acute hypotensive event as a result of haemorrhage from the live twin into the dead one. Fetal cerebral lesions may result and antenatal magnetic resonance imaging (MRI) studies may prove useful in evaluating the extent of neurological damage to aid parental counselling.

Discordant abnormalities

Dizygotic twins are no more likely than any other sibling pair to have concordant anomalies, whereas monozygotic twins have the same genetic material and so may be concordant for chromosomal or genetic abnormalities. However, the consequence of cleavage of a single zygote may result in an uneven distribution of cells increasing the risk of discordant structural anomalies such as neural tube defects. Abnormal placentation may also increase the risk for some fetal anomalies as a result of altered blood flow to the fetus during early development.

Selective reduction of DC twins that are discordant for fetal abnormality is achieved with an injection of KCl into the fetal heart, whereas the shared placental circulation precludes this in MC twins. Alternative cord-occlusion techniques such as interstitial laser and bipolar cord occlusion may be considered.[45]

Conjoined twins

These occur as a result of splitting of the embryonic mass after day 12 following fertilisation. The prognosis for conjoined twins depends on the site of conjoining and shared organs. Studies have suggested that about two-thirds of such twins are stillborn, and for those born alive, surgery may not be possible in a third of cases.

TABLE 1.14 Diagram of types of conjoined twins[46]

Type	Incidence %	Organs potentially involved	
Thoracopagus	74%	Heart, liver, intestine	
Omphalopagus	1%	Liver, biliary tree, intestine	
Pyopagus	17%	Spine, rectum, genitourinary tract	

(continued)

Type	Incidence %	Organs potentially involved	
Ischiopagus	6%	Pelvis, liver, intestine, genitourinary tract	
Craniopagus	2%	Brain, meninges	

FETAL INFECTIONS

Maternal infections in pregnancy have long been known to have the potential for fetal effects such as fetal abnormalities, and infection in early pregnancy can increase the risk of pregnancy loss through miscarriage.

Rubella

Rubella is a mild disease characterised by a transient red rash and raised lymph glands, and used to be a very common childhood illness. Fetal infection in the first 12 weeks of pregnancy has profound consequences. In the era before mass immunisation for rubella, it is estimated that in the UK about 200–300 babies per year were born with congenital rubella, causing significant problems such as sensorineural deafness, cataracts, microphthalmia, congenital glaucoma, congenital heart defects, and microcephaly. A far greater number of pregnancies were terminated because of the risk of fetal effects.

TABLE 1.15 Risks of intra-uterine infection with rubella depending on stage of pregnancy[47]

Stage of pregnancy	Risk of intra-uterine transmission
4–11 weeks	90%
11–16 weeks	20%
16–20 weeks	Risk of deafness only
>20 weeks	No increased risk

In the UK, vaccination has been offered in childhood since 1971, with a corresponding decrease in the number of confirmed cases. Only 27 confirmed cases of rubella were recorded in England and Wales in 2007. It is a notifiable disease. All pregnant women are offered serological testing for rubella immunity, and those who are found to be susceptible are advised to avoid contact with rubella in pregnancy and seek immunisation following the birth of their baby. There still remains a risk for those women who were born in parts of the world where universal vaccination is not offered, or if those women who are susceptible travel to parts of the world where rubella is still common.

Parvovirus B19

Also known as slapped-cheek syndrome, Fifth disease, or erythema infectiosum, parvovirus B19 is a single-stranded-DNA virus belonging to the parvoviridae group of viruses which include the animal parvoviruses such as canine parvovirus and feline panleukopenia virus. It is characterised by a facial rash usually preceded by a mild flu-like illness, and may be asymptomatic in 20–30% of cases. It is a common childhood illness. Occasionally parvovirus in pregnancy can cause adverse consequences associated with viral replication in the fetal bone marrow. This causes suppression of red blood cell production, leading to fetal anaemia and hydrops formation. Parvovirus infection before 20 weeks of pregnancy can be associated with fetal loss, and about 3% of those pregnancies that are infected between 9 and 20 weeks may develop hydrops. Surveillance using ultrasound to detect fetal signs of anaemia (by measuring the middle cerebral artery peak systolic velocity, *see* page 32) may be used, with a potential for fetal treatment with intra-uterine transfusion if anaemia is confirmed before the fetus is severely hydropic.

Cytomegalovirus (CMV)

CMV is a member of the herpes virus family. It is so called because it causes enlargement of the cells it infects. It is very common and it has been estimated that 60–90% of the population have come in contact with CMV by adulthood. Once a person has been infected, the virus remains dormant in the body throughout life.

Most primary maternal infections are sub-clinical. It is a relatively common primary infection during pregnancy, and 60–70% of babies will not acquire the infection from their mother. Of those that do become infected, most babies (85–90%) are not affected and do not develop disease associated with the virus. However, those babies that are affected with congenital CMV can have significant long-term complications such as hearing loss, mental retardation and chorioretinitis. Growth retardation, microcephaly and seizures may be apparent and mental retardation is common. Intra-uterine death may occur. Ultrasound features such as echogenic bowel or microcephaly may prompt investigations including maternal serology and also consideration of amniocentesis or fetal blood sampling to determine if the fetus has been infected to aid management decisions.

Congenital CMV accounts for as much disability in the population as Down's syndrome or spina bifida, and whilst no vaccine exists, women can be given information about the importance of good hand hygiene in reducing the chance of primary infection in pregnancy.

Toxoplasmosis

Toxoplasmosis is a disease caused by a common parasite called *Toxoplasma gondii*. Symptoms in healthy people are mild and non-specific and so the disease often goes unreported. The parasite can form microscopic cysts in muscle tissue and remain in the body for many years with no ill effect. The parasite can be transmitted through contact with infected cats faeces, contaminated soil, livestock such as sheep, or uncooked meat. Pregnant women should be advised to avoid contact with these sources.

If the mother becomes infected for the first time during pregnancy, the fetus may have effects, depending on the gestation at infection. It is most severe if contracted during the first trimester but only 15% of babies will become infected even if the mother is infected during this time. Babies born after contracting the disease in the first trimester can have symptoms including brain damage, jaundice, fever, rash, convulsions, enlarged liver and spleen, microcephaly, hydrocephalus, and impaired vision. There is a significant mortality rate for affected fetuses.

If it is contracted in the second trimester, about 25% of babies will be infected, but with less severe disease, and if it is contracted in the third trimester, 65% of babies may become infected. This group of babies will have fewer effects at birth, but may have eye problems in later life.

If a mother has a confirmed new toxoplasmosis infection in pregnancy, administration of spiramycin may reduce transmission to the fetus. Spiramycin will not reduce the severity of an acquired fetal infection. Amniocentesis should be considered to obtain evidence of fetal infection before treatment commences.

Varicella

Varicella zoster virus causes a common childhood illness, characterised by mild cold-like symptoms followed by the development of an itchy vesicular rash, typically over the trunk and limbs. Transmission is via droplet infection from an infected person. Varicella infection in pregnancy has risks both for the fetus and for the mother. Women who develop chickenpox during pregnancy are at risk of varicella pneumonia, whilst the fetus may acquire congenital varicella. Congenital varicella causes a range of symptoms including limb abnormalities, skin scarring, cataracts and growth restriction, depending on the gestation at infection. Ultrasound scanning may detect fetal limb anomalies, but other features except growth retardation are unlikely to be detected antenatally. The chance of fetal infection is thought to be 1% in the first 12 weeks of pregnancy, 2% between 13 and 20 weeks and negligible from 20–28 weeks. The risks increase at later gestations with a risk of preterm delivery or neonatal chickenpox, particularly if maternal disease occurs between 7 days before and 7 days after birth. Women who have a confirmed varicella infection in pregnancy should be offered oral antiviral treatment such as acyclovir if they present within 24 hours of the onset of rash. Prophylaxis against infection may be considered using VZIG for women who are not immune and at high risk of contracting the virus (e.g. child within the household already infected).

BLOOD GROUP ANTIBODIES AND HAEMOLYTIC DISEASE OF THE NEWBORN (HDN)

Fetal HDN caused by maternal blood-group antibodies continues to be a significant cause of perinatal morbidity and occasionally mortality, despite advances in antenatal prevention, monitoring and treatment.

Maternal blood-group antibody formation is due to an immune response to antigens found on red blood cells that are not present in the mother. This is usually due to sensitisation with fetal red blood cells during pregnancy or at delivery, or occasionally from blood transfusion. The initial response to a foreign antigen is to produce IgM antibodies, which do not cross the placenta, but subsequent exposure (typically during a second pregnancy) stimulates the rapid production of IgG antibodies, which can cross the placenta and enter the fetal circulation. These antibodies can bind to the antigen on the fetal red cell surface and cause destruction by phagocytosis. This produces fetal anaemia, the degree of which is determined by the type and amount of antibody production.

Antigens most likely to cause this response include those of the Rh class, particularly D, although C, c, E and e can also produce a response. Other blood-group antigens can cause antibody production but with more minimal effects on the fetus, including those of the Kell, Fy (Duffy) and Kidd (Jka and Jkb) groups. Typically a mother who is RhD-negative with a fetus that is RhD-positive is at risk of development of anti-D antibodies. Anti-D immunoglobulin is given prophylactically during pregnancy, following sensitising events and at delivery to destroy any fetal red cells before the maternal immune system can mount a response. There is no prophylaxis available to reduce sensitisation to Rhc, RhE and Kell antigens and so morbidity associated with these antigens accounts for an increasing proportion of the total.

Identification of those women at risk of HDN includes routine determination of the maternal blood group and antibody status when women present initially for maternity care. Those women who are RhD-negative should be offered prophylactic anti-D immunoglobulin during pregnancy.[48]

Women who are found to have relevant blood group antibodies should be monitored using serial antibody titres although there is not always good correlation with antibody levels and the severity of fetal disease. The trend in antibody levels may be more significant than the actual value. For anti-D antibodies a level over 4 iu should prompt increased surveillance for fetal anaemia, whilst the level for anti-c is 7 iu, and for other antibodies a titre of 1 in 32 should be used. Severe anaemia is unlikely at anti-D levels of less than 15 iu.[49] Assessment of the fetal blood group is of value particularly when the father of the pregnancy is heterozygous for the RhD gene or is unknown. Free fetal DNA in the maternal plasma can be genotyped as early as 8–10 weeks to predict the fetal Rh or Kell group. If the fetus is RhD-negative, no further testing or invasive interventions would be needed.[50]

Severe HDN is characterised by fetal anaemia and hydrops (the development of fluid within fetal body cavities such as ascites, pleural or pericardial effusions and skin oedema) *in utero*, and also by hyperbilirubinaemia post-natally. The aim of surveillance is to detect fetal anaemia before the development of hydrops, so that intra-uterine treatment or delivery can be planned whilst the fetus is still well. For women with a previous history of HDN, the severity of the disease tends to increase in subsequent pregnancies and so surveillance should be started from an early gestation.

Antenatal surveillance for fetal anaemia primarily now uses ultrasound techniques. The fetal circulation responds to a degree of anaemia by making cardiovascular adjustments. Initially, to maintain oxygenation, cardiac output is increased through a combination of decreased blood viscosity and a fall in peripheral vascular resistance. This increased cardiac output can be monitored using Doppler sonography to measure the arterial peak systolic velocity, typically in the middle cerebral artery

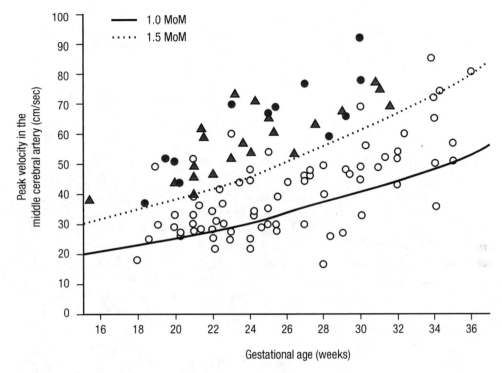

FIGURE 1.17 Chart showing plotting of MCApsv against gestational age. Values above 1.5 MoM may indicate fetal anaemia (Mari *et al.* 2000)

(MCApsv). Studies have shown a direct correlation with MCApsv and the degree of fetal anaemia.[51]

Serial assessment of the MCApsv is used, along with ultrasound imaging to look for hydrops and the assessment of fetal movements to provide an overall picture of fetal well-being. If the MCApsv rises above 1.5 MoM, in association with hydrops or a reduction in fetal movements, consideration should be given to invasive assessment of fetal anaemia, or delivery, depending on gestation.

Invasive assessment of fetal anaemia is achieved by fetal blood sampling – a 20–2 g needle is inserted under ultrasound control into either the placental insertion of the umbilical vein, (cordocentesis) or the intrahepatic portion of the umbilical vein. 1–5 mL fetal blood is aspirated and the haemoglobin concentration determined. Donor packed red blood cells can be administered through the same needle, following initial sampling, to correct the fetal anaemia. *In utero* transfusions carry a small risk of fetal compromise and possible fetal loss. Repeated fetal blood transfusion can be used as directed by evaluation of the MCApsv.

FETAL THERAPIES

The potential for fetal therapies to reduce the severity of existing fetal disease or even treat abnormalities is exciting and holds great promise for the future. The reality at present, however, is that there are limited options to treat fetuses *in utero*, not least because of adverse maternal effects and the difficulty in obtaining clinical evidence of benefit from randomised studies. Ethical debates about the role of experimental treatments and fetal versus maternal rights have influenced progression of some treatment options, and at present many fetal therapies are only undertaken in those fetuses who are predicted to have a poor prognosis; the risk-benefit analysis must be considered before any intervention occurs. NICE interventional procedures guidance has been produced for some fetal therapies.[52]

In utero treatments fall into several categories which are considered below.

Medical therapies (including maternal or fetal pharmacological administration)

For conditions such as fetal tachyarrhythmias, which may lead to cardiac failure and hydrops, administration of anti-arrhythmic agents such as flecainide or digoxin to the mother would be the first line of treatment. Transplacental transfer of the drug may have an effect on the FHR, although there is a risk of maternal side effects. If treatment by maternal administration fails, direct intravenous or intraperitoneal injection to the fetus may improve cardiac rate and function and allow resolution of hydrops prior to delivery.

Direct fetal (either intravenous or intra-amniotic) administration of other therapeutic agents such as thyroxine has been used for the treatment of fetal goitre to reduce the risk of post-delivery airway obstruction.

Drug therapy is used to reduce the vertical transmission of infections, such as drug regimens used in HIV-positive women, and spiramycin therapy for those women who acquire toxoplasmosis in pregnancy.

Maternal administration of indomethacin constricts the smooth muscle in fetal blood vessels, particularly those supplying the kidneys and so can be used to lessen polyhydramnios by reducing the fetal urine output. Because it can also constrict the ductus arteriosus, this treatment is used with caution particularly at later gestations.

Maternal dexamethasone is used to reduce the virilising effects of high levels of circulating hormones on female fetuses affected by congenital adrenal hyperplasia.

Administration of intravenous immunoglobulins to the mother may also reduce the thrombocytopenic effects of antibodies to the fetal platelets where fetal allo-immune thrombocytopaenia is present and it has been used in other rare conditions such as hereditary haemochromatosis.

Other medical therapies include the administration of maternal corticosteroids to improve maturation of fetal lungs prior to preterm delivery, and the use of folic acid periconceptually to reduce the incidence of neural tube defects.

Invasive intra-uterine therapy

Invasive therapies require the use of ultrasound to guide the placement of a needle or other instrument through the maternal abdominal wall and into the fetus or placenta.

Transfusion

As previously described, intra-uterine blood transfusions are used to treat fetuses who are predicted to be anaemic as a result of maternal blood group antibodies or infection (parvovirus B19) and platelets may be transfused to treat fetuses with thrombocytopaenia.

Amnioreduction

Amniotic fluid volumes may be manipulated by amnioreduction using a needle to aspirate large volumes of fluid to reduce polyhydramnios. The excess amniotic fluid may result from either obstruction within the gastrointestinal tract (for example in fetuses with duodenal atresia, compression of the oesophagus in diaphragmatic hernia) or from neuromuscular conditions such as congenital myotonic dystrophy or from increased fetal urine output, e.g. fetuses with a high cardiac output such as the recipient twin in TTTS. By reducing the amniotic fluid volume, the operator reduces the intra-uterine pressure and hence improves the mother's comfort and reduces the risk of preterm labour. This benefit, however, is gained at the risk of precipitating labour.

Amniotic fluid infusions

Amniotic fluid infusions may be used to improve the diagnostic ability of ultrasound scanning in cases of oligohydramnios or anhydramnios, but its role in reducing the risk of lung hypoplasia is not proven.

Vesico-amniotic shunts

Fetal vesico-amniotic shunts have been used to drain fluid from the bladder that has accumulated as a result of lower urinary tract outflow obstruction (commonly posterior urethral valves). It is thought that fetuses most likely to benefit from the insertion of a pig-tailed catheter are those with obstruction severe enough to compromise renal and pulmonary development, but not so severe that renal damage is irreversible even if the obstruction is relieved. A randomised controlled trial is currently underway in the UK to evaluate this intervention (the PLUTO trial, www.pluto.bham.ac.uk).

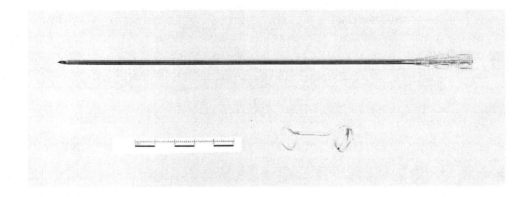

FIGURE 1.18 A Harrison Fetal Bladder Stent (Shunt)

Pleuro-amniotic shunts

Ultrasound guided placement of a pleuro-amniotic shunt may be used in cases of fetal pleural effusion, to allow decompression of the lung and allow normal lung growth and development.

Fetoscopic procedures
Laser ablation of placental vessels

This is used for the treatment of TTTS and is carried out with maternal sedation and local anaesthesia.

Insertion of endotracheal balloons

Animal models have suggested that occlusion of the trachea using a fetoscopically guided balloon may be a potential treatment for antenatally diagnosed diaphragmatic hernia. When the trachea is blocked the fluid that is made within the fetal lung cannot escape into the amniotic fluid and so it builds up, causing potential expansion of the lungs, stimulation of their growth and the pressure pushes the abdominal content (liver, intestines, stomach) out of the chest and back into the abdomen. This treatment is currently being evaluated.

Open surgical procedures

These have largely been superseded by less invasive endoscopic and needle-guided procedures, but are still carried out in certain situations despite significant maternal effects. Surgical repair of meningomyelocele following hysterotomy is the subject of a randomised controlled trial in the USA (the MOMS study). The study is designed to see if surgical repair before birth protects the exposed neural tissue from damage.

EXIT procedures

Ex utero intrapartum treatment ('EXIT') may be used to partially deliver a fetus and allow stabilisation of an airway or surgery whilst the fetus is still attached to the placental circulation.

Other treatments such as *fetal stem cell transplants* and *ablation of stenosed fetal cardiac valves* are rare. The potential, however, for treatment of conditions *in utero* holds great promise, as the fetus has biological advantages over an adult, particularly at the immunological and cellular level, perhaps allowing restoration of organ development and function.

All fetal intervention is really maternal-fetal intervention, and the most important consideration is the safety of the mother and her reproductive potential. The intervention is designed to benefit the fetus that has a problem, but the mother is an innocent bystander who assumes some risk for the sake of her unborn fetus.

REFERENCES

1 Pijnenborg R, Vercruysse L. Shifting concepts of the fetal-maternal interface: a historical perspective. *Placenta.* 2007; **22:** S20–5.
2 Barker DJP. *Mother, Babies and Health in Later Life.* 2nd ed. Edinburgh: Churchill Livingston; 1998.

3 Lyall F. The placenta bed revisited. *Placenta.* 2002; **23**: 555–62.

4 Pijnenborg R, Vercruysse L, Hanssens M, *et al.* Incomplete trophoblast invasion: the evidence. In: Critchley H, MacLean A, Poston L, *et al.*, editors. *Pre-eclampsia.* London: Royal College of Obstetricians and Gynaecologists; 2003. pp. 15–26.

5 Blackburn ST. *Maternal, Fetal and Neonatal Physiology: a clinical perspective.* Edinburgh: Saunders Elsevier; 2003.

6 Lyall F. Mechanisms underlying failure of trophoblast invasion. In: Critchley H, MacLean A, Poston L, *et al.*, editors. *Pre-eclampsia.* London: Royal College of Obstetricians and Gynaecologists; 2003. pp. 27–48.

7 Knöfler M, Simmons DG, Lash GE, *et al.* Regulation of trophoblast invasion: a workshop report. *Placenta.* 2008; **22**(Suppl. A): S26–8.

8 Abramowicz JS, Sheiner E. Ultrasound of the placenta: Part 1: Imaging. *Placenta.* 2008; **29**: 225–9.

9 Mazouni C, Gorincour G, Juham V, *et al.* Placenta accreta: a review of current advances in prenatal diagnosis. *Placenta.* 2007; **28**: 599–603.

10 Godfrey KM. The role of the placenta in fetal programming: a review. *Placenta.* 2002; **23**(Suppl. A – Trophoblast Research): S20–7.

11 Quinton AE, Cook C-M, Peek MJ. The relationship between cigarette smoking, endothelial function and intrauterine growth restriction in human pregnancy. *BJOG.* 2008; **115**: 780–4.

12 Godfrey KM, Walker- Bone K, Robinson S, *et al.* Neonatal bone mass: influence of parental birth weight and maternal smoking, body composition, and activity during pregnancy. *Journal of Bone Mineral Research.* 2001; **16**: 1694–703.

13 Jansson T, Powell TL. Human placental transport in altered fetal growth: does the placenta function as a nutrient sensor? A review. *Placenta.* 2006; **27**(Suppl. A): S91–7.

14 Samangaya RA, Haezell AP, Baker PM. Hypertension in pregnancy. In: Greer IA, Nelson-Piercy C, Walters B, editors. *Maternal Medicine: medical problems in pregnancy.* Edinburgh: Churchill Livingston Elsevier; 2007. pp. 40–52.

15 Wallis AB, Saftlas AF, Hsia J, *et al.* Secular trends in the rates of preeclampsia, eclampsia, and gestational hypertension, United States, 1987–2004. *Am J Hypertens.* 2008; **21**(5): 521–6.

16 Knight M. Eclampsia in the United Kingdom 2005. *BJOG.* 2007; **S114**(9): 1072–8.

17 Mütze S, Rudnik-Schöneborn S, Zerres K, *et al.* Genes and the pre-eclampsia syndrome. *J Perinat Med.* 2008; **36**(1): 38–58.

18 Redman CW, Sargent IL. Pre-eclampsia, the placenta and the maternal systemic inflammatory response: a review. *Placenta.* 2003; **24**(Suppl. A): S21–7.

19 Redman CW, Sargent IL. Pre-eclampsia as an inflammatory response. In: Critchley H, MacLean A, Poston L, *et al.*, editors. *Pre-eclampsia.* London: Royal College of Obstetricians and Gynaecologists; 2003. pp. 101–12.

20 Wareing M, Baker PN. The role of the endothelium. In: Critchley H, MacLean A, Poston L, *et al.*, editors. *Pre-eclampsia.* London: Royal College of Obstetricians and Gynaecologists; 2003. pp. 113–33.

21 Wild S, Roglic G, Green A, *et al.* Global prevalence of diabetes: estimates for the year 2000 and projections for 2030. *Diabetes Care.* 2004; **27**: 1047–53.

22 Buimer M, Keijser R, Jebbink JM, *et al.* Seven placental transcripts characterize HELLP Syndrome. *Placenta.* 2008; **29**: 444–53.

23 Confidential Enquiries into Maternal and Child Health (CEMACH). *Pregnancy in Women with Type 1 and Type 2 Diabetes in 2002–03, in England, Wales and Northern Ireland.* London: CEMACH; 2005.

24 Wild S, Roglic G, Green A, *et al.*, op. cit.

25 Cheung NW, Walter BNJ. Type 1 and type 2 diabetes in pregnancy. In: Greer IA, Nelson-Piercy C, Walters B, editors. *Maternal Medicine: medical problems in pregnancy.* Edinburgh: Churchill Livingston Elsevier; 2007. pp. 82–97.

26 National Institute for Health and Clinical Excellence. *Diabetes in Pregnancy: management of diabetes and its complications from pre-conception to the postnatal period: NICE guideline 63.* London: NIHCE; 2008. www.nice.org.uk/nicemedia/pdf/CG063FullGuideline.pdf (accessed 14 April 2009).

27 Savander M, Ropponen A, Avela K, *et al.* Genetic evidence of heterogeneity in intrahepatic cholestasis of pregnancy. *Gut.* 2003; **52**: 1025–9.

28 Williamson C, Girling J. Hepatic and gastrointestinal disease. In: James DK, Steer PJ, Weimer CP, *et al.*, editors. *High Risk Pregnancy: management options.* 3rd ed. Philadelphia: Saunders Elsevier; 2006. pp. 1037–40.

29 Royal College of Obstetricians and Gynecologists. *Obstetric Cholestasis: guideline no. 43*; 2006. Available at: www.rcog.org.uk/resources/Public/pdf/obstetric_cholestasis43.pdf (accessed 14 April 2009).

30 Billington M, Heptinstall T. Medical disorders and critically ill women. In: Billington M, Stevenson M, editors. *Critical Care in Childbearing for Midwives.* Oxford: Blackwell; 2007. pp. 30–64.

31 Burrows RF, Clavisi O, Burrows E. Interventions for treating cholestasis in pregnancy. *Cochrane Database Syst Rev.* 2001; **4**: CD000493.

32 National Screening Committee. *Consent Standards for Screening Fetal Anomalies during Pregnancy.* London: UK National Screening Committee; 2007. Available at: www.fetalanomaly. screening.nhs.uk/images/Fetal/Publications/Consent%20Standards%20Booklet_final.pdf (accessed 14 April 2009).

33 National Collaborating Centre for Women's and Children's Health, on behalf of National Institute for Health and Clinical Excellence. *Intrapartum Care: care of healthy women and their babies during childbirth: NICE guideline 55.* London: NIHCE; 2007. Available at: www. nice.org.uk/CG055 (accessed 14 April 2009).

34 Alfirevic Z, Devane D, Gyte GML. Continuous cardiotocography (CTG) as a form of electronic fetal monitoring (EFM) for fetal assessment during labour. *Cochrane Database Syst Rev.* 2006; **3**: CD006066.

35 Neilson JP. Fetal electrocardiogram (ECG) for fetal monitoring during labour. *Cochrane Database Syst Rev.* 2006; **3**: CD000116.

36 Office for National Statistics. *Birth Statistics 2006 FM1.* Available at: www.statistics.gov.uk (accessed 14 April 2009).

37 Dodd JM, Crowther CA. Reduction of the number of fetuses for women with triplet and higher order multiple pregnancies. *Cochrane Database Syst Rev.* 2003; **2**: CD003932.

38 Taylor MJ, Fisk NM. Prenatal diagnosis in multiple pregnancy. *Baillières Best Pract Res Clin Obstet Gynaecol.* 2000; **14**(4): 663–75.

39 Dahoun S, Gagos S, Gagnebin M, *et al.* Monozygotic twins discordant for trisomy 21 and maternal 21q inheritance: a complex series of events. *Am J Med Genet A.* 2008; **146A**(16): 2086–93.

40 Mari G, Roberts A, Detti L, *et al.* Perinatal morbidity and mortality rates in severe twin–twin transfusion syndrome: results of the international registry. *Am J Obstet Gynecol.* 2001; **185**(3): 708–15.

41 Quintero RA, Morales WJ, Allen MH, *et al.* Staging of twin–twin transfusion syndrome. *J Perinatol.* 1999; **19**(8 Pt 1): 550–5.

42 Senat M, Deprest J, Boulvain M, *et al.* Endoscopic laser surgery versus seral amnioreduction for severe twin-to-twin transfusion syndrome. *New Engl J Med.* 2004; **351**: 135–44.

43 Crombleholme TM, Shera D, Lee H, *et al.* A prospective randomised multicenter trial of amnioreduction vs selective fetoscopic laser photocoagulation for the treatment of severe twin–twin transfusion syndrome. *Am J Obstet Gynecol.* 2007; **197**(4): 396.

44 Pasquini L, Wimalasundera RC, Fichera A, *et al.* High perinatal survival in monoamniotic twins managed by prophylactic sulindac, intensive ultrasound surveillance, and Cesarean delivery at 32 weeks' gestation. *Ultrasound Obstet Gynecol.* 2006; **28**(5): 681–7.

45 Rustico MA, Baietti MG, Coviello D, *et al.* Managing twins discordant for fetal anomaly. *Prenat Diagn.* 2005; **25**(9): 766–1.

46 Spitz L. Conjoined twins. *Br J Surg.* 1996; **83**: 1028–30.

47 Health Protection Agency. *Rashes in pregnancy – HPA guidelines, information and advice.* Available at: www.hpa.org.uk/web/HPAweb&HPAwebStandard/HPAweb_C/1195733745858 (accessed 14 April 2009).

48 National Institute for Health and Clinical Excellence. *Routine Antenatal Anti-D Prophylaxis for Women who are Rhesus D Negative.* London: NIHCE; 2008. Available at: www.nice.org.uk/Guidance/TA156 (accessed 14 April 2009).

49 Nicolaides KH, Rodeck CH. Maternal serum anti-D antibody concentrations and assessment of rhesus isoimmunisation. *BMJ.* 1992; **304**: 1155–6.

50 Finning K, Martin P, Summers J, *et al.* Effect of high throughput RHD typing of fetal DNA in maternal plasma on use of anti-RhD immunoglobulin in RhD negative pregnant women: prospective feasibility study. *BMJ.* 2008; **336**: 816–18.

51 Mari G, Deter R, Carpenter R, *et al.*, for the Collaborative Group for Doppler Assessment of the Blood Velocity in Anemic Fetuses. Noninvasive diagnosis by Doppler ultrasonography of fetal anaemia due to maternal red-cell alloimmunization. *N Engl J Med.* 2000; **342**: 9–14.

52 National Institute for Health and Clinical Excellence. Interventional procedures guidance. Available at: www.nice.org.uk/guidance/index.jsp?action=byTopic&o=7261 (accessed 18 May 2009).

IPG	Title	Date published
175	Percutaneous fetal balloon valvuloplasty for aortic stenosis	May 2006
176	Percutaneous fetal balloon valvuloplasty for pulmonary atresia with intact ventricular septum	May 2006
180	Percutaneous laser therapy for fetal tumours	June 2006
190	Insertion of pleuroamniotic shunt for fetal pleural effusion	Sept 2006
192	Amnioinfusion for oligohydramnios in pregnancy	Dec 2006
198	Intrauterine laser ablation of placental vessels for the treatment of twin–twin transfusion syndrome	Dec 2006

CHAPTER 2

An overview of genetics

Bruce Castle

CONTENTS

DNA, THE GENETIC CODE AND ALTERATIONS

DNA (deoxyribonucleic acid) and RNA (ribonucleic acid) are the macromolecules of information of the genetic code. DNA is the informative structure of the chromosomes and is contained within the nucleus of almost all cells. An additional package of DNA is also present in the mitochondria, which will be dealt with later in the chapter.

DNA is made up of four types of base – the purines adenine (A) and guanine (G), and the pyrimidines cytosine (C) and thymine (T). These are attached to a five-carbon sugar, deoxyribose, which is, in turn, linked by phosphodiester (phosphate) bonds in succession (*see* Figure 2.1). The base, sugar and phosphate group constitutes a **nucleotide** – the building unit of DNA.

RNA molecules are similar to those of DNA but contain the sugar ribose, and the base thymine is replaced by uracil (U).

The common structure of DNA is that of the double helix described in 1953 by Watson and Crick[1] (*see* Figure 2.2). The nucleotides have specific relationships within

41

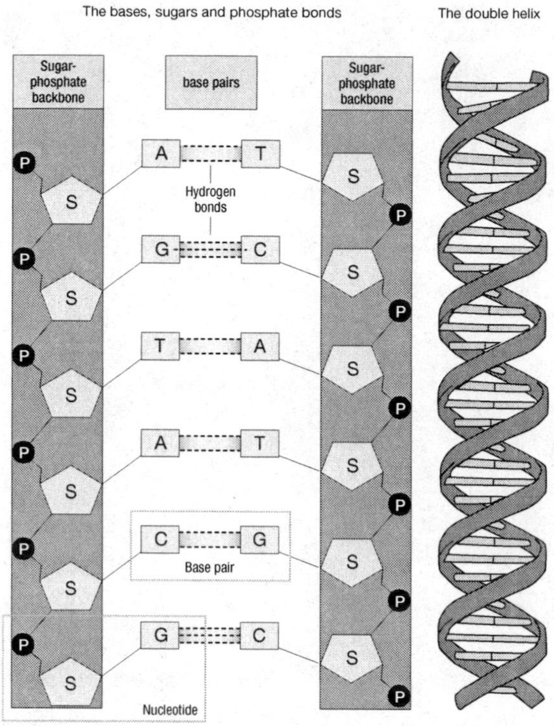

The bases, sugars and phosphate bonds

The double helix

Sugar-phosphate backbone

base pairs

Sugar-phosphate backbone

A ┈┈┈┈ T

Hydrogen bonds

G ┈┈┈┈ C

T ┈┈┈┈ A

A ┈┈┈┈ T

C ┈┈┈┈ G

Base pair

G ┈┈┈┈ C

Nucleotide

FIGURE 2.1 The structure of DNA

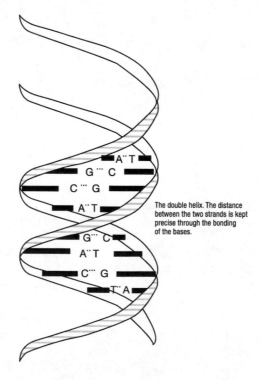

A ̈ T
G ⋯ C
C ⋯ G
A ̈ T

The double helix. The distance between the two strands is kept precise through the bonding of the bases.

G ⋯ C
A ̈ T
C ⋯ G
T ̈ A

FIGURE 2.2 DNA

the structure due to chemical affinity such that adenine (A) pairs with thymine (T) and cytosine (C) with guanine (G). These are held together by weak chemical bonds. This has been important in making possible the development of the very useful tool in molecular analysis, the polymerase chain reaction (PCR), where these weak bonds are broken easily by heat.

The helical structure of DNA is kept constant in dimension (width) due to this pairing of the nucleotides, and the particular order in which they are arranged is the genetic code. Additionally, the faithful replication whereby these nucleotides pair up enables DNA to:

(a)   act as a template for the replication necessary for cell division, and

(b)   be copied for the production of RNA – the process of **transcription.**

A gene is simply a recipe, as in cooking, and is a section of DNA which has a unique sequence of bases. The sequence provides the code for the production of an individual protein. It functions through the products it produces. The initial product is a molecule of RNA, which is faithfully copied off the DNA template by transcription using the base codes in a **reading frame** for each amino acid and an **open reading frame** of the sequence. The amino acids join together to form a protein, which has a precise structure, or **conformation**. Not all RNAs are so used and a small number are involved in the regulation of other RNA production.

The process of protein production is as shown in Figure 2.3 below.

The DNA molecule containing the gene involved separates into its two strands. This acts as a template for the production of the new strand of RNA called messenger RNA (mRNA). This is an exact complementary copy of the original DNA through the complementarity of the base pairs (uracil replacing thymine). Not all of a gene's

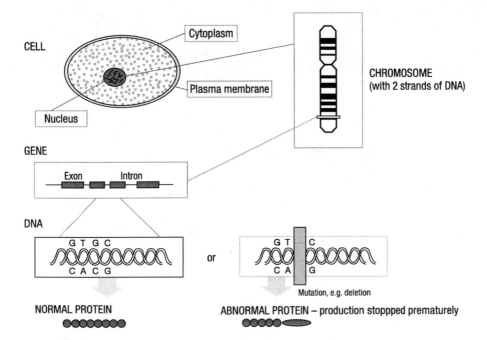

FIGURE 2.3 Cellular and molecular organisation

DNA is coding – that is, not all of the DNA is used to make the protein – so the **non-coding** DNA needs to be removed. This post-transcriptional processing removes the non-coding portions or **introns** and joins together the coding portions or **exons** through a process called *splicing*.

The mRNA so formed now moves from the nucleus of the cell into the cytoplasm and becomes attached to **ribosomes**. These are large RNA-protein molecular complexes found in the cytoplasm of cells and in mitochondria. A protein molecule is formed of **amino acids,** which determine its structure and function depending on their sequence. This sequence, initially determined from the gene's DNA and thereafter through mRNA, relies on a precise coding system so that the correct amino acid is attached in the protein-building process. Each 'letter' of the original recipe in the DNA is formed by a sequence of three nucleotide bases, which is called a *triplet* or *codon*. Through the mRNA this codon is **translated** into the protein by another form of RNA called transfer RNA (tRNA). Each tRNA codon specifies which amino acid corresponds to the codon on the mRNA, thus faithfully replicating the original code of the gene into a protein product.

There are 20 different amino acids. As there are four bases and a codon contains three of them, there are 43 or 64 possible different combinations of bases available. Three codons constitute STOP codons, which terminate the translation process in protein production. This leaves 61 codons for the amino acids. Therefore most amino acids are coded for by more than one codon and the term used to describe this state of affairs is *degenerate*.

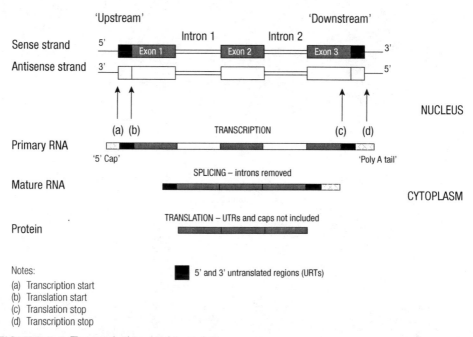

FIGURE 2.4 Transcription and translation

Mutations

A change in the genetic code is called a mutation. This may occur by chance (spontaneously) or through the influence of environmental factors such as chemical exposure or radiation. These changes can occur in both the germ cells in the gonads and in somatic cells (non-germ cells) but it is only those in the germline which can be passed on to the next generation and are therefore heritable. These are important in evolution as well as in disease, since some mutations create advantages. An example of this is the mutation for sickle-cell disease, which conveys some protection against malaria and so carriers of this mutation will have an advantage over those who don't in areas of the world affected by this disease.

Types of mutation: stable mutations

SILENT MUTATIONS

Silent mutations are those changes where the amino acid is not altered. With the degenerate amino-acid code (*see* above) this may occur such that a substitution, although altering the codon, doesn't change the amino acid. An example might be where a CG**T** becomes a CG**C**, both coding for arginine. Of importance, however, is that some substitutions may affect a splice site, thus affecting the post-translational process leading to an altered gene product.

MISSENSE MUTATIONS

Missense mutations are those from which an altered amino-acid sequence in the protein results. This alteration may have no effect on the function of the protein and so the function is conserved and is termed a *conservative mutation*. If the function is altered, this is called a *non-conservative mutation*. The change in function will be determined by the position of the altered amino acid within the protein and whether the alteration changes its three-dimensional structure by altered electrical charge.

TRUNCATING MUTATIONS

Truncating mutations result in premature termination of production and a shortened protein may arise in various ways.

▶ **Nonsense mutations** cause loss of the reading frame of the gene. These occur when a single nucleotide substitution occurs creating a premature STOP codon.
▶ **Insertions/deletions.** Altering the reading frame through insertion or deletion of bases will depend on whether these are in multiples of three. If it is not a multiple of three it is known as a *frameshift mutation* and the reading frame is lost with a downstream STOP codon being produced. (If it is, then an *inframe alteration* occurs lengthening or shortening the protein, which may or may not have functional effects.)

SPLICE-SITE MUTATIONS

These occur where the sequence at the splicing junction between intron and exon is altered. This often occurs at the mandatory dinucleotides at the beginning of an intron – GT (splice donor site) or the end – AG (splice acceptor site) but may also occur in sequences flanking these. This may lead to reading through the intron as well as the exons resulting in a protein with far too many amino acids in it. Alternatively, due to an alteration in the splice region, one or more exons may be lost resulting in a shortened protein due to fewer amino acids. Both situations result in malfunctioning proteins. An example of these mutations is given in Figure 2.5 below.

Normal								
sense strand	ATG	TCA	GCA	TTT	CGT	TAT	AAC	TTA
antisense strand	TAC	AGT	CGT	AAA	GCA	ATA	TTG	AAT
amino acid	Met	Ser	Ala	Phe	Arg	Tyr	Asn	Leu
Silent mutation through substitution								
sense strand	ATG	TCA	GCA	TTT	CCT	TAT	AAC	TTA
antisense strand	TAC	AGT	CGT	AAA	GGA	ATA	TTG	AAT
amino acid	Met	Ser	Ala	Phe	Arg	Tyr	Asn	Leu
Missense mutation through substitution								
sense strand	ATG	TCA	GCA	TTT	CAT	TAT	AAC	TTA
antisense strand	TAC	AGT	CGT	AAA	GTA	ATA	TTG	AAT
amino acid	Met	Ser	Ala	Phe	His	Tyr	Asn	Leu
Nonsense mutation through substitution								
sense strand	ATG	TCA	GCA	TTT	CGT	TAA	AAC	TTA
antisense strand	TAC	AGT	CGT	AAA	GCA	ATT	TTG	AAT
amino acid	Met	Ser	Ala	Phe	Arg	STOP		
Frameshift mutation through deletion								
sense strand	ATG	TCA	GCA	TTT	CGT	ATA	ACT	TA
antisense strand	TAC	AGT	CGT	AAA	GCA	TAT	TGA	AT
amino acid	Met	Ser	Ala	Phe	Arg	Ile	Thre	

FIGURE 2.5 Examples of types of mutation

How do we know that a mutation is significant?

Truncating mutations are nearly always pathogenic. Splice-site mutations usually are significant. However, some genes have alternative splice products in that different products occur in different tissues so this may not affect a particular tissue's product. Missense mutations are more difficult. The nature of the amino-acid change determines whether the structure and function of the protein is altered. Amino acids have different characteristics particularly with respect to electrical charges and whether they are polar or non-polar. Polar amino acids are hydrophilic (attract water) and tend to be on the surface of molecules that interact with the aqueous environment. Non-polar amino acids tend to be hydrophobic (repel water). These properties, amongst others, help determine the three-dimensional structure of proteins and alterations between the different groups of amino acids may lead to this structure (or conformation) being altered. Such alterations change the shape of the protein and therefore how it functions.

Factors which may increase the prospect of a mutation being pathogenic are:

1 Whether it is *de novo* in a patient (not found in either parent) or whether it tracks, or segregates, with the disease of interest in a family.
2 Whether the alteration changes the conformation of the protein as outlined above.
3 Whether it affects an important part of the protein such as a binding site or transmembrane region.
4 Whether it has been reported before in other families with the disease in question.
5 Whether it occurs in the general population unaffected by the disease.

How do mutations cause their phenotypic effect?
LOSS-OF-FUNCTION MUTATIONS
These are also termed *inactivating mutations* and include the truncating mutations delineated above. The majority of the recessively inherited disorders are in this category.

GAIN-OF-FUNCTION MUTATIONS
Also termed *activating mutations*, these alterations result in activation of a specific protein function.

DOMINANT-NEGATIVE MUTATIONS
Here, the mutation gives rise to an altered protein which not only does not function but also prevents the normal protein from the normal copy of the gene from functioning, too. This is seen in proteins where there are complex building blocks requiring assembly, such as collagen, where a helical structure fails to form.

HAPLOINSUFFICIENCY
This occurs when one copy of the gene fails to function and the system requires the product from both copies of the gene involved. This reduction by 50% of the gene product is insufficient for normal function.

Dynamic repeat mutations
TRIPLET REPEAT MUTATIONS
These are mutations involving a triplet or codon, which has, above a threshold number of repeats of the codon, the ability to expand. This expansion may take place in the coding sequence of the gene (exons) or in the untranslated flanking regions at the beginning (the five prime untranslated region, or 5'UTR) or end (the three prime untranslated region or 3'UTR) of the gene. The mechanism for this instability is still unclear but may involve replication slippage during meiosis and mitosis and/or incompetent DNA repair mechanisms. Several diseases have now been found to be due to this form of mutation.

Those expansions affecting exons are the CAG repeats coding for glutamine, which form polyglutamine tracts. These include Huntington's disease, Kennedy's spinobulbar muscular atrophy and the spinocerebellar ataxias.

Expansions in the 5'UTR occur in Fragile X syndrome, and expansions in the 3'UTR occur in myotonic dystrophy.

These disorders demonstrate a phenomenon called **anticipation** where the age of onset decreases and the severity of the disease increases with subsequent generations.

TETRAREPEAT MUTATIONS
Recently a quad-repeat mutation has been discovered to cause myotonic dystrophy type 2 or proximal myotonic myopathy (PROMM). This, too, is an unstable repeat in intron 1 of the zinc finger gene ZNF9 on chromosome 3. It is to be expected that further disorders of this nature may be found.

Mitochondrial DNA
The only places that contain DNA outside the nucleus of a cell are the mitochondria. There are thousands of mitochondria in each cell and they are the energy batteries of the cell, producing high-energy molecules such as ATP. The mitochondria contain their own ribosomes for translation of their own protein-coding genes. The mitochondrial genome is a single circle of double-stranded DNA (mtDNA) of 16.6 kb in length. It encodes 37 genes of which 13 are protein-producing for subunits of the respiratory chain complexes. Two are for ribosomal RNA and the rest (22 genes) encode transfer RNAs. There are no introns and almost the entire DNA is coding sequence; each mitochondrion contains several copies of mtDNA. The bulk of mitochondrial proteins are encoded for by nuclear genes and synthesised on cytoplasmic ribosomes after which they are imported into the mitochondria for energy production.

PATTERNS OF INHERITANCE
Autosomal dominant (AD) inheritance
AD disorders occur through mutations in genes on the autosomes (non-sex chromosomes). They manifest through heterozygotes which means that one copy of the gene is mutated and the other is normal. AD disorders show both intrafamilial and interfamilial variability which may be due to the modifying action of other genes, environmental factors, or chance.

Characteristics of AD inheritance
PENETRANCE
This refers to the clinical expression of the gene and is the *proportion* of people with the gene who express the disorder to any degree. That is, in what percentage of people who carry a mutation in the gene does it show, from the most minor to the most severe degree? A mutation may not show itself in all individuals who carry it, thus demonstrating *reduced* or *incomplete penetrance* as in many of the cancer-predisposition genes. Many AD disorders show an *age-related penetrance* where the disorder is not present at birth but evidences itself over time. Huntington's disease is an example of this.

EXPRESSIVITY
Expressivity is the variation in the severity of the disorder in people who carry the mutant gene. It refers to the degree of expression of the physical manifestations of the disorder and there may be significant inter- and intrafamilial variation. For example,

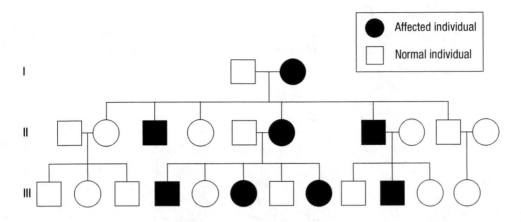

Characteristics of autosomal dominant inheritance

a. Multiple generations affected
b. Male and females are affected in equal proportion
c. Male to male transmission does occur
d. Each offspring of an affected parent has a 50% chance of being affected, 50% of being unaffected

FIGURE 2.6 Autosomal dominant inheritance, e.g. myotonic dystrophy

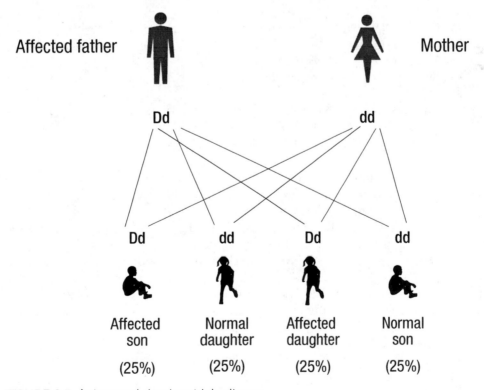

FIGURE 2.7 Autosomal dominant inheritance

in the disorder of Marfan's syndrome (a connective tissue disorder which may affect the skeletal, ocular and cardiovascular systems), some may show abnormalities in some systems but not in others. Many AD disorders demonstrate this.

MOSAICISM

Mosaicism occurs when there is both a normal cell line and one carrying an abnormality present in an individual.

▶ **Somatic mosaicism** occurs when a new mutation in a dominant condition arises during early embryo development causing a partial manifestation of the physical effect. This is a private situation occurring only in that individual. This cannot be passed on to a child unless the mosaicism includes gonadal mosaicism (*see* below).

▶ **Germline (gonadal) mosaicism** occurs when a group (or clone) of cells within the ovary or testis carries a mutation, which has arisen during spermatogenesis or oogenesis. The person shows no sign of this and it is not present in the blood or other tissues but can be passed on to a child. This may cause a recurrence of a condition, e.g. Duchenne muscular dystrophy, where the gene mutation is not present in the blood of the parent on testing.

In summary

— Multiple generations are affected, apart from when the disorder arises as a new mutation.

— Beware the minimally or non-penetrant person in a family who may be missed.

— Males and females are affected in equal proportions (except where a gene change is expressed differently in the sexes, e.g. breast and ovarian cancer).

— Male-to-male transmission occurs.

— Offspring of an affected parent have a 50% chance of being affected.

Autosomal recessive inheritance

In autosomal recessive (AR) conditions the manifestations of the disorder only occur in homozygotes (this means that both copies of the gene have the same mutation) or compound heterozygotes (where each copy of the gene has a different mutation). The person must therefore have inherited a mutated gene from each parent. This will mean that both parents are carriers of the condition but show no effects of this as the normal copy of the gene compensates. If they do show some effect, then it is very mild, e.g. sickle-cell trait. There is seldom a family history of the condition other than in a brother or sister. The exception to this is where consanguinity exists. Here a mutant gene can come down both sides of the family and so the risk of the condition is far higher than may be apparent from the carrier rate in the general population. The risk that a carrier of a particular recessive condition will have an affected child depends on the carrier frequency in the population. The lower the carrier frequency, the less likely it is that a carrier will meet another carrier through random selection. Cystic fibrosis is a good example of this where the carrier rate for the condition in northern European peoples is 1 in 25, giving a risk of 1 in 2500 of having an affected child.

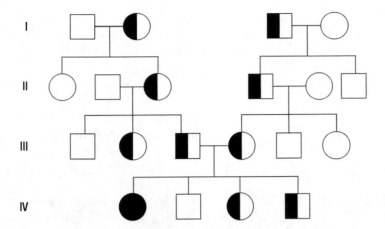

Characteristics of autosomal recessive inheritance

a. Male and females are equally likely to be affected
b. Both parents must be carriers of a single copy of the responsible gene in order for a child to be affected.
c. There is a one-in-four risk of the condition (25%) for each offspring of carrier parents
d. Certain autosomal recessive conditions are more common in specific ethnic groups
e. Inquire about consanguinity, particularly if the condition is very rare

●	Affected individual
□	Normal individual
◑	Non-affected carrier

FIGURE 2.8 Autosomal dominant inheritance

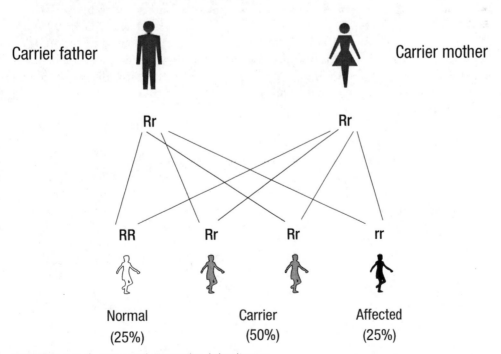

FIGURE 2.9 Autosomal recessive inheritance

Characteristics of AR

Males and females affected equally.

❱ Both parents must be carriers of the mutated gene for a child to be affected.
❱ The recurrence risk is 1 in 4 (25%) for each child of carrier parents.
❱ Consanguinity suggests AR inheritance, particularly if the condition is very rare.

A word of warning regarding carrier testing in AR conditions is necessary. Testing may reveal non-paternity and this issue should be raised in the counselling process beforehand.

X-linked inheritance

These are disorders where the gene lies on the X-chromosome and may follow X-linked dominant (XLD) and X-linked recessive (XLR) patterns. The difference between these two patterns revolves around whether a heterozygote (carrier female) demonstrates the disorder or not. XLD manifests severely in males and may be lethal *in utero* or lead to neonatal death, whereas there is mild affectation in females by comparison. Examples are Rett's syndrome (MeCP2 mutations) and incontinentia pigmenti (mutations in the NEMO gene).

During normal embryogenesis, as the Y-chromosome has significantly fewer genes on it than does the X, compensation for this gene dosage imbalance is achieved by X-inactivation of one of the X-chromosomes in a female. This occurs very early in development when the female embryo is at the 64-cell stage. It is controlled by the X-inactivation centre and involves activation of the XIST gene. This process involves counting the number of Xs and leaving only one active in a cell. Thus, all additional X-chromosomes are largely inactivated (there are small areas which are not inactivated leading to effects when there are more than two Xs). This is usually a random process. If not, and skewed X-inactivation occurs, this may be an indication of an X-linked disorder. The relative proportion of cells with, for example, the normal X inactivated may be different in different tissues. This will lead to a disproportionate representation of the abnormal X and the disorder may manifest in a female with this situation.

Characteristics of X-linked inheritance

Males severely affected (leading to spontaneous pregnancy loss or neonatal death in XLD).

❱ Female carriers are either unaffected or far less affected than males (degree dependent on pattern of X-inactivation).
❱ Male-to-male transmission is never seen but all daughters of an affected man will be carriers.
❱ Males born with a normally lethal XLD condition may have survived because they have Klinefelter's syndrome (XXY)
❱ Females born with a severe form of XLD disorder may have Turner's syndrome (XO), have very unfavourably skewed X-inactivation, or have an X-autosome translocation.

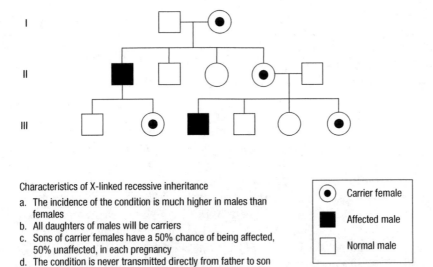

Characteristics of X-linked recessive inheritance

a. The incidence of the condition is much higher in males than females
b. All daughters of males will be carriers
c. Sons of carrier females have a 50% chance of being affected, 50% unaffected, in each pregnancy
d. The condition is never transmitted directly from father to son

- Carrier female
- Affected male
- Normal male

FIGURE 2.10 X-linked recessive pedigree, e.g. Duchenne muscular dystrophy

Mitochondrial inheritance

As described earlier, these organelles are the only part of the cell containing DNA outside the nucleus. The feature of mitochondrial inheritance is that it is exclusively *matrilineal*; that is, we all get all our mitochondria from our mothers. Although sperm do contain mitochondria at fertilisation, only the head/nucleus of the sperm enters the ovum. Thus men affected by a mitochondrial disorder cannot pass this on to their offspring. Women who carry a mitochondrial mutation may not do so in all their mitochondria and have a mixture of normal and mutant mitochondrial DNA

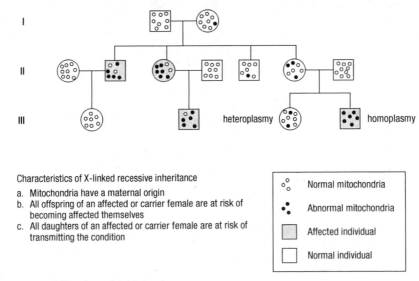

Characteristics of X-linked recessive inheritance

a. Mitochondria have a maternal origin
b. All offspring of an affected or carrier female are at risk of becoming affected themselves
c. All daughters of an affected or carrier female are at risk of transmitting the condition

- Normal mitochondria
- Abnormal mitochondria
- Affected individual
- Normal individual

FIGURE 2.11 Mitochondrial inheritance

in their cells. The proportion of mutant DNA will determine whether the disorder is expressed or not and some disorders have a threshold effect where, below a certain level, all is normal and above it the disorder occurs. The phenomenon whereby a mixture of mutant and normal mitochondrial DNA is found is called *heteroplasmy*. If all the mitochondria have mutant DNA this is called *homoplasmy*.

CHROMOSOMES

As genes are the recipes of instruction, so chromosomes are the recipe books into which these are packed. They were so named in the nineteenth century when they were seen as brightly staining bodies and were thus given this name combining two Greek words meaning 'coloured bodies'. Chromosomes are a complex arrangement of DNA more or less tightly wound round itself and structures of proteins called histones. They are situated in the nucleus of the cell and passed on during the process of cell division at meiosis in the gonads during the production of the gametes (ova or sperm), and mitosis during cell replication. Numerous structural alterations may take place involving the chromosomes and will be dealt with here.

Human cells have 46 chromosomes made up of 23 pairs, one of each pair being inherited from each parent, and these constitute the genome. Of these pairs, 22 are the same in both female and male and are called *autosomes*. The remaining pair are the **sex chromosomes** in which XX is found in females and XY in males. A woman will always pass on an X to any child whereas a man will pass on either an X – thereby fathering a girl – or a Y – and thus fathering a son. A pair of chromosomes are termed *homologues* or *homologous chromosomes*.

Chromosome morphology

Chromosomes are linear structures, which have a narrow part, or constriction, called a **centromere** and two arms. The short arm is called **p** (for petite) and the long arm **q** (letter after p). Chromosomes are classified according to the position of the centromere and are numbered according to size (from largest to smallest, 1 to 22).

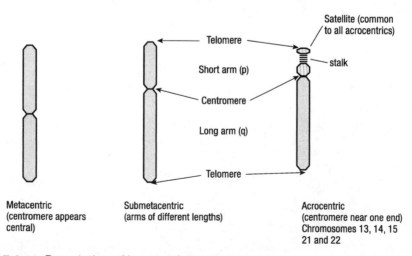

FIGURE 2.12 Description of human chromosomes

Chromosome analysis is usually performed by scientists called cytogeneticists who are able to identify chromosomes according to their size, shape and banding pattern, when stained by Giemsa (G) staining. The position of the centromere determines shape and may be central, off-centre or near one end. Chromosomes so structured are called *metacentric, submetacentric* and *acrocentric* respectively.

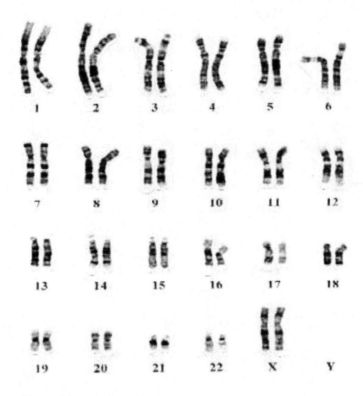

FIGURE 2.13 Normal female karyotype

The routine method of analysis of chromosomes is to photograph the spread, identify the pairs and paste them p, or short arm, up. This is called a *karyotype* and the word is also used as a general term signifying a person's chromosome makeup.

Cell division
It is important to remember that there are two types of cell division, namely **meiosis** and **mitosis.**

Meiosis
This is the specialised cell-division process that involves two cell divisions but only one chromosomal replication, which takes place only in the gonads and is responsible for the production of the gametes, i.e. ova and sperm. This occurs only in the germline, the heritable part of us, and only once per cell progenitor. It is a reduction division such that only one of each pair of homologues ends up in the gamete, which

thus has half the chromosome complement of all other cells – this is called the *haploid* set. Of great significance is the fact that, in the process of cell division in meiosis, there is swapping of material between the individual chromosomes of a pair. This process is called *recombination* or *crossover* and there are approximately 40 such crossovers in each meiosis involving one to three per chromosome pair. In this way, DNA from the paternal and maternal line of an individual is mixed. This is a vital part of making us unique beings and is the central aspect of variation within the species. It is during this process, and the original duplication of the chromosomes that mistakes happen and can be passed on to the next generation. The process is illustrated and explained in Figures 2.14 and 2.15.

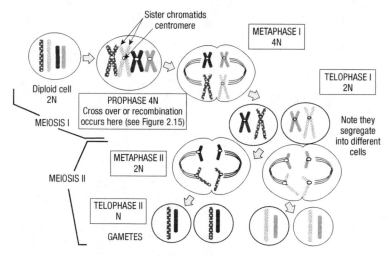

FIGURE 2.14 Meiosis (this is a reduction division)

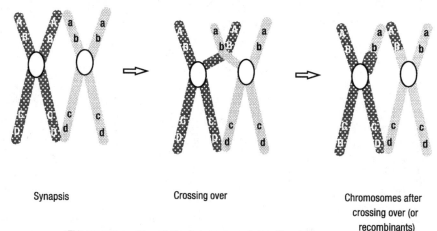

Synapsis   Crossing over   Chromosomes after crossing over (or recombinants)

This process creates variation between us and gives the species the opportunity to adapt to change in evolution through the swapping of different copies of many genes.

FIGURE 2.15 Crossing over and recombination in meiosis I

Mitosis

This is the process of ordinary cell division of the rest of the cells in the body (or soma) and is therefore the somatic division necessary for cell growth and repair. This process produces two identical cells from the original parent cell with both of each pair of chromosomes being present – the **diploid** complement. In order to achieve this, a cell will grow to approximately twice its original size thereby duplicating much of its content. This includes its DNA. The duplication of the DNA of its chromosomes means that each of the chromosomes are double their normal structure with duplicates called *sister chromatids*. These are attached to the centromere which is a crucial structure necessary for chromosome survival and division. When cell division occurs, the duplicated centromeres separate and the sister chromatids migrate to opposite ends of the cell. Completion of division leaves each daughter cell with the same chromosome content as the original cell (*see* Figure 2.16). Should a mistake occur in the process of duplication then, assuming it is not fatal to the cell's function, this will be perpetuated through further cellular divisions and result in a group, or **clone,** of cells with the same error. This results in two lines of cells in an individual, one normal and the other carrying an error (whether chromosomal or mutational) and this situation is called *mosaicism.*

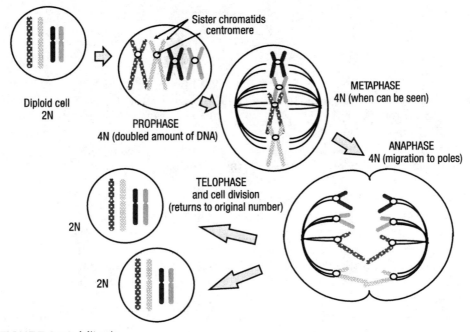

FIGURE 2.16 Mitosis

Chromosome analysis

In order to analyse chromosomes, the cells must be dividing. These cells are commonly lymphocytes from peripheral blood but could also be fibroblasts from a skin biopsy; bone-marrow cells; or cells from a chorionic villus sample or from amniocentesis. They are cultured in a culture medium and then arrested in division by the addition of the drug **colchicine**. This blocking of mitosis takes place in metaphase and allows the chromosomes to be stained, usually using Giemsa stain, and analysed. Giemsa (or G-banding) creates a series of light and dark bands characteristic for each chromosome and these conform to an internationally recognised convention of numbering.

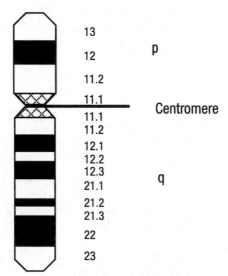

FIGURE 2.17 Chromosome nomenclature using G-banding on chromosome 18

The resolution of this light microscope technique is of the order of 5 Mb. That is, a loss or gain of material on a chromosome is visible only if it involves 5 million base pairs or more. Anything smaller will be missed, which is a large chunk of DNA usually containing many genes. More sophisticated techniques using molecular technology are now available allowing more accurate analysis involving very much smaller amounts of DNA. These include the following.

Fluorescent in situ hybridisation (FISH)

An area of interest, for example on chromosome 22q11 involved in DiGeorge syndrome, is investigated using a DNA probe. This sequence of DNA is specific to that region and unique to it so binds there exclusively. Attached to the probe is a tag, which fluoresces under ultraviolet light. When the probe is applied to the chromosome preparation it binds to the specific sequence of interest and may be seen using a special microscope due to its fluorescence. If the piece of DNA is missing from one chromosome then only one fluorescent signature is seen from the normal chromosome, signifying a deletion on the other.

Multiplex ligation probe amplification (MLPA)

This uses molecular technology to detect deletions or duplications of whole genes or large parts of genes. It may also be used to detect deletions or duplications of parts of chromosomes such as the sub-telomere gene-rich areas near the ends of chromosomes. It is an efficient, cheap and reliable technique allowing gene dosage (number of copies) to be assessed relative to control samples.

Comparative genome hybridisation (CGH) array

This is the newest of the techniques and uses a FISH-based technology. This involves many hundreds to thousands of DNA probes some 44 Kb to 1 Mb apart across the whole genome being spotted onto a slide with a fluorescent label of a specific colour – green. This is the control DNA, which has been analysed to ensure that it is normal. The test DNA is labelled with a different colour – red – and then mixed on the slide. All these specific sequences bind to one another, mixing their colours at each specific site. If the ratio is 1:1 then the spot fluoresces orange. If, however, a particular sequence in the 'test' DNA is missing, i.e. deleted, then the spot will fluoresce green. Alternatively, if there is a duplication of an area then there will be more 'test' DNA and the spot will fluoresce red. In this way the whole genome can be interrogated at intervals for deletions and duplications, which would otherwise be invisible. This process is computerised and automated. A simplified diagram is given in Figure 2.18 below.

Examples of conditions caused by deletions detectable by FISH are given in Table 2.1.

Despite the advances in technology, a 'normal' chromosome result does not mean that a patient's chromosome analysis is entirely normal. It simply means that within the limits of our current technology that is the case. This new technology brings with it more complexity. As the genome has significant variation amongst us, so variants called 'copy number variants' are found. These may not be important or may signify causative changes. Delineating this is a continuing process and is similar to the 'unknown variants' found with missense mutations.

COMPARATIVE GENOMIC
HYBRIDISATION ARRAY

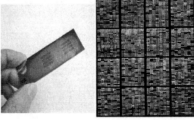

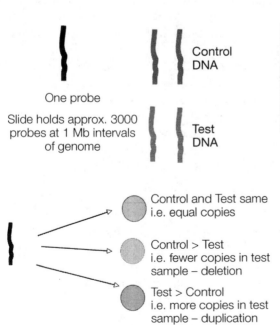

High-throughput detection of large-scale copy number changes (deletions and duplications)

Control DNA

One probe

Slide holds approx. 3000 probes at 1 Mb intervals of genome

Test DNA

Control and Test same i.e. equal copies

Control > Test i.e. fewer copies in test sample – deletion

Test > Control i.e. more copies in test sample – duplication

FIGURE 2.18 Comparative genome hybridisation array

TABLE 2.1 Some chromosome microdeletions detectable by FISH

Syndrome	Some clinical features	Deletion
DiGeorge/ Velocardiofacial	Cardiac outflow tract anomalies, cleft palate, thymus hypoplasia, straight nose	22q11
Smith Magenis	Tented upper lip, sleep disturbance, self-destructive behaviour, unusual mannersims, hoarse voice	17p11.2
Williams	Mental retardation, supravalvular aortic stenosis, hypercalcaemia, 'jowled facies', overfriendly manner	7q11.23
Miller Dieker	Lissencephaly (smooth brain), severe mental retardation, characteristic facies	17p13
Rubinstein-Taybi	Beaked nose, broad thumbs and great toes, mental retardation	16p13.3

Chromosomal abnormalities

Given the complex nature of human development it is not surprising that an incorrect amount of genetic material will disturb normal patterns of growth and formation. Chromosome abnormalities are common and occur in around 1 in 120 live-born babies. Of these, approximately 50% will demonstrate an effect from this. The effects are due to gain or loss of genetic material and the human system is more able to cope with gain than with loss. Other than for Turner's syndrome (*see* below), monosomy for other chromosomes is almost always non-viable. Chromosomal abnormalities may be due to numerical, structural or functional alterations.

Chromosome terminology

This follows an internationally agreed nomenclature of which the following is a brief summary. The karyotype always begins with the total number of chromosomes present, followed by the sex chromosomes seen. Thus a normal male will be denoted **46XY**.

An abnormal number of chromosomes is immediately obvious. A mosaic karyotype in which there are two cell populations will be documented as a normal followed by abnormal notation, e.g. **46XX/47XX+21** denoting a mosaic Down's syndrome.

Rearrangements follow the sex chromosome notation, e.g. **46XX,t(1:6)(q24q21)** signifies a balanced translocation between chromosomes 1 and 6 with the exchange occurring between the two long arms and the numbers q24 and q21 give the exact breakpoints. Robertsonian translocations (see below) are written as, for example, **rob(13q14q)**.

Numerical alterations

Aneuploidy is the term used to describe gain or loss of one or more chromosomes. Gain of one chromosome is called *trisomy* and loss, resulting in a single chromosome, is called *monosomy*. There are eight common numerical chromosomal conditions. These are the commonly known trisomies (extra chromosome) 13, 18 and 21, mosaic trisomy 8 and the sex chromosome aneuploides. These are summarised in Table 2.2 below.

TABLE 2.2 Common numerical chromosomal conditions

Aneuploidy	Incidence	Description of some clinical features
Trisomy 13 (Patau syndrome)	1/9500 births	Growth retardation, holoprosencephaly, micro/anopthalmia, cleft lit/palate, postaxial polydactyly, cardiac anomalies
Trisomy 18 (Edwards syndrome)	1/8000	Growth retardation, prominent occiput, simple ears, overriding fingers, rocker-bottom feet, cardiac anomalies, exomphalos
Trisomy 21 (Down's syndrome)	Maternal age dependent 1/1500 at 18, 1/80 at 40	Characterstic facies, hypotonia, cardiac defects, duodenal atresia, developmental delay
Mosaic Trisomy 8	1/30,000	Mental retardation, high forehead, finger and toe contractures, deep palmar and plantar creases, spinal difficulties
XXX (Triple X syndrome) Maternal age effect	1/1000 female births	Normal appearance, tall stature, IQ average of 10–15 points below siblings. Majority never detected due to normality
XYY	1/1000 male births	Normal appearance, tall stature, IQ average of 10–15 points below siblings, some speech/learning difficulties, some behaviour difficulties, Majority never detected due to normality
XXY (Klinefelter's syndrome) Maternal age effect	1/2500 at 33 to 1/300 at 43	Normal appearance, tall stature, gynaecomastia, hypogonadotrophic hypogonadism, IQ 10–15 points below siblings but large range. Majority never detected
45X and variants (Turner's syndrome)	1/2500 female live births 99% abort	Short stature, webbed neck, gonadal dysgenesis, cardiac anomalies particularly coarctation and VSD, renal anomalies, IQ 10–15 points below siblings

The autosomal trisomies have significantly more severe phenotypic effects than that of the sex chromosome aneuploidies. These aneuploidies are usually caused by failure of the chromosome pair to separate into separate cells during meiosis, which is called *non-disjunction*, with both going into one daughter cell. A complete extra set of chromosomes making 69 is called *triploidy*. Rarely infants with this may be live-born, but survive for only a short time.

DOWN'S SYNDROME
As this is a disorder very commonly encountered in clinical practice, the chromosomal basis is summarised here:
- 95% are due to non-disjunction causing trisomy 21.
- 2% arise from Robertsonian translocations (*see* below) – in particular 14/21 (50% are familial).
- 2% are due to mosaicism.
- 1% result from various chromosome rearrangements involving trisomy for 21q22 causing the phenotype.

Structural alterations

Rearrangement of chromosome material results from breakage and reconstitution of the fragment in an abnormal way. You will recall that, in meiosis, the process of crossing over is normal and occurs across the genome. In this process, were a piece of chromosome to break off and then reattach in a different way to either the same or a different site, then a variety of situations may arise. Should the fragment be lost altogether, a **deletion** results. If the fragment detaches, turns round and then rein-serts, an **inversion** occurs. Should the piece of chromosome reattach to a different part of the original chromosome then an **insertion** has occurred. If the fragment unites with a different chromosome, then this is called a **translocation.**

These rearrangements may take place with no loss or gain of genetic material in which case they are called **balanced.** Such situations normally do not give rise to any difficulties unless the breakpoints of the segment which has been altered go through a vital gene – a rare situation but one which allows genes, hitherto undiscovered, to be found. Should chromosome material be gained or lost, however, then an **unbalanced** rearrangement has occurred with probable clinical repercussions for the individual.

Unbalanced rearrangements result from a variety of situations. Deletions of part of a chromosome lead to partial monosomy of that region. The clinical effects of this will depend on the size of the deleted segment and the number and function of the genes contained therein. The larger the deletion, the more genes will be lost and the less likely a conceptus is to survive. Survival with smaller deletions usually results in significant phenotypic effect and severe abnormalities of structure and function. This loss of material may occur *de novo* or from a balanced translocation in meiosis in a parent. Many deletion syndromes have been found and characterised both through the findings of visible deletions and through the use of FISH. Details of some of the more common in both categories are given in Tables 2.1 and 2.3.

TABLE 2.3 Some cytogenetically visible chromosome deletions

Syndrome	Some clinical features	Deletion
Angelman	Seizures, microcephaly, mental retardation, inappropriate laughter, little or no speech, ataxia	15q11–12 (the maternal copy is deleted)
Prader-Willi	Severe hypotonia at birth, feeding difficulties as infant followed by hyperphagia and obesity as children, mental retardation	15q11–12 (the paternal copy is deleted)
Wolf-Hirschorn	Low birthweight, failure to thrive, hypotonia, seizures, 'greek helmet' profile, coloboma, severe mental retardation	4p-
Cri-du-chat	Cat-like cry from an underdeveloped larynx, failure to thrive, severe mental retardation	5p-

Duplications of part of a chromosome appear to cause less in the way of pheno-typic effects, which follows the principle stated earlier that we are able to tolerate more easily a gain of genetic material than we tolerate a loss. More duplications of a submicroscopic nature are being found with the new technology of CGH array analysis, requiring characterisation to see whether they are related to pathology.

A form of deletion disorder occurs with the formation of a ring chromosome. In this situation, the ends of both the short and long arms are lost and the two arms join to form a ring. As the ends of the chromosomes are gene-rich, this often gives rise to serious repercussions. There is a common phenotype, related to ring-chromosome formation, of growth deficiency, mental retardation, microcephaly and dysmorphism. The majority of ring-chromosome abnormalities arise sporadically (by chance) but some rare instances of familial ring-chromosome transmission have been reported.

Translocations

These may be balanced or unbalanced and frequently the latter arises in a fetus with a parent who has the former. There are two forms of translocation, **reciprocal translocation** and **Robertsonian translocation**. Reciprocal translocations occur between any two non-homologous chromosomes whereas Robertsonian translocations, which may homologous or non-homologous, involve only the acrocentric chromosomes 13, 14, 15, 21 or 22 (*see* karyotype earlier).

RECIPROCAL TRANSLOCATIONS

In balanced form these occur in approximately 1 in 400 newborns and in unbalanced form in 3 in 10 000 newborns. The familial balanced translocation is usually unique to the family and will run down through the generations. There is one form of balanced translocation which is common in man, between chromosomes 11 and 22 written as t(11:22)(q23:q11).

In order to understand how imbalances occur from a parental balanced translocation it is necessary to construct a diagram to illustrate the situation. The laboratory can assist you in doing this by giving you a diagram drawn to scale. A useful counselling tool is to do this with different coloured pencils. This enables you to see how the chromosomes will come together during meiosis and what possibilities exist for unbalanced products to occur (*see* Figures 2.19 and 2.20).

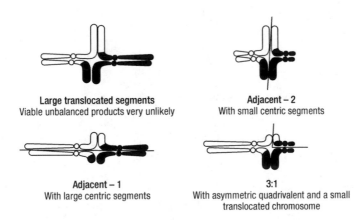

Large translocated segments
Viable unbalanced products very unlikely

Adjacent – 2
With small centric segments

Adjacent – 1
With large centric segments

3:1
With asymmetric quadrivalent and a small translocated chromosome

FIGURE 2.19 Predicted segregation

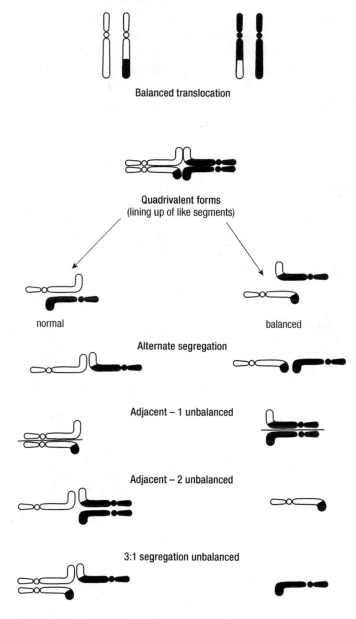

Balanced translocation

Quadrivalent forms
(lining up of like segments)

normal

balanced

Alternate segregation

Adjacent – 1 unbalanced

Adjacent – 2 unbalanced

3:1 segregation unbalanced

FIGURE 2.20 Translocation quadrivalent segregation

During meiosis it is necessary for homologous chromosomes to align in order to achieve crossover as described earlier. If there is a piece of another chromosome attached, then it isn't possible either for that chromosome to align with its partner, or for the other chromosome with which it has swapped material to do so either. They therefore come together as a **quadrivalent,** which occurs when the four chromosomes align with their respective pieces and one another. How big the swapped segments are will determine the degree of imbalance and whether a viable baby might occur.

Using the diagram drawn to scale as suggested above, one may now predict what segregations might give rise to a viable offspring. The first thing to say is that the large majority of children from balanced translocation parents are normal. That is to say that alternate segregation is common so that either normal or balanced products occur. Should imbalance occur then the least imbalance with the least monosomic content is the most likely one to be viable (remembering that we tolerate loss of material far less than we tolerate gain).

There are tables available to ascertain the risk for various translocated segments, which may be consulted when necessary.

ROBERTSONIAN TRANSLOCATIONS

These occur in approximately 1 in 1000 individuals. They may be **homologous** or **non-homologous**. The homologous translocations involve fusion of the long arms of a pair of acrocentrics, e.g. chromosome 21, where they become joined. The individual has 45 chromosomes and the karyotype is written as 45 rob(21q21q). This is very rare.

The great majority of Robertsonian translocations involve different acrocentric chromosomes and are non-homologous translocations. The most common is that involving chromosomes 13 and 14 which occurs in approximately 1 in 1300 people. In both forms, the loss of the short arms of the chromosomes does not cause any difficulty. They do not carry unique genes so the other acrocentric chromosome short arms will compensate for those genes lost.

The difficulties that may arise in Robertsonian translocations relate to the following. A translocation involving chromosomes 13 and 21 gives rise to the risk of **trisomy 13 or 21** respectively. Those translocations involving chromosomes 14 and 15 produce the risk of **uniparental disomy (UPD)** and this occurs when both chromosomes of a pair are inherited from the same parent. As chromosomes 14 and 15 have areas of **imprinting** (*see* below), this inheritance leads to difficulties.

The risk of having a child with an unbalanced chromosome makeup depends on which parent is carrying the translocation. Maternal transmission carries a higher risk than does paternal, and both are generally a higher risk than for unbalanced products from a reciprocal translocation carrier. Maternal transmission of trisomy 13 from a non-homologous Robertsonian translocation involving chromosome 13 is 1%, whereas the risk of trisomy 21 from a translocation involving this chromosome is 10–15%. Paternal transmission risk is less than 1% for both trisomies. This risk of a **translocation Down's syndrome** is the explanation for the small number of Down's syndrome cases which are familial (Figure 2.22).

In those parents who carry a **homologous** Robertsonian translocation involving chromosome 13 or 21, virtually all offspring will be trisomic unless there is trisomic rescue during mitosis. This is where the cell rejects the extra normal chromosome thus bringing it back to the normal chromosome complement.

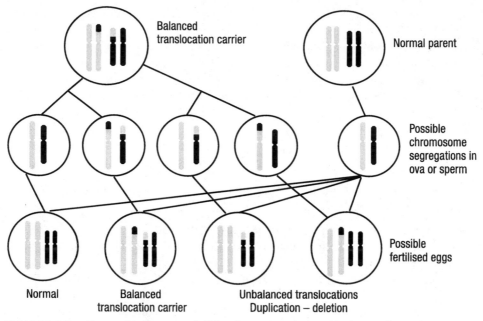

FIGURE 2.21 Reproductive possibilities from a reciprocal balanced translocation carrier

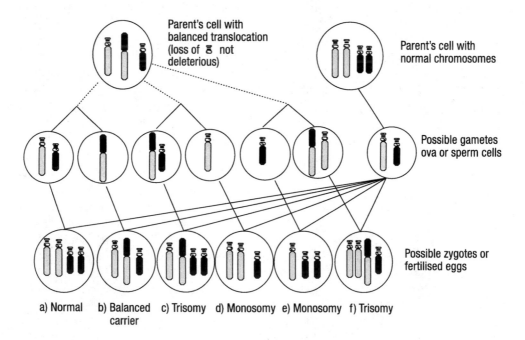

Remember that monosomy is tolerated less than trisomy and would be non-viable

FIGURE 2.22 Reproductive possibilities from a Robertsonian translocation carrier

Genomic imprinting and uniparental disomy (UPD)

Genomic imprinting is the phenomenon whereby particular genes are expressed (active) depending on which parent they are inherited from – that is, the '**parent of origin**' effect. This mechanism distinguishes between the maternal and paternal homologue and will switch 'off' or 'on' these particular genes according to imprint. This signal is maintained throughout the life of the individual but is 'reset' in the germ cells so that the imprint is transmitted during reproduction. For example, a woman will inherit a copy of such a gene from each parent but only the one from her *mother* is active. When she reproduces she will 'reset' the copy from her father (which has been silent) so that it becomes active as the *maternal* copy for her child, so maintaining the imprint. These imprinted genes are important in growth and development of the child and also have a role in tumour suppression. The two best-known imprinting disorders are Prader-Willi and Angelman syndromes.

As 'parent of origin' imprint is important in those chromosomes with imprinted genes, it is easy to appreciate why UPD of chromosomes 14 and 15 from Robertsonian translocations may be problematic. UPD may arise from a variety of mechanisms. The first is as described for such translocations where the whole of both chromosomes is inherited from the same parent. Alternatively the **imprinting centre**, the organisational area of the chromosome, which contains the 'switch' mechanism necessary for maintaining the imprint, is either deleted or mutated, so removing it. Finally, one copy of the imprinted gene may be deleted thus leaving only one copy available for transcription. This is the common mechanism involved in the Prader-Willi and Angelman syndromes where a deletion of the same part of chromosome 15 causes both. If the paternal copy is lost, then Prader-Willi syndrome results. If the maternal copy is the one deleted, then Angelman syndrome occurs.

Any translocation involving chromosomes 14 or 15 should be examined for UPD in order to detect such problems.

Supernumerary marker chromosomes (SMC)

This is extra chromosome material which is separate from the other chromosomes. Different terms have been used to describe these, including *extra structurally abnormal chromosomes* (ESAC). I will use SMC to denote this finding. They may be found at prenatal analysis when a pregnancy is being assessed, either because congenital anomalies have been found or to exclude aneuploidy. Alternatively, this finding may arise during investigation of a child for developmental delay. They are found in 1 in 2000 live births. Seventy per cent of SMCs are of acrocentric origin and, of these, 50% are derived from chromosome 15.

When a SMC is found, the first question at diagnosis is whether the finding is of clinical significance. As with all such questions relating to chromosomes, it is important to analyse the parental karyotype, particularly regarding mosaicism. Inheritance from a normal, non-mosaic parent almost always means it is inconsequential. If found *de novo* – i.e. the SMC is not present in either parent – then it will depend on where it comes from and whether it contains euchromatin (the genetically active chromosome material seen as a light band). The origin is determined by G-banding and FISH analysis using chromosome-specific probes. If the origin is from an imprinted chromosome, then UPD studies should be carried out.

There are two well-characterised SMCs with established phenotypes. The first is **isodicentric** (containing two centromeres from the same chromosome) **(idic).15** containing the Prader-Willi/Angelman critical region determined by FISH. This causes developmental delay and seizures. The second is **idic.22**, causing Cat-eye syndrome, in which the phenotype includes coloboma, anal, cardiac and renal anomalies and variable developmental delay.

KEY POINTS FOR PRACTICE
Chromosomal abnormalities should be suspected:
- When there is significant growth retardation (both pre- and post-natal growth retardation).
- Where there are congenital anomalies present, including ambiguous genitalia.
- Where there is a family history of recurrent miscarriages, intra-uterine deaths/stillbirths, and mental retardation.
- Where dysmorphism is apparent.
- Where there is a family history of a specific chromosomal abnormality such as a translocation.

REFERENCE
1 Watson JD, Crick FHC. A structure for deoxyribose nucleic acid. *Nature.* 1953; **171**: 737–8.

FURTHER READING
Firth H, Hurst J, editors. *Oxford Desk Reference: Clinical genetics.* Oxford: Oxford University Press; 2005.
Turnpenny P, Ellard S, editors. *Emery's Elements of Medical Genetics.* 13th ed. London: Churchill Livingstone; 2007.
Strachan T, Read A, editors. *Human Molecular Genetics.* 2nd ed. Oxford: Bios Scientific Publications; 1999.
Harper P. *Practical Genetic Counselling.* 6th ed. London: Hodder Arnold; 2004.
Gardner R, Sutherland G. *Chromosome Abnormalities and Genetic Counseling.* 3rd ed. Oxford: Oxford Universtity Press; 2004.

CHAPTER 3

Inherited biochemical disorders

Valerie Walker

CONTENTS

INTRODUCTION

Inherited biochemical disorders are genetic defects which cause a biochemical abnormality. The term is applied rather loosely and is not restricted to defects which disturb metabolic pathways.

'Genetic' implies an abnormality of the DNA code. This interferes with the production of a protein normally directed by a gene and results in:

▶ deficiency of a normal protein, or
▶ production of an abnormal protein which does not function properly.

The classes of proteins which may be deficient or defective include the following.

(1) *Enzymes*, which are catalysts which convert one substance into another. They have a range of important functions. Some help to produce active compounds which

69

are essential to the body, some break down large unwanted structural components of the body, and others convert potentially harmful substances into safe waste products which can be excreted. Examples of inherited enzyme disorders are: **phenylketonuria**, **galactosaemia** and the **glycogen storage disorders** which affect metabolic processes, and the **mucopolysaccharide disorders** in which large components of the connective tissues are not degraded and accumulate, often causing an abnormal appearance.

(2) *Transport proteins*, which carry substances into and out of cells. In cystic fibrosis, for example, the chloride transporter of cell membranes (CFTR; cystic fibrosis transmembrane regulator) is defective.

(3) *Receptor proteins*, which recognise and bind with substances on the surface or inside of cells and through this activate cellular processes. Deficiency of the intracellular receptor for testosterone and dihydrotestosterone is one example encountered neonatally as a baby of uncertain sex: severely affected boys have normal testes and can make testosterone, but it cannot masculinise them and they have apparent female external genitalia.

(4) *Structural proteins*, which are essential for normal construction of the body. One example is osteogenesis imperfecta, due to production of abnormal bone collagen which leads to deformed, weak and fragile bones.

This chapter will focus on **enzyme** defects which may lead to acute illness neonatally. Those which upset metabolic processes are also called inborn errors of metabolism. After an overview, important classes of disorders will be discussed, focusing on those where urgent diagnosis and intervention are crucial for the baby and family.

Disorders presenting in newborns are generally severe defects. In some, early intervention leads to a good outcome with normal development. In others, even a delay of a few days results in death, or irreversible damage in survivors. Sometimes there is no treatment, and the natural outcome is early death or severe developmental problems. Establishment of a firm diagnosis in these babies is extremely important to facilitate genetic counselling and enable prenatal diagnosis for future pregnancies.

The early presenting signs of inherited disorders are seldom diagnostic, and are indistinguishable from much commoner problems including sepsis, perinatal compromise, or intracranial bleeds. The types of presentation will be overviewed and alerting clues highlighted.

Preliminary diagnosis rests on the results of appropriate, urgent biochemical tests. These will be discussed. Scriver *et al.*[1] have edited an authoritative text on inherited biochemical disorders, and Fernandes *et al.*[2] a clinically orientated textbook for those involved in the diagnosis and management of these disorders. Published detailed UK guidelines for the management of acutely presenting disorders are accessible on the website of the British Inherited Metabolic Disease Group.[3]

EXAMPLES OF INHERITED ENZYME DEFECTS

Biochemical conversions in the body are catalysed by single enzymes or, more often, by several enzymes acting sequentially in a pathway. Often intermediates in the pathway are shunted along another track, where a different set of enzymes makes a different product which may be useful, or harmful, to the body. The clinical consequences of an enzyme defect may result from deficiency of a product which is essential for health, or from accumulation of intermediates which are damaging.

Congenital adrenal hyperplasia (CAH)

A good example is deficiency of the enzyme **21-hydroxylase** which causes the commonest form of **congenital adrenal hyperplasia** (CAH). This decreases the production of the essential steroids **cortisol** and **aldosterone** from **cholesterol** (*see* Figure 3.1). The low level of cortisol in the blood stimulates the hypothalamus to increase ACTH secretion. This drives the adrenal glands to produce more cortisol (but they still cannot make enough), and the glands enlarge. Large amounts of steroids before the enzyme block build up. Some of these are diverted into pathways that make the male sex hormones, including testosterone.

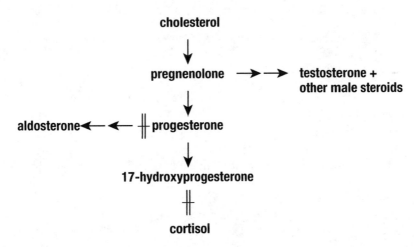

+|+ and 21-hydroxylase defect blocking the pathways to cortisol and aldosterone

FIGURE 3.1 The consequences of 21-hydroxylase deficiency in congenital adrenal hyperplasia

This all starts *in utero* from around six weeks of gestation. The extra testosterone is not important for the male fetus, but it causes masculinisation of the external genitalia of female fetuses, who may be mistaken for boys at birth. The high blood levels of one precursor, 17-hydroxyprogesterone, are used as a diagnostic test. This steroid can be measured urgently in blood spots after the first 48 hours of life, making rapid diagnosis possible. Deficiencies of the essential products, cortisol and aldosterone, may cause a severe hypotensive salt wasting crisis in both boys and girls with dehydration, high potassium and sometimes hypoglycaemia, and collapse, often in the second week of life.

Galactosaemia

The main sugar in both human and full-term formula milk is lactose. In the intestinal mucosa, this is split into its two components, glucose and galactose, by the enzyme lactase. These are then absorbed and transported to the liver. In order to be used to make energy, galactose has then to be converted into glucose. This is brought about in the liver through the action of a series of enzymes, one of which is galactose-1 phosphate uridyl transferase, commonly referred to as GAL-1-PUT or GALT. This enzyme is deficient in galactosaemia, an autosomal recessive disorder with an incidence of around 1 in 50 000 live births. As soon as affected babies start milk-feeding after birth, there is a progressive build-up of galactose and its metabolite, galactose-1-phosphate (*see* Figure 3.2).

GALACTOSE + ATP ⟶ **GALACTOSE-1-PHOSPHATE** + ADP

GALACTOSE-1-PHOSPHATE + UDP GLUCOSE — ‖ ‖ ⟶ UDP GALACTOSE + GLUCOSE-1-PHOSPHATE

UDP GALACTOSE ⟶ ⟶ ⟶ GLUCOSE-1-PHOSPHATE

‖ ‖ Galactose-1-phosphate uridyl transferase (GAL-1-PUT; GALT)

FIGURE 3.2 The enzyme defect in galactosaemia

Clinical features

The only clinical damage caused by the increased **galactose** is in the lens of the eye, where it causes cataracts. These may be found as early as three or four weeks of life. **Galactose-1-phosphate**, however, is much more toxic, affecting the liver, brain and kidneys.

Typically, babies with a severe enzyme deficiency have normal birth weight and are well for the first three or four days. However, galactose-1-phosphate accumulates with feeding and, from around day four, they become increasingly unwell: there is an acute liver disturbance with jaundice, hepatomegaly, possibly bleeding and gram-negative septicaemia, and progressive brain disturbance (encephalopathy) with refusal to feed, increasing lethargy, abnormal tone and movements (cycling and fisting).[4] Hypoglycaemia is rare, unless the liver fails. Unless diagnosed and treated quickly, babies die or sustain irreversible brain damage. Damage continues during childhood, causing severe learning problems, poor growth, dense cataracts and liver damage (cirrhosis) with portal hypertension and oesophageal varices which may cause fatal haemorrhage.

Diagnosis

The initial diagnosis is made from ward urine tests: urine collected whilst the baby is having normal milk feeds gives a positive reaction with a Clinitest (a Bayer® chemical test for reducing sugars including glucose, galactose and fructose) and a negative Multistix (Bayer®) or BM-stick test (Boehringer Mannheim) reaction for glucose. These findings indicate a sugar in the urine which is not glucose. The diagnosis is galactosaemia until proven otherwise and treatment must be started at once. The positive urine sample must be sent to the laboratory for galactose analysis. Definitive confirmation is by measuring GAL-1-PUT in blood. This may be done on blood spots at a referral laboratory. Treatment must not be delayed until the results of these tests come back. NOTE: If a baby has been transfused, GAL-1-PUT cannot be measured for three months. Galactose-1-phosphate can still be measured in plasma. If this is normal, and galactosaemia is a strong possibility, it may be helpful to test the parents' blood, since they should both be carriers.

Treatment

The treatment is to remove the 'toxin' – i.e. galactose – from the diet. Breast or standard milk feeds are stopped and replaced with a lactose-free milk. When the baby is weaned, lactose must be excluded as far as possible. This includes excluding all dairy products and many other foods. With care, the children develop well, and have a normal IQ, although some have delayed speech and mild learning problems. The majority of girls, however, have ovarian failure with primary amenorrhoea, need oestrogens for secondary sexual development, and are infertile.[4]

INHERITED ORGANIC ACID DISORDERS

Organic acids are acids that contain carbon atoms. They include well-known compounds such as lactic acid and the ketone body acetoacetic acid, and many others. They are produced continuously in the body as intermediates in the metabolism of amino acids, carbohydrates and fats, and of drugs and food additives. They do not normally accumulate, since most are rapidly converted to non-acidic end-products. Small amounts are excreted in urine.

In the inherited organic acid disorders there is an enzyme deficiency in one of the metabolic pathways which normally break down one or more acids. These therefore accumulate and often (but not invariably) cause metabolic acidosis. In addition, deficiencies of the end-products of the enzyme sequence may cause problems. Characteristically, large amounts of organic acids are excreted in the urine at acute presentation. More than 45 different disorders are known. Many of them have atypical, or variant, forms.

The most severe defects present neonatally and may cause death or permanent neurological damage. Unfortunately very few have clear, diagnostic, clinical features – they may closely resemble, for example, illness after perinatal asphyxia or septicaemia.

With a few exceptions, inherited organic acid disorders fall into three groups:

▶ defects of amino acid metabolism
▶ defects of fatty acid oxidation
▶ congenital lactic acid disorders in which there is an abnormal accumulation of lactic acid.

Defects of amino acid metabolism

There are many such defects. In general they present with a severe acute illness with metabolic acidosis. The clinical problems are caused by the acidosis and often, also, by toxic intermediates that accumulate.

Several defects occur in the pathways by which the branched-chain amino acids – valine, leucine and isoleucine – are broken down. The best known is **maple syrup urine disease** (*see* Figure 3.3).

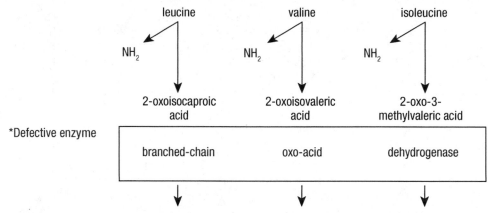

FIGURE 3.3 Deficiency of the enzyme (branched-chain oxo-acid dehydrogenase*) which causes maple syrup urine disease

The first step in the breakdown of these amino acids is loss of an amino group which happens as normal. This leaves three oxo-acids, also known as keto-acids (*see* Figure 3.3). In maple syrup urine disease, the large enzyme that should break these down is missing or defective. The abnormal acids accumulate very quickly and so do some side-products which are also acids.

Clinical features

Severely affected newborns are usually well during the first few days, but as feeds are established, there is increasing exposure to the branched-chain amino acids which they cannot metabolise and the oxo-acids derived from them build up. Generally towards the end of the first week, severe metabolic acidosis develops with acidotic breathing, dehydration, and electrolyte imbalance. There is an acute brain disturbance (encephalopathy), manifest as irritability, poor feeding and often abnormal movements and handling. Without intervention, death results.

Diagnosis

The urine has a characteristic sugary smell and gives a strong positive reaction for ketones. The diagnosis is made by analysis of plasma amino acids and urine amino acids and organic acids. It is confirmed by analysis of the enzyme in fibroblasts cultured from a skin biopsy.

Treatment

1 The emergency treatment is to stop feeds that contain protein because they contain leucine, valine and isoleucine.
2 Intravenous glucose is given to supply calories to limit breakdown of body proteins, another source of the toxic amino acids.
3 Acidosis is corrected with bicarbonate.
4 Very sick babies may require haemodialysis, haemofiltration, or peritoneal dialysis.

Once the condition has stabilised, protein feeding is re-introduced: all the daily requirements for amino acids **except** valine, leucine and isoleucine are provided as a special milk. Very small amounts of natural protein are given as well by adding small amounts of breast milk or a standard formula milk, to provide the small quantities of branched-chain amino acids essential for life. Life-long dietary management is essential. A good outcome is achievable, with normal growth and development but, at any age, intercurrent infections may trigger decompensation, resulting in neurological damage.[5]

Defects of fatty acid oxidation

In these disorders, energy is not made efficiently from long-chain fatty acids in the body's fat stores because one of the key enzymes concerned with their breakdown, by the process of fatty acid oxidation, is lacking. Long-chain fatty acids have from 14 to 22 carbon atoms in them – palmitic acid, for example, has 16. Their oxidation is essential to provide energy for contraction of heart muscle and skeletal muscle and, during fasting, to supply ketones for use as an alternative to glucose as a source of energy. With fasting, long-chain fatty acids are released from the fat stores and transported to the liver, where they are carried into the mitochondria. Here, they are broken down step-wise, by a series of enzymes working in sequence. The fatty acids go round and round this sequence. Each time they complete a circuit, two carbons are removed from them as acetyl-CoA, and they are two carbons shorter. Each circuit is started by a dehydrogenase enzyme. At first, this is very long-chain acyl-CoA dehydrogenase (VLCAD), but when the fatty acids have been shortened to 12–14 carbons, medium-chain acyl-CoA dehydrogenase (MCAD) takes over until they have been shortened to 6 carbons, when short-chain acyl-CoA dehydrogenase (SCAD) completes the degradation (*see* Figure 3.4). This process releases large amounts of acetyl-CoA which provides ATP for the numerous functions undertaken by the liver. Some acetyl-CoA is also made into the ketone bodies, acetoacetic acid and 3-hydroxybutyrate. These are not used by the liver, but are exported to provide energy for the brain, muscles and kidneys.

Medium-chain acyl-CoA dehydrogenase deficiency (MCADD)

Inherited deficiencies of all of the enzymes involved in fatty acid oxidation occur. They are all autosomal recessive disorders. The commonest is MCADD (MCAD deficiency). From neonatal screening figures, the incidence in England is around 1 in 1400 live births. This disorder has now been added to the national newborn screening programme in England.

Clinical features

Babies homozygous for MCADD are generally healthy, normal babies with no perinatal or neonatal problems. They develop normally, and some never have problems from the disorder. However, others present with an acute, life-threatening, illness, typically in early childhood (median age 14 months), after feeding poorly for 24–36 hours because of an intercurrent infection. They soon use up their body reserves of glucose (stored as glycogen). Normal children then make enough energy and ketone bodies from fats to tide them over until they start to eat properly again. Children with

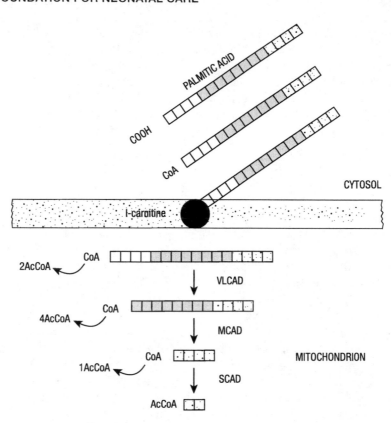

FIGURE 3.4 Oxidation of long-chain fatty acids in the mitochondria

MCADD cannot do this. They become ill very quickly. They present with an acute brain disturbance (encephalopathy) with vomiting and increasing drowsiness, which progresses rapidly to coma and brain-stem failure as the brain becomes oedematous. There is also a serious liver upset. The blood glucose falls. Of 47 children in England and Scotland presenting clinically with their first acute episode from March 1994 to March 1996, 22% died and 13% had neurological sequelae.[6]

Presentation in the neonatal period
Fatty acid defects may present neonatally with acute encephalopathy, cardiomyopathy, liver disturbance and hypoglycaemia, which may be quite a late feature. MCADD only rarely presents in the first week, and then often with cardiomyopathy.

Diagnosis
The diagnosis is made from organic acid abnormalities in urine collected at presentation, and from an unusual pattern of fatty acids circulating in the blood as **acylcarnitines**. Acylcarnitines are measured in blood spots and are generally diagnostic, even when well. If the diagnosis is confirmed, DNA is analysed for mutations. Siblings must be tested for the disorder.

Management

At acute presentation, intravenous glucose is the emergency treatment to supply energy for the brain, but not in large volumes of fluid because of the risk of cerebral oedema. If the diagnosis is made quickly, children with MCADD make a full recovery and develop normally, providing they eat regularly and have glucose enterally or intravenously when off feeds. The parents are provided with an emergency protocol for 'sick days' when the children are refusing feeds and/or vomiting, and there is open access to the hospital if this persists. After age 5 or 6 years, the risk of acute episodes falls, but even young adults have presented in crisis. In some of the other fat oxidation defects, there are long-term complications, including cardiomyopathy, muscle problems or chronic liver damage.

Congenital lactic acid disorders

This is a large group of different inherited disorders in which the common feature is accumulation of lactic acid. This indicates that there is a problem at one of several key sites in the metabolism (*see* Figure 3.5).

Lactic acidosis is very common as an **acquired** disorder in newborns, because of circulatory failure, hypoxia, and liver damage, and these causes must be considered before looking for an inherited defect.

Clinical features

The clinical features of genetic lactic acidosis will depend upon the site of the enzyme defect and its severity. Severe lactic acidosis will contribute to the disease presentation. However, often the increase in lactic acid is not sufficient to produce acidosis, but it is a clue to a serious problem in energy-producing processes. Defects of pyruvate dehydrogenase, of the respiratory chain and of the Krebs cycle, may cause brain damage *in utero*, and affected newborns may also be dysmorphic.

Glycogen storage disease type 1 (glucose-6-phosphatase deficiency)

In this disorder, glucose production both from glycogen and from gluconeogenesis is blocked at the very last step which frees glucose from glucose-6-phosphate, allowing it to be released from the liver into the blood.

Clinical features

Babies have severe, recurrent hypoglycaemia which may develop in as little as 2 hours after a feed, lactic acidosis and a large liver packed with unused glycogen.

Diagnosis

A provisional diagnosis is made by measuring glucose and lactate in the blood before and after feeds and can now be confirmed by DNA analysis of white blood cells, avoiding the need for liver biopsy.

Treatment

This demands rigorous dietary control to ensure an uninterrupted provision of glucose round the clock, supplied overnight via a nasogastric tube.

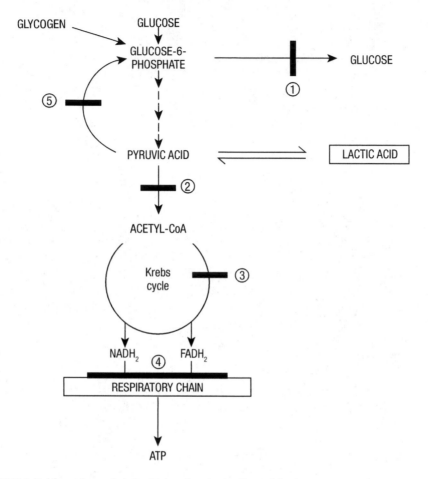

FIGURE 3.5 Key sites of defects leading to lactic acidosis

1 Glycogen storage disease Type 1 (glucose-6-phosphatase deficiency).
2 Pyruvate dehydrogenase (PDH) deficiency.
3 Defects of the Krebs tricarboxylic acid cycle.
4 Defects of the mitochondrial respiratory chain which makes ATP. Some of these are caused by mutations in mitochondrial DNA.
5 Defects in producing glucose from pyruvic acid, i.e. of gluconeogenesis.

Inherited disorders of the respiratory chain

These may be from mutations in nuclear DNA (then generally autosomal recessive) or in mitochondrial DNA (maternally transmitted). They may affect any metabolically active tissue and cause numerous different clinical problems.[7] The most commonly affected organs are the central nervous system, heart and skeletal muscles, and the eyes.

Clinical features

Babies with a neonatal presentation often have a severe multi-system disorder with persistent lactic acidosis, poor muscle tone, severe neurological disturbance (possibly with structural abnormalities of the brain, including agenesis of the corpus callosum), liver disease, nephropathy with a Fanconi syndrome, cardiomyopathy, most often hypertrophic, and sometimes cataracts.

Diagnosis

Diagnostic tests include measurement of lactic acid in plasma and cerebro-spinal fluid (CSF), plasma creatine kinase (CK), plasma and urine amino acids, urine organic acids, and generally a muscle biopsy and skin biopsy (to culture fibroblasts) for analysis of the respiratory chain enzymes and possibly mitochondrial DNA. Sometimes defects of mitochondrial DNA can be detected from a blood sample, but this is unusual in neonatally presenting disorders. There is no specific treatment.

INHERITED UREA CYCLE DEFECTS

The main purpose of the urea cycle is to remove waste nitrogen and ammonia from the body. Ammonia is produced by the catabolism of dietary and body proteins and by bacterial activity on gut contents. It is toxic to the nervous system. It is detoxified in the liver by conversion to urea via the urea cycle, which is operated by five enzymes working in sequence (*see* Figure 3.6). A sixth enzyme (not shown) makes an activator (N-acetylglutamate; NAG) which is essential for the first step.

Inherited deficiencies of all six enzymes occur,[8] but they are rare. The damaging effects of five of these disorders are due to the large amounts of ammonia which accumulate. The blood levels become particularly high in catabolic illnesses, generally infective, when large amounts of amino acids are released from destruction of body proteins. Levels are also increased by a high protein intake, or by bleeding into the bowel.

Clinical features

The most severe disorders present acutely in the first week of life, when plasma ammonia usually exceeds 300 µmol/L and plasma urea may be low. Generally the babies are born without problems after an uneventful pregnancy, and are apparently well at first. From around 24 hours to 72 hours, they become lethargic, feed poorly, vomit, may be hypothermic and are irritable. The encephalopathy progresses rapidly, manifest as abnormal movements, seizures, loss of reflexes, apnoeas and coma, requiring full intensive care. Ammonia stimulates respiration and respiratory alkalosis is often present in the early stages. Severe, recurrent or chronic elevation of ammonia causes permanent brain damage.

Diagnosis

1 Very high levels of plasma ammonia, not explained by liver failure, provide a provisional diagnosis.
2 Analysis of plasma and urine amino acids helps to identify the site of the defect, since the intermediates in the urea cycle are all amino acids. In addition, plasma alanine and glutamine are usually increased non-specifically.
3 In those disorders of the cycle after carbamyl phosphate synthetase, urinary excretion of **orotic acid** is increased (*see* Figure 3.6). This is a very useful diagnostic marker for urea cycle defects.

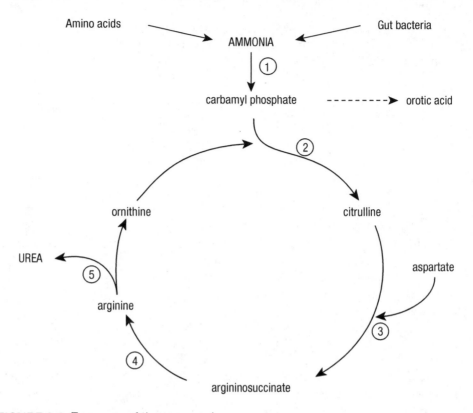

FIGURE 3.6 Enzymes of the urea cycle

    1 CPS1: carbamylphosphate synthetase1; this is activated by NAG
    2 OTC: ornithine transcarbamylase
    3 AS: argininosuccinate synthetase
    4 AL: argininosuccinate lyase
    5 arginase

4 Confirmation of the enzyme defect. Depending on the defect, this is done on white blood cells or cultured fibroblasts from a skin biopsy. For the commonest OTC (ornithine transcarbamylase) deficiency, a liver biopsy is needed – but this may be avoided by a DNA test, which is helpful in around 80% of cases.
5 If a urea cycle defect is confirmed, DNA is now usually analysed for mutations, but may require gene sequencing because there are many mutations for each defect.

Acute treatment[3,8]

It is essential to recognise and respond to hyperammonaemia quickly, before cerebral oedema and vasomotor instability develop. The mainstays are to reduce production of nitrogenous waste and to lower plasma ammonia as quickly as possible. Arginine is essential to replenish low levels.
1 All protein intake is discontinued for 24–48 hours and glucose is given intravenously to minimise the catabolism of body proteins.
2 **L-arginine** is infused intravenously.

3 Sodium benzoate and sodium phenylbutyrate are given intravenously. These 'alternative pathway remedies' remove excess nitrogen from the body by using pathways which do not require the urea cycle. They help lower the plasma ammonia quickly.

4 If plasma ammonia is >350 µmol/L, dialysis is considered. Haemodialysis (or of this is impractical, peritoneal dialysis) is more effective than haemofiltration. When the plasma ammonia has fallen, the baby is started on low protein feeds supplying enough calories for growth and sodium phenylbutrate and arginine are given enterally. The outcome of neonatally presenting urea cycle defects with severe hyperammonaemia is poor. Around half the babies die. A normal cognitive outcome is very unlikely if ammonia exceeds 400 µmol/L, and the neurological prognosis is very poor if hyperammonaemic coma exceeds 72 hours.[9] In these cases, aggressive treatment may not be appropriate. Delays in diagnosis and instituting treatment increase the risk. Newborns diagnosed within hours of birth because of an affected sibling, and treated prospectively, have a better outcome. However, there is an on-going risk of episodes of decompensation with recurrent infections and brain damage. Liver transplantation is now recommended as definitive corrective therapy for babies in good condition after the neonatal period.

NON-KETOTIC HYPERGLYCINAEMIA (NKH)

This autosomal recessive disorder has a characteristic presentation in neonates, and is one of the commoner defects seen in the UK.

The cause is a defect in a large enzyme complex, the **glycine cleavage system**, which degrades glycine in the liver, brain and kidneys. It is the accumulation of glycine within the central nervous system which causes the problems. Glycine is an inhibitory neurotransmitter in the brain stem, and high levels cause early hypotonia and apnoeas. Within the brain, glycine binds to some of the glutamate receptors (NMDA receptors) of neurons and helps to open them up, causing excitation, and eventually neuronal destruction. This accounts for the increase in tone and seizures which develop.

Clinical features

Typically babies appear normal at birth and there are no perinatal problems. Within the first two days or so, however, a progressive encephalopathy develops. The babies are sleepy and not interested in feeds, and develop gross hypotonia, lie in a frog's leg posture and are extremely floppy on handling. They develop apnoeas and need ventilation, and become unresponsive. After day four or five, they become hypertonic and have seizures. Hiccoughs are a striking feature. The EEG is grossly abnormal with a burst-suppression pattern. Babies presenting neonatally do badly. Most die between 6 days and 5 years. Generally survivors have severe neurological problems with seizures.[10,11] There is no treatment which slows the progression of the illness.

Diagnosis

The diagnosis is made by analysis of amino acids in CSF and blood collected simultaneously, and in urine. Glycine levels are very high, but the other amino acids are normal. The concentration of glycine in plasma is *normally* 10 to 30 times higher than in CSF and so blood contamination leads to spuriously high CSF glycine levels – a bloody tap is no use.

OTHER DISORDERS CAUSING SEVERE SEIZURES

Other defects present with a severe seizure disorder. Two which disturb pyridoxine (vitamin B6) metabolism, are treatable and must be considered.[12]

Pyridoxine dependent epilepsy is due to a defect in the metabolism of the amino acid lysine. It presents with intractable seizures perinatally, sometimes starting *in utero*. The EEG is very abnormal. Seizures stop dramatically with 50–100 mg (rarely 500 mg) of intravenous pyridoxine, and the EEG becomes normal within 24 hours. Seizures can then be controlled with oral pyridoxine, but recur if this is stopped.

Another vitamin B6 disorder, **PNPO (pyridox(am)ine-5'-phosphate oxidase) deficiency**, is caused by deficiency of the enzyme needed to convert vitamin B6 into its active form, pyridoxal phosphate. These babies present with intractable seizures which are controlled by giving pyridoxal phosphate (orally), but not by pyridoxine. Biochemical tests are available to diagnose both conditions, and DNA tests if confirmed.

There are no specific treatments for most other seizure disorders due to metabolic defects (*see* Table 3.1 for a list). One is **sulfite oxidase deficiency** for which there is a urine dip-stick test which picks up increased sulfite (Merckoquant Sulfi-Test®). The urine must be sent to the laboratory as soon as voided and tested when very fresh. Even then it may give false negative results. Another is the group of disorders due to deficiencies of enzymes present in **peroxisomes**. These are tiny packages of around 40 enzymes found in all cells except red blood cells. They have numerous functions, but among the most important are their roles in the removal and synthesis of various lipids in the nervous system. More than 20 different peroxisomal disorders are known, with single or multiple enzyme deficiencies. Those presenting neonatally may involve the brain, liver and kidneys, and affected babies are often dysmorphic. Seizures are just one of a range of presentations. The initial diagnostic test is measurement of very long-chain fatty acids (VLCFAs) in plasma.

DIAGNOSIS OF INHERITED METABOLIC DISORDERS
Clinical clues

With a few exceptions, such as NKH, the neonatal presentations of inherited metabolic disorders are non-specific and are similar to those of much commoner, and hence more likely, disorders – such as sepsis. There are some clues which should alert suspicion; a very strong pointer, which must not be ignored, is a normal baby who was well for the first 24–72 hours and then becomes acutely ill for no obvious reason.

KEY POINTS FOR PRACTICE (1)
Alerting clues in an acutely ill baby
▶ Family history of similar or of unexplained infant deaths
▶ Parents consanguineous
▶ Unexplained vomiting
▶ Dysmorphic

TABLE 3.1 Clinical presentations of inherited biochemical disorders and relevant first-round tests

Presentation†	Possible disorders†	Biochemical tests		
		Plasma/blood	Urine	CSF
Encephalopathy	NKH	glycine	glycine	glycine
	urea cycle defects	ammonia amino acids	amino acids orotic acid	
	organic acidurias	amino acids	organic acids amino acids	
+ hypoglycaemia	fat oxidation defects	acylcarnitines (blood spots)	organic acids	
+ lactic acidosis	lactic acidoses	lactic acid amino acids	organic acids amino acids	lactic acid
+ dysmorphic	peroxisome defects	VLCFAs*		
	lactic acidoses	lactic acid amino acids	organic acids amino acids	lactic acid
Seizures	NKH	glycine	glycine	glycine
	urea cycle defects	ammonia amino acids	amino acids orotic acid	
	vitamin B6 disorders: PNPO deficiency (pyridox(am)ine-5′-phosphate oxidase deficiency)	amino acids	organic acids	amino acids pyridoxal phosphate neurotransmitter metabolites
	pyridoxine dependency (response to pyridoxine demonstrated)		α-aminoadipic semialdehyde	
	sulfite oxidase deficiency (isolated) in molybdenum co-factor deficiency	amino acids uric acid	sulfite stick test purines	
	some organic acidurias	amino acids	organic acids amino acids	
	peroxisome defects	VLCFAs*		

(continued)

Presentation†	Possible disorders†	Biochemical tests		
		Plasma/blood	Urine	CSF
	magnesium malabsorption	magnesium calcium	magnesium	
	3-phosphoglycerate dehydrogenase deficiency	amino acids		amino acids
Recurrent or severe hypoglycaemia	glycogen storage disorders	pre- + post-feed glucose + lactate		
	disorders of gluconeogenesis	glucose + lactate + amino acids (pre-feed)	organic acids	
	fatty acid oxidation defects	acylcarnitines (blood spots)	organic acids	
	persistent hyperinsulinism	insulin + C peptide when glucose low ammonia		
Hepatomegaly +/– liver failure	galactosaemia	GAL-1-PUT**	Clinitest; glucose stick test; sugar chromatography (if having lactose)	
	fatty-acid oxidation defects	acylcarnitines (blood spots)	organic acids	
	tyrosinaemia type 1	amino acids	organic acids amino acids	
	α-1-antitrypsin deficiency	α-1-antitrypsin		
	respiratory chain defects	lactic acid amino acids	organic acids	lactic acid
	peroxisome defects	VLCFAs*		
	congenital disorders of glycosylation (CDGs)	transferrin isoforms		

(continued)

Presentation†	Possible disorders†	Biochemical tests		
		Plasma/blood	Urine	CSF
Hepatosplenomegaly +/– coarse features or dysmorphic; +/– hydrops	some storage disorders	white cell enzymes	glycosaminoglycans = mucopolysaccharides	
	peroxisome defects	VLCFAs*		
	congenital disorders of glycosylation (CDGs)	transferrin isoforms		
Cardiomyopathy	respiratory chain disorders	CK, lactic acid, amino acids, blood count	organic acids	lactic acid
	fatty-acid oxidation defects	acylcarnitines (blood spots)	organic acids	
	some organic acidurias	amino acids	organic acids, amino acids	
	mucopolysaccharidoses		glycosaminoglycans = mucopolysaccharides	
	Pompe disease	white cell α-glucosidase, vacuolated lymphocytes		
	congenital disorders of glycosylation (CDGs)	transferrin isoforms		

† This is an incomplete list of presentations and disorders; see Chakrapani et al.[13] and Saudubray et al.[14] for more comprehensive summaries.

* VLCFAs: very long-chain fatty acids.

** GAL-1-PUT: galactose-1-phosphate uridyltransferase.

❱ Hepatomegaly
❱ Onset with fasting/poor feeding
❱ Persistent metabolic acidosis
❱ Abnormal smell
❱ **A normal baby who was well for the first 24–72 hours, then becomes unwell for no obvious reason.**

Investigation

The dominant clinical features are a guide to possible underlying defects. Table 3.1 presents a brief summary, but the list is incomplete and lacks detail. For more comprehensive lists, *see* Chakrapani *et al.*[13] and Saudubray *et al.*[14] . Most babies will have features from more than one category.

Table 3.1 also lists a selection of first-round tests relevant to presentation. Positive results generally require subsequent enzyme confirmation on blood or skin, muscle or, infrequently, liver biopsies, and/or DNA tests. In general, the initial sweep will include:

❱ plasma and urine amino acids
❱ urine organic acids
❱ plasma lactate
❱ plasma ammonia (seizures, encephalopathy, hepatomegaly)
❱ blood acylcarnitines (hypoglycaemia, hepatomegaly, cardiomyopathy).

Plasma VLCFAs are the screen for peroxisomal disorders, which have a broad presentation. After 21 days of age, plasma transferrin isoforms (carbohydrate-deficient transferrin) may be analysed to look for a congenital glycosylation disorder (CDG), in which there is a defect in adding carbohydrate chains (oligosaccharides) to proteins. These have a broad presentation neonatally.

Not infrequently, a baby has a catastrophic illness thought likely to be due to a metabolic disorder, but will die before this can be investigated. It is crucial to obtain appropriate samples before death, which will cover a wide range of possibilities, to try to establish a diagnosis in hindsight. This is essential for accurate genetic counselling. For confirmed defects, if the biochemical abnormalities of the dead baby are known, prenatal diagnosis can often be offered for subsequent pregnancies. After discussion with the parents, and obtaining consent, the following samples should be taken:

❱ plasma lactate
❱ plasma ammonia
❱ plasma amino acids
❱ blood acylcarnitines
❱ blood to extract for DNA for mutation analysis if needed and to store for VLCFAs and other tests if required later
❱ urine (at least 10 mL if available) for amino acids, organic acids, orotic acid (if indicated), and to store for other tests if needed.

A **skin biopsy** should be taken to culture fibroblasts which may be needed for special enzyme analyses, a **muscle biopsy** if the baby is hypotonic or if a respiratory chain disorder is possible and, exceptionally, a **liver biopsy** if NKH or certain rare liver disorders are suspected.

GOOD SAMPLES FOR BIOCHEMISTRY TESTS

To make a rapid diagnosis of inherited metabolic disorders, it is essential to have reliable biochemistry test results and to alert the laboratory early. The first step is to provide good samples. Some metabolites in blood increase rapidly after venesection, giving spuriously high results. For this reason, samples for lactate, if not measured on a blood gas analyser, must reach the laboratory within 15 minutes; and samples for ammonia within 20 minutes (preferably transported in water ice). Levels of both these compounds are increased if the baby is struggling during venesection and in haemolysed samples. A minimum of 5 mL of blood is required for white cell enzyme analyses – even from very small babies. This is because only the white cells in blood are used for this test, and there are not many of them. Good-quality urine samples are important for measurement of organic acids and amino acids, and must be without faecal contamination, which can alter the profiles. A bag urine sample is preferred, but if this proves difficult, unsoiled urine collected into a cotton wool ball may be the only option – it is essential that urine is analysed. The dip-stick test for sulfite must be done quickly on freshly voided urine. Samples collected at the time of an acute illness are the most informative. Abnormal metabolites may disappear after treatment is started, with a risk of missing the diagnosis. This is particularly important in galactosaemia, since galactose will not be detectable in urine when lactose is removed from the feeds. Similarly, in fatty acid oxidation defects, the urine profiles change rapidly when babies are given calories as glucose, and hence fatty acid turnover is suppressed. CSF for glycine analysis in suspected NKH must be clear: blood contamination makes the result uninterpretable. There is a protocol for collection of CSF for neurotransmitters, which includes immediate freezing. Analysis of samples for DNA, and collection of skin and tissue biopsies require informed parental consent.

SUMMARY

Inherited biochemical defects are rare, but important, disorders. The most severe present neonatally, sometimes with a severe life-threatening illness. Prompt recognition and precise diagnosis are essential.

KEY POINTS FOR PRACTICE (2)

▶ Some defects are treatable and have a good outcome with early intervention. Treatment may be by dietary manipulation, specific medications or by both. Examples are galactosaemia, treated by altering the feeds; congenital adrenal hyperplasia, treated by giving replacement steroids; intractable seizures responsive to pyridoxine or pyridoxal phosphate; urea cycle defects treated by combination of a low protein diet, a dietary supplement (arginine) and medications (sodium benzoate and phenylbutyrate).

▶ Some conditions which respond poorly to treatment or are untreatable, cause early death or severe handicap. However, accurate diagnosis:
   — Helps the parents – the condition and its likely course can be explained to them and they can be supported through a distressing illness.
   — Facilitates genetic counselling for subsequent pregnancies.
   — Is essential if prenatal diagnosis is to be offered for subsequent pregnancies. Tests of fetal tissue using enzyme or DNA analysis are available for an

increasing number of serious defects and can be done on chorionic villus samples, collected at 9–11 weeks of gestation. The parents can be reassured if the result is normal (three out of four chance for autosomal recessive disorders) or the pregnancy terminated if the fetus is affected. Knowing this, more couples who have had a child with an inborn error are prepared to embark on a second pregnancy.

REFERENCES

1 Scriver CR, Beaudet AL, Sly WS, *et al.*, editors. *The Metabolic and Molecular Bases of Inherited Disease.* 8th ed. New York: McGraw-Hill; 2001.

2 Fernandes J, Saudubray J-M, van den Berghe G, *et al.*, editors. *Inborn Metabolic Diseases.* 4th ed. Heidelberg: Springer; 2006.

3 British Inherited Metabolic Disease Group. Available at: www.bimdg.org.uk/guidelines.asp (accessed 18 May 2009).

4 Berry GT, Segal S, Gitzelman R. Disorders of galactose metabolism. In: Fernandes J, Saudubray J-M, van den Berghe G, *et al.*, op. cit. pp. 123–30.

5 Morton DH, Strauss KA, Robinson DL, *et al.* Diagnosis and treatment of maple syrup urine disease: a study of 36 patients. *Pediatrics.* 2002; **109**: 999–1008.

6 Pollitt RJ, Leonard JV. Prospective surveillance study of medium chain acyl-CoA dehydrogenase deficiency in the UK. *Arch Dis Child.* 1998; **79**: 116–19.

7 Munnich A, Rötig A, Cormier-Daire V, *et al.* Clinical presentation of respiratory chain deficiency. In: Scriver CR, Beaudet AL, Sly WS, *et al.*, editors. *The Metabolic and Molecular Bases of Inherited Disease.* 8th ed. New York: McGraw-Hill; 2001. pp. 2261–74.

8 Leonard JV. Disorders of the urea cycle and related enzymes. In: Fernandes J, Saudubray J-M, van den Berghe G, *et al.*, op. cit. pp. 263–72.

9 Wilcken, B. Problems in the management of urea cycle disorders. *Mol Gen Metab.* 2004; **81**(Suppl.1): S86–91.

10 Hoover-Fong JE, Shah S, Van Hove JLK, *et al.* Natural history of nonketotic hyperglycinaemia in 65 patients. *Neurology.* 2004; **63**: 1847–53.

11 Dulac O, Rolland M-O. Nonketotic hyperglycinaemia (glycine encephalopathy). In: Fernandes J, Saudubray J-M, van den Berghe G, *et al.*, op. cit. pp. 307–13.

12 Clayton PT. B6-responsive disorders: a model of vitamin dependency. *J Inherit Metab Dis.* 2006; **29**: 317–26.

13 Chakrapani A, Cleary MA, Wraith JE. Detection of inborn errors of metabolism in the newborn. *Arch Dis Child. Fetal and Neonatal Edition.* 2001; **84**(3): F205–10.

14 Saudubray J-M, Desguerre I, Sedel F, *et al.* A clinical approach to inherited metabolic diseases. In: Fernandes J, Saudubray J-M, van den Berghe G, *et al.*, op. cit. pp. 3–48.

CHAPTER 4

Fundamental physiological concepts

Alan Noble

CONTENTS

INTRODUCTION

General textbooks of physiology and of adult medicine are written with a rather specific type of individual in mind. The textbook person is male, 70 kg in weight and 20–25 years old. Although many of the physiological processes in fetal and neonatal individuals have much in common with those in the textbook person, there are also crucial differences. The aim of this chapter is to review some fundamental physiological processes but also to highlight the important differences between fetal and neonatal subjects on the one hand and mature individuals on the other. These differences do not relate purely to differences in body size.

BODY FLUID COMPARTMENTS

The textbook person has about 42 L of total body water, 60% of total body weight. The distribution of this body water is approximately 25 L (60% of total body water) in the intracellular compartment and 17 L (40% of total body water) in the extracellular compartment. Even in respect of this very simple physiological parameter there are surprising differences within the population at large. Women typically have only 50% of their total body weight as water. This reflects the relatively greater distribution of adipose tissue in adult females compared with that in men. In people of both genders, water contributes a smaller proportion of total body weight as we get older. This is attributable to both a true reduction in total body water and also to an increase in the amount of adipose tissue with advancing years. An average elderly male might have only 50% of body weight as water.

In term infants, water typically contributes about 75% of total body weight and this percentage is even higher in premature neonates. In a child with a gestational age of 32 weeks, water contributes about 83% of body weight and in even less mature neonates this may rise to 90%. Total body water distribution into fluid compartments is also different. In a term neonate, this is typically 55% intracellular and 45% extracellular, figures which are similar to those of an adult. However, a 30-week neonate has a different distribution, with 60% of body water in the extracellular compartment and only 40% in the intracellular spaces. Newborn babies also have a daily water turnover rate which is three to four times higher than it is in adults. Low birth weight babies lose about 10% to 12% of their extracellular fluid in the first five days of life.

Movement of water between compartments

The fluid compartments of the body are not 'watertight'. There is free movement of water across capillary walls and through cell membranes if there is an appropriate driving force. These 'driving forces' are fundamentally of two types: *hydrostatic pressure gradients* and *osmotic pressure gradients*. There are no active 'pumps' which move water between fluid compartments in the body. All cells are porous and water can move through the lipid bilayer in the cell membrane. These membranes are not identical in all cell types, however, and the water permeability depends on the lipid composition of individual cell walls. Those cells which are relatively rigid have lower water permeability than those in which the lipid composition leads to a higher membrane fluidity. In some cell types, such as those in the collecting duct of the kidney which require a capacity for high water permeability, this is provided by the insertion of water channels, called aquaporins (*see* page 150), in the membrane. The driving forces to move water through these channels are still provided by hydrostatic and osmotic gradients.

Hydrostatic pressure gradients

The concept of a hydrostatic pressure gradient is perhaps most easily understood in relation to a blood capillary. The blood pressure inside a capillary is higher than the pressure in the interstitial fluid outside the capillary. There is, therefore, a tendency for water to move out of capillaries down a hydrostatic pressure gradient. This concept is further developed later in this book in the section on the cardiovascular system in relation to capillary dynamics and the formation of oedema (*see* Chapter 5, page 137). The idea of a hydrostatic pressure gradient driving water movement is not confined to capillary function.

Any tendency for water to move into a cell would tend to inflate it like a balloon and this would result in an increase in the hydrostatic pressure inside the cell. This would progressively oppose further water influx driven by either an osmotic or a hydrostatic gradient. However, under normal conditions, the hydrostatic pressure gradient across a cell membrane is close to zero. Only osmotic gradients are therefore of prime importance in determining water movement across cell membranes.

Osmotic pressure gradients

An osmotic gradient is, simplistically, the movement of water down its concentration gradient. Thus, we may imagine two theoretical situations, a 'strong' and a 'weak' solution. A 'strong' solution, in which there is a high concentration of dissolved solute, will mean that there is relatively less space for the water molecules and so the concentration of water molecules is lower. In a 'weak' solution, there is a low concentration of dissolved solute and the concentration of water molecules would be correspondingly higher. If we placed the 'weak' solution (e.g. pure water) and the 'strong' solution (e.g. blood plasma) on either side of a semipermeable membrane, a structure through which water molecules can pass, water would move down its concentration gradient by the process of diffusion from the 'weak' solution to the 'strong' solution (*see* Figure 4.1). This is the process of osmosis.

Visualising the concentration of water molecules is quite difficult and so it is easier to think in terms of the solute concentration gradient generating an osmotic pressure gradient. It is useful to have ways for quantifying the osmotic strength of a solution and this depends on the number of solute particles.

A 1 molar solution of a substance is made by dissolving one relative molecular mass in grams (one molecular weight in grams) of a solute in water and then making the volume up to 1 L. If the solute does not dissociate into smaller particles when dissolved, then, by definition, the 1 molar solution is also a 1 osmolar solution. An example of such a solute is glucose.

A solute which, when dissolved in water, dissociates completely into two ions exerts twice the osmotic strength compared with a solute which does not dissociate. A 1 molar solution would therefore become a 2 osmolar solution. Sodium chloride does dissociate into a sodium ion (Na^+) and a chloride ion (Cl^-) in solution. Sodium chloride is the constituent of 'physiological saline solution', and is the major contributor to the osmotic strength of blood plasma. A 1 molar solution of NaCl is actually slightly less than 2 osmolar. This is because electrostatic attraction between the Na^+ ions and Cl^- ions in solution means that some of them transiently re-form undissociated NaCl molecules, thus reducing the total number of particles in solution. Dissociation of the NaCl occurs again instantly. The practical units in which osmolarity is expressed are mosmoles/L.

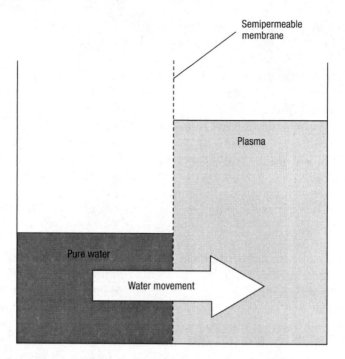

FIGURE 4.1 Model to illustrate osmosis

The left-hand compartment contains pure water and on the right is blood plasma, a solution containing dissolved solutes. Water movement by osmosis is from left to right, from a high concentration of water molecules to a lower concentration.

Source: Noble *et al. The Cardiovascular System*. Elsevier Health Sciences; 2005.

When body-fluid samples such as blood plasma and urine, which contain many different osmotically active solutes, are sent for laboratory analysis of osmotic strength, this is measured using the physical principle of depression of freezing point. Thus, the more dissolved solute there is in a solution, the lower the temperature at which the solution freezes. This general principle can be illustrated by the fact that freshwater ponds and puddles on pavements freeze at 0 °C in winter but the sea, which has more dissolved solute, will only freeze at a lower temperature. The depression of freezing point technique provides a measurement not of osmolarity but of *osmolality* and the units are mosmoles/kg. The term osmolality can be explained as follows.

If one relative molecular mass in grams (one molecular weight in grams) of a solute is dissolved in 1 kg (1 L) of water, this produces a 1 molal solution. The total volume of the solution produced is slightly more than 1 L because of the volume occupied by the dissolved solute. A 1 molal solution is therefore slightly weaker than a 1 molar solution. The difference under physiological conditions is small, of the order of 2% to 3%, usually a negligible difference for clinical considerations.

The different sets of units applied to measurements of osmotic strength sometimes cause confusion. Osmolarity and osmolality are useful concepts when used in the assessment of the osmotic strength of body fluid samples or replacement fluids but they are not appropriate when it comes to considering the balance between the two sets of forces concerned with water movement, a hydrostatic pressure gradient versus an osmotic gradient. This is where the concept of osmotic pressure becomes useful.

A simple model to illustrate the concept of osmotic pressure is shown in Figure 4.2.

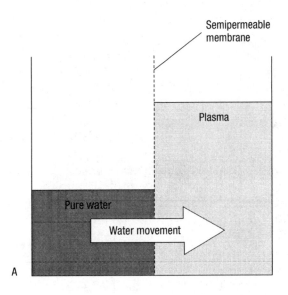

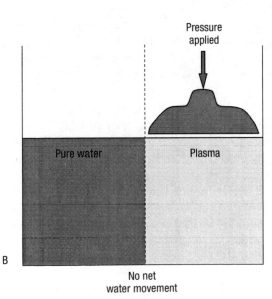

FIGURE 4.2 Model to illustrate the concept of osmotic pressure

Source: Noble A *et al.*, op. cit.

The two compartments in each of the containers are separated by a semipermeable membrane through which only water molecules can pass. In the top model, water molecules can pass by osmosis from the pure water compartment to the compartment containing blood plasma. If, however, a pressure is applied to the plasma, it would be possible to stop the water movement. The applied pressure which would just stop water movement from the pure water compartment is called the osmotic pressure of the solution.

Typically, the total osmotic pressure exerted by all the dissolved components in blood plasma is about 7.6 atmospheres (5800 mmHg). Most of the osmotic pressure of plasma is generated by the small particles which have the highest concentration in plasma, especially sodium and chloride ions. The contribution of large molecules, the plasma proteins, to the total osmotic pressure of plasma is relatively small – of the order of 28 mmHg out of the total osmotic pressure of 5800 mmHg. The plasma protein which is of the greatest significance quantitatively is albumin because it is relatively small (relative molecular mass (RMM) 69 000) compared with other plasma proteins and has a high concentration (35–39 g/L) in relation to total plasma protein concentration (70–78 g/L).

There is frequently a misunderstanding regarding the contribution of the colloid osmotic pressure to the total osmotic pressure of plasma. The basis for the misunderstanding comes from models of capillary function. Blood capillaries are quite leaky and so the small dissolved components of plasma (Na$^+$, Cl$^-$, glucose, urea, etc.) are equally distributed inside and outside capillaries. There is, therefore, effectively no osmotic gradient produced by the small molecules. Capillary walls have only a limited permeability to plasma proteins so there is a higher protein concentration inside the capillary than there is outside. The osmotic gradient produced by the plasma proteins is referred to as either a gradient of colloid osmotic pressure or of oncotic pressure.

Clinically, exogenous colloids can be administered to boost the colloid osmotic pressure of plasma and thus pull water from the interstitial space into the intravascular (plasma) volume. Examples of colloids used include human albumin, polygelatin solutions, hydroxymethyl starches (HES) and dextrans but these all have limitations on their uses.

The half-life of exogenous albumin is short: 10% of the albumin administered leaves the circulation within 2 hours, and 95% of it within 2 days. Polygelatin solutions are polypeptides but they are comparatively small (RMM 35 000) and can therefore pass through the glomerular filter in the kidney to be excreted. Their half-life in the circulation is only about 4 hours. HES are highly branched glucose polymers with a half-life of about 17 days. They do have some unwanted side effects, including disruption of aspects of the clotting cascade. Dextrans are large polysaccharide molecules with a half-life of 2 to 12 hours. Dextrans also have some side effects including interference with the cross-matching of blood and, in some patients, anaphylaxis.

MOVEMENT OF SUBSTANCES ACROSS CELL MEMBRANES

The outer (plasma) membrane of cells consists primarily of a double layer of phospholipid molecules with a series of proteins embedded in it. The presence of variable amounts of lipids such as cholesterol, in addition to the phospholipid, in the lipid bilayer can have important effects on membrane fluidity and hence on membrane permeability. The plasma (outer) membrane of cells is not a rigid structure and has been described as having a consistency similar to that of olive oil. For this reason, the model of membrane structure is often called the 'Fluid Mosaic Model'. The 'mosaic' part of this description refers to the proteins which are embedded in the lipid bilayer.

This membrane structure determines what may pass through the membrane and how passage of ions and molecules can be achieved. There are fundamentally four groups of mechanism.

- *Diffusion* through the lipid bilayer, a route which is only available for small uncharged molecules such as oxygen and carbon dioxide.
- *Passage through ion channels*, a route mainly for ions which are both small and carry an electric charge.
- *Carrier-mediated* mechanisms which promote the movement of small molecules across the cell membrane. These mechanisms may either assist movement down a concentration gradient (facilitated diffusion) or, by the use of energy in the form of ATP, promote movement against a concentration or electrical gradient (active transport).
- *Endocytosis and exocytosis* are processes which involve the formation of vesicles derived from the cell membrane to make it possible for a variety of items ranging from neurotransmitters to small pieces of foreign matter such as bacteria to cross cell membranes.

Each of these processes will now be described in more detail.

Diffusion

The lipid bilayer in the cell membrane is essentially impermeable to anything other than very small non-polar (uncharged) molecules. Charged ions, such as Na^+, K^+ Cl^-, are soluble in water but not in lipid and effectively cannot cross the bilayer without the assistance of a specific mechanism. Oxygen and carbon dioxide, which are not charged, can cross cell membranes freely through the lipid bilayer.

Diffusion is the movement of a molecule or ion down its concentration gradient from a region of high concentration to an area of lower concentration. Thus, oxygen diffuses into cells and carbon dioxide diffuses out of cells. The rate of diffusion depends on temperature (slower at low temperature); molecular size (small molecules diffuse quicker than large molecules), and solubility in the 'solute'. What may be regarded as the solute can either be the lipid environment of a cell membrane or water on both the inside and the outside of cells.

In 1905, Einstein showed that the time taken for a molecule to diffuse between two points varies as the square of the distance between the points. In the case of oxygen, the time taken to diffuse the width of a typical cell, about 10 μm, would be a few milliseconds. The time to diffuse 1 mm (a hundred times 10 μm) would be 10 000 times as long. This represents a substantial oxygen supply problem for the approximately 100 million million cells in the body of the textbook person, but it is also of immense importance in a tiny neonate.

Oxygen is really not very soluble in water. This rather simple statement conditions the design structure of all multi-cellular animals. The poor solubility of oxygen means that we cannot rely on oxygen diffusion over anything other than very small distances in the body to occur at a rate which would be adequate to supply tissues. We have therefore evolved with a highly prolific circulatory system. It is estimated that cells in the body can rarely be more than two or three cell widths (20–30 μm) away from a blood capillary. This means that the textbook person (70 kg male, 20 to 25 years old) has a circulatory system which, if stretched out end to end, would measure approaching 60 000 miles (96 000 kilometres) – enough to encircle the world three times. Even a neonate will have a surprisingly large amount of blood vessel measured in units of thousands of miles/kilometres.

Interruption of blood flow will lead to tissue damage very quickly. For example, disruption of blood flow to the brain leads to loss of consciousness in 8–10 seconds and permanent brain damage in 5–10 minutes. Although carbon dioxide is about 20 times as soluble in water as oxygen, and will therefore diffuse more rapidly, it is crucially important to clear CO_2 from cells and tissues very quickly. Oxidative metabolism generates acidic products, particularly CO_2, and removal of these acidic products is essential for the maintenance of life. Aspects of the regulation of acid-base balance are dealt with later in this chapter (*see* page 112).

The poor solubility of oxygen in water also means that it is essential to have haemoglobin as an oxygen carrier in blood in order to ensure adequate delivery of oxygen to the tissues. Thus, physiologically, diffusion is a process for moving molecules over only very short distances. For larger distances a transport system, the circulation containing haemoglobin, is essential.

Ion channels

Ion channels are membrane proteins which span the complete width of the lipid bilayer. A water-filled hole through the protein provides a channel through which ions, which are water-soluble, can move by diffusion. Water can also move through the channels in either direction. The water pressure (hydrostatic pressure) inside and outside cell membranes is normally similar, so this is not a major consideration but changes in the osmotic strength of the interstitial fluid outside a cell can alter water flux across cell membranes.

Water-filled channels in membranes that are always open are sometimes referred to as 'pores'. Some of these are also found in intracellular membranous structures such as mitochondria. In the kidney, water pores are stored in the epithelial cells of the distal parts of the nephron ready to be inserted into either the luminal or baso-lateral membranes under the influence of anti-diuretic hormone (ADH) (*see* page 150). These channels, called aquaporins, provide the mechanism for increasing the water permeability of the nephron in conditions of increased plasma osmolarity or dehydration. These are the major stimuli for ADH secretion and these mechanisms provide for an increase in water retention in the body. Some other types of pore can allow quite large molecules to cross the membrane. Insertion of large-diameter pores (called perforins) is one of the mechanisms by which cytotoxic T lymphocytes kill their target cells. In this way, the cell membrane is made freely permeable to water and small molecules.

Many ion channels have a 'gating' mechanism. This is a part of the channel protein which can move to allow the channel to be either opened or closed. Almost all channels for ions such as Na^+, K^+, Cl^- are gated. An ion channel is therefore a gated pore and conversely, a pore is an ungated channel.

Ion channel gates may be opened by one of two types of mechanism.

▶ *Voltage-gated channels* (also called potential-operated channels) are opened and closed by a change in the electrical potential (charge difference) across the cell membrane. The generation of a membrane potential and the role played by voltage-gated ion channels in nerve cells, is described later in this chapter (*see* page 101).

▶ *Ligand-gated channels* (also called receptor-operated channels) are linked to a membrane protein referred to as a receptor (*see* page 105). When a specific chemical messenger (e.g. a hormone or neurotransmitter) binds to the receptor, the response is a change in channel gating.

Genetically determined alterations in the structure of ion channels form the basis for a number of disease mechanisms. These are sometimes referred to by the rather ungainly term 'channelopathies'. Among a rather long list of channelopathies are cystic fibrosis (a Cl^- channel defect). Some forms of either over- or under-secretion of insulin which become apparent in infancy and some skeletal muscle disorders are associated with altered function of Na^+ channels. Genetically determined alterations in either sodium or potassium channel function are the basis for the cardiac dysrhythmias known as the long QT syndrome. This is a cause of sudden cardiac death.

Some drugs are targeted towards blocking selective ion channels. These include calcium channel blocking drugs, such as nifedipine. In addition to its use as an anti-hypertensive, this drug is sometimes used to suppress uterine contractility and hence reduce the risk of premature labour. A range of drugs is used to modify Na^+ channel function. These include lidocaine and flecainide which are anti-cardiac dysrhythmia drugs. Local anaesthetic agents which block sodium channels, including bupivicaine, are used for superficial administration but also for epidural anaesthesia. Other drugs which block sodium channels are used in the management of epilepsy. Entry of Na^+ into neurones contributes the rising phase of nerve action potentials (*see* page 102) and so Na^+ channel blockers will reduce the repetitive neuronal firing associated with epilepsy.

Carrier-mediated mechanisms

A wide range of both ions and molecules such as glucose are transferred across cell membranes by carrier-mediated mechanisms. These transmembrane proteins have specific binding sites for one or more solutes and when these binding sites are all occupied, the carrier protein changes shape (called a conformational change) depositing the solutes on the other side of the membrane. The rate at which carrier mechanisms function is determined partly by the number of transporters available but also by the number of molecules each carrier protein can bind. However, a generalisation is that the number of ions which can cross a membrane in a given time via an ion channel is greater than can be moved by a carrier protein. Typical transport rates for a single carrier molecule are about 100 to 1000 molecules a second although it can be up 10 000 molecules a second. Some K$^+$ ion channels permit 10 million ions to cross a cell membrane per second.

Some of the jargon which is used to describe carrier proteins is as follows. A carrier which is only concerned with the movement of a single ion or molecule is called a **uniport mechanism**. When two ions or molecules are transported in the same direction, this is a **symport mechanism**, and when two ions or molecules are transported in opposite directions, this is called an **antiport mechanism**.

In a large number of cases, the drive to make a symport mechanism function is provided by the normal sodium gradient across a cell membrane. The extracellular [Na$^+$] is approximately 140 mmoles/L whilst intracellular [Na$^+$] is of the order of 10–20 mmoles/L. There is, therefore, a substantial diffusive gradient which would tend to move Na$^+$ into a cell. In addition, there is a net negative charge inside cells which will tend to attract in positively charged Na$^+$ ions (*see* page 102). This concentration and electrical gradient tending to move Na$^+$ into cells can be used to drive a symport mechanism and therefore to transport another chemical species, such as glucose, into a cell (*see* Figure 4.3).

Na$^+$-glucose co-transporter mechanisms exist in tissues such as the gut for the absorption of glucose and in the kidney tubule for the reabsorption of filtered glucose. The fact that the number of Na$^+$-glucose carrier proteins in the nephron is limited is the basis for the development of glycosuria when plasma [glucose] rises.

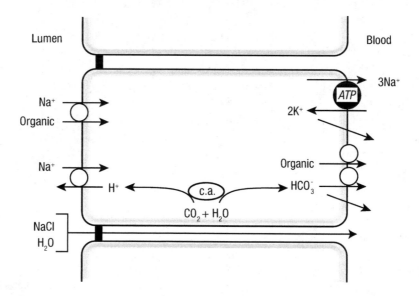

FIGURE 4.3 Sodium gradient driven movement of substances into a cell

The 'sodium/organic' symport mechanism on the lumen side of this model of a cell in the proximal tubule of the nephron drives entry of, for example, glucose or amino acids into the cell. The Na$^+$/H$^+$ antiport mechanism is involved in the reabsorption of filtered bicarbonate ions (*see* section in this chapter called 'Acid-base balance'). Expulsion of Na$^+$ into the blood at the basolateral side of the cell is against a concentration gradient and needs energy in the form of ATP.

Source: Field M, Pollack C, Harris D. *The Renal System*. Elsevier Health Sciences; 2001.

When the carrier mechanism for glucose in the proximal tubule of the nephron is saturated, not all of the filtered glucose can be reabsorbed and the remainder must appear in the urine (*see* page 149).

The functioning of co-transport mechanisms as described so far does not have any involvement of ATP as an energy source. If leakage of Na^+ into cells or transport of Na^+ into cells on carrier proteins were to proceed unopposed, then intracellular $[Na^+]$ would rise and the $[Na^+]$ gradient across the cell membrane would be dissipated. Co-transport processes would cease to work and it is essential, therefore, to have a mechanism for actively expelling Na^+ from the cells. A rise in intracellular $[Na^+]$ would also have an effect on membrane potentials (*see* page 102).

The sodium pump is illustrated in Figure 4.4.

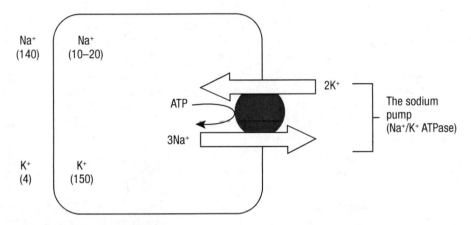

FIGURE 4.4 The sodium pump

Entry of Na^+ and efflux of K^+ from the cell both occur down a concentration gradient and are passive processes. The sodium pump (Na^+/K^+ ATPase) on the right-hand side of the diagram is an active, ATP-consuming process working against the concentration gradients for both ions.

Source: Noble A *et al.*, op. cit.

This active transport mechanism expels Na^+ from the cell against a concentration gradient and in this counter-transport (antiport) mechanism, K^+ is also moved against its concentration gradient into the cells. This is driven by the hydrolysis of ATP. For each ATP molecule consumed, three Na^+ are expelled and two K^+ are pumped into the cell.

The imbalance in the numbers of Na^+ and K^+ ions moved is important in maintaining the intracellular fluid volume of cells. As there is a tendency for Na^+ to move into cells down their concentration and electrical gradients, this will tend to provide an osmotic gradient by which water will move into cells. Cell swelling is therefore a characteristic of hypoxic tissues which have an inadequate ATP synthesis capacity. The cell swelling is accompanied by loss of normal cellular function.

The overall energy cost of keeping the sodium pump (Na^+/K^+ ATPase) functioning is enormous. Although textbook diagrams frequently show a single sodium pump mechanism in a cell membrane, the true situation is more complex. For some cells there may be about a million sodium pump molecules, each operating at a frequency of about 30 times a second. A molecule of ATP is hydrolysed every time the pump operates and so keeping the sodium pumps running accounts for of the order of 30% of our lifetime energy intake.

Pump mechanisms can be selectively inhibited by drugs. A well-known example of this is the cardiac glycoside drug digitalis, an inhibitor of the sodium pump.

Endocytosis and exocytosis

Uptake of material into the cell from the extracellular fluid (*endocytosis*) and release of chemicals from the cell (*exocytosis*), both involve the formation of intracellular vesicles. The wall structure for these vesicles is the same as the plasma membrane of a cell.

Endocytosis involves the development of an invagination of the plasma membrane which eventually separates into the cytosol of the cell as a complete sphere. In its simplest form, the vesicle contains only a small volume of the extracellular fluid and this process is called *pinocytosis*. There are more sophisticated versions of this basic process. Binding of chemicals to a specific membrane receptor may be followed by the formation of an intracellular vesicle, a process known as receptor-mediated endocytosis. An example of this is the mechanism by which protein-cholesterol complexes (low-density lipoproteins) are absorbed into cells.

Phagocytosis is a special form of endocytosis. Cells which perform this function (neutrophils and macrophages) are called phagocytes. This process results in larger particles, such as bacteria and cell debris, entering into cells. The vesicle produced in this way, called a *phagosome*, can then fuse with a lysosome in the cell. Lysosomes contain a number of enzymes which can promote the digestion of the foreign material. This process is also important in scavenging the body's dead and dying cells so that their contents may be recycled. As an example of this, the average lifespan of a red blood cell in an adult is 120 days and therefore approaching 1% of all red cells are turned over each day. In the neonate, the lifespan of red blood cells is shorter – probably about 60–80 days – and the process of the replacement of fetal red cells is occurring; this contributes to an increased formation of bilirubin from the metabolism of haem resulting in jaundice in many neonates. Phagocytic mechanisms also contribute to bodily defence mechanisms by engulfing bacteria.

Exocytosis is a process whereby products such as digestive enzymes, hormones and neurotransmitters, which are synthesised inside a cell, are exported out of the cell. Some of these secretory mechanisms occur continuously in a relatively unregulated fashion. This is referred to as a *constitutive pathway*. Vesicles fuse spontaneously with the plasma membrane and release their contents. The alternative scenario, a *regulated pathway*, means that the vesicle contents are only released following the arrival of a neural or hormonal signal. Examples of this type of mechanism are the release of pancreatic enzymes into the pancreatic ducts following stimulation by cholecystokinin (CCK) or the release of a neurotransmitter such as acetylcholine (ACh) in the parasympathetic nervous system (*see* page 110).

In all cases, the composition of the vesicle membrane is the same as that of the plasma membrane of the cell. When the vesicles fuse with the membrane and disgorge their contents, the vesicle membrane is incorporated into the plasma membrane. There is therefore a continuous trafficking of membrane segments between the plasma membrane and internal structures in the cell by the processes of endocytosis and exocytosis.

MEMBRANE POTENTIALS
Movement of ions across cell membranes takes place through ion channels (*see* page 96). There are two possible driving forces for such movement.
- *Diffusive gradient*, where ions move down their concentration gradient (*see* page 95).
- *Electrical gradient* produced by the existence of a charge imbalance (electrical potential) across the cell plasma membrane.

The fundamental mechanisms involved with the generation of an electrical gradient recall the simple experiments which can be carried out with two bar magnets. These lead to the conclusion that like charges repel, unlike charges attract. The mechanisms leading to the generation of a membrane potential can be understood by considering the concept of equilibrium potentials. These are purely theoretical concepts which involve imaginary cells and the effects of imbalances in the distribution of cations inside and outside cells. The major cations to consider are sodium ions (Na^+) and potassium ions (K^+) but similar principles could be applied to other cations, such as calcium (Ca^{++}) or magnesium (Mg^{++}) and to the anion chloride (Cl^-).

Potassium equilibrium potential
A typical intracellular $[K^+]$ is 150 mmoles/L and extracellular $[K^+]$ is about 4 mmoles/L. We will consider a theoretical cell with this concentration gradient and initially no charge imbalance; that is, an equal number of positive and negative charges inside the cell.

If this theoretical cell becomes permeable only to K^+ ions, they will move out of the cell down a concentration gradient leaving the inside of the cell with a net negative charge. These negative charges are largely carried by proteins and by phosphate groups which are too big to follow the exodus of K^+ ions from the cell. The increasingly negatively charged environment inside the cell caused by the outward K^+ movement will attract K^+ ions back into the cell down an 'electrical gradient'.

At equilibrium, the tendency for K^+ to leave the cell down a concentration gradient will be balanced by the tendency to pull K^+ into the cell down an electrical gradient. The charge imbalance at this situation is called the 'potassium equilibrium potential'. It is measured in units of millivolts (mV), is abbreviated to E_K, and can be calculated by putting the intracellular and extracellular $[K^+]$ into the Nernst equation. The logic behind the derivation of the Nernst equation is simply that, at equilibrium, the diffusion gradient for an ion equals the electrical gradient generated by the diffusion of the ion.

For physiological concentrations of K^+ inside and outside cells, and assuming a temperature of 37 °C, a typical value for the E_K is −90 mV. Note, the convention is that if the inside of a cell carries a net negative charge, then the membrane potential is regarded as negative.

Sodium equilibrium potential

Typical extracellular [Na$^+$] is about 140 mmoles/L and intracellular [Na$^+$] is 10–20 mmoles/L. In another theoretical cell, starting again with an equal number of positive and negative charges inside the cell, which becomes permeable this time just to Na$^+$, the sodium ions would tend to move into the cell down their concentration gradient. This would generate a net excess of positive charges inside the cell. This positive charge would tend to repel Na$^+$ ions back out of the cell down an 'electro-chemical gradient'.

At equilibrium, the tendency for Na$^+$ to diffuse into the cell down its diffusive (concentration) gradient will be just matched by the movement of Na$^+$ out of the cell down an electrochemical gradient. The charge imbalance at this time is known as the 'sodium equilibrium potential' which is abbreviated to E$_{Na}$.

Given the usual concentrations of Na$^+$ inside and outside a cell, a typical value for E$_{Na}$ is +60 mV. Again, this figure can be calculated by inserting the figures for [Na$^+$] inside and outside the cell into the Nernst equation. The logic behind the Nernst equation is still the same: at equilibrium the diffusion of Na$^+$ into the cell is equal to the movement of Na$^+$ out of the cell down an electrical gradient.

Resting potential of a cell

Initially, we will consider the situation which exists in excitable tissues such as nerves and muscles. The membranes of these cells are very permeable to K$^+$ ions and also, to a much lesser extent, permeable to Na$^+$ ions. The difference in permeability to the two ions is about twentyfold to fortyfold.

A typical value for a nerve cell resting potential is –70 mV. This is relatively close to E$_K$ at –90 mV. If the cell at rest was only permeable to K$^+$, then the resting potential would be –90 mV. However, the resting nerve or muscle cell is a little permeable to Na$^+$ as well. In this circumstance, there is a tendency for Na$^+$ ions to enter the resting cell, moving down both a concentration gradient for Na$^+$ and also an electrical gradient with the negative charge on the inside of the cell generated primarily by the [K$^+$] gradient. Limited entry of Na$^+$ ions will have the effect of reducing E$_K$ (–90 mV) to the typical resting potential value of –70 mV. The ionic gradients which determine the resting potential are maintained by the activity of the sodium pump (*see* page 99).

Cells which do not have the differential permeability to K$^+$ and Na$^+$ ions which characterises nerve and muscle cells will not have a resting potential of –70 mV. A cell which is equally permeable to K$^+$ and Na$^+$ ions but which has the same ionic gradients as other cells would have a resting membrane potential which is half way between E$_K$ (–90 mV) and E$_{Na}$ (+60 mV), i.e. –15 mV. Cells which behave in a similar way to this include adipose cells and red blood cells. These are described as non-excitable cells as they cannot generate action potentials.

Action potentials in nerve and muscle cells

A simple description of the events associated with nerve and muscle action potentials will first be described. This concept for nerve cells will be modified a little in order to explain some of the events described subsequently under the heading of 'Cell-to-cell communication mechanisms' (*see* page 109).

As described above, the resting potential of a nerve cell is determined by the ionic gradients for potassium and sodium ions (high [K$^+$] inside cells and low [K$^+$] outside cells; high [Na$^+$] outside cells and low [Na$^+$] inside cells) and by the relative permeability to the two ions at rest (high permeability to K$^+$ and low permeability to Na$^+$). If the resting cell membrane becomes a little more permeable to Na$^+$ (i.e. some more Na$^+$ ion channels open) then Na$^+$ ions will enter the cell down their concentration gradient and also down an electrical gradient because the inside of the cell has a net negative charge. This will result in the inside of the cell being less negatively charged; that is, the cell is said to have been partially depolarised.

What normally causes the initial opening of sodium ion channels is the effect of neurotransmitter chemicals released from other nerve cells and which bind to ligand-gated (receptor-operated) ion channel complexes (*see* page 97). If the number of Na$^+$ channels opened in response to neurotransmitter release is insufficient to raise the membrane potential from the resting potential (–70 mV) to a critical point, the threshold or trigger potential, which is about –55 mV, then the ion channels will close again and the membrane potential will return to the resting potential. This concept is further explored later in this chapter under the heading 'Cell-to-cell communication mechanisms' (*see* page 109).

If the membrane potential is reduced (depolarised) to a critical point (the trigger or threshold potential), then a population of voltage-gated ion channels will be opened and much more Na$^+$ will enter the cell, a faster depolarisation will occur and an '***action potential***' will be generated. This is illustrated in Figure 4.5.

The number of Na$^+$ ions entering a nerve cell during one action potential is quite impressive, about 40 million. However, this large number is small compared with the total number of Na$^+$ ions inside a cell, about 200 000 million. The change in [Na$^+$] inside a nerve cell during one action potential is therefore small, only about 0.02%. The important fundamental concept here is that effectively the [Na$^+$] inside a nerve cell does not change during a single action potential.

Eventually, as a result of the entry of Na$^+$ into nerve cells during an action potential, the membrane potential reaches a positive value of between +10 mV and +40 mV. At this point, the voltage-gated Na$^+$ channels close (*see* page 97) and the cell is in a state where it is effectively only permeable to K$^+$ ions. The potassium (K$^+$) ions will move out of the cell down their concentration gradient but also, initially, they will be repelled out of the cell because the inside of the cell now carries a net positive charge. This is, of course, the result of the inward movement of Na$^+$ ions. Outward movement of K$^+$ will mean that the membrane potential will return towards the resting potential. This is called ***repolarisation***. The number of K$^+$ ions which will move out is the same as the number of Na$^+$ ions moving into the cell during depolarisation, i.e. about 40 million. As intracellular [K$^+$] is about ten times as great as intracellular [Na$^+$], the change in intracellular [K$^+$] during the repolarisation phase of one action potential is correspondingly even smaller – about 0.002%.

At the end of an action potential there is a delay before some of the sodium channels reopen. Therefore, the membrane potential temporarily moves even closer to E_K. This is called the ***hyperpolarisation phase*** of the action potential (*see* Figure 4.5). With the reopening of some of the sodium channels the resting potential is re-established. All of these events in an action potential take place in only 1–2 milliseconds.

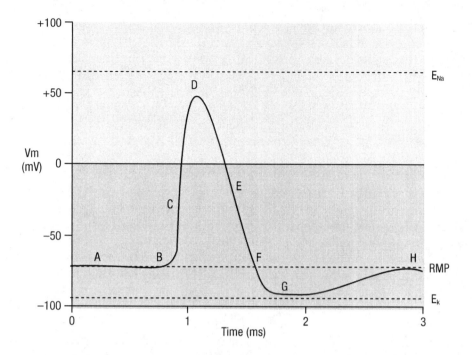

FIGURE 4.5 A typical nerve action potential

Resting membrane potential (RMP) is shown as a dashed line. At position B, Na⁺ channels open, and during phase C there is entry of Na⁺ ions into the cell. At D, the Na⁺ channels close and in phase E efflux of K⁺ from the cell is the key event. At G, the cell is hyperpolarised and the membrane potential gradually returns to the resting potential level at position H. The period B to F is the absolute refractory period during which the cell cannot produce a further action potential. During the relative refractory period (F to H), stimulation above threshold intensity levels is needed to generate an action potential.

Source: Michael-Titus A, Revest P, Shortland P. *The Nervous System*. Elsevier Health Sciences; 2007.

After one action potential, the nerve cell contains about 40 million more Na⁺ ions and about 40 million fewer K⁺ ions. This situation is corrected by the activity of the sodium pump (*see* page 99). As the relative changes in [Na⁺] and [K⁺] inside the cell during one action potential are quite small, a nerve or muscle can function for some time even if the sodium pump is not fully operational. This is illustrated by the effect of sitting cross-legged on the floor, which sometimes results in a 'dead-leg'. What happens is that the blood supply into the leg is compressed and hence oxygen delivery to make ATP is reduced. The sodium pump is unable to expel all the Na⁺ and put the K⁺ ions back into the nerve cell and so the resting ionic gradients run down. The resting potential rises and the cells eventually become unable to generate further action potentials. The problem is getting the membrane potential back to a sufficiently negative level so that the voltage-gated sodium pumps can reopen. These ion channels, of course, have closed at the top of the action potential. When the owner of the 'dead-leg' suddenly realises and moves, the blood flow is re-established,

ATP is generated and the ionic gradients returned to normal along with the resting membrane potential. All of these events only take a few seconds.

Transmission of action potentials (nerve impulses) is dealt with below.

CELL-TO-CELL COMMUNICATION MECHANISMS

The textbook 70 kg person consists of approximately 10^{14} cells, i.e. 100 million million cells. Although neonates are clearly going to have proportionately fewer cells, this is still going to be a very large number. The fundamental mechanisms by which these cells communicate with each other are the same in adults and in neonates. These can be summarised as:

- gap junctions
- paracrine communication
- endocrine communication
- nervous communication.

Of these possibilities, gap junctions bear some resemblance to large ion channels (*see* page 96). The other three types have a common factor in that they are all receptor-mediated events. General concepts regarding gap junctions and receptor-mediated events will be dealt with before returning to the specifics of paracrine, endocrine and nervous communication.

Gap junctions

Gap junctions provide a low-resistance form of electrical and chemical communication between adjacent cells and are particularly important in sheets of tissue which contract as a single entity, such as the heart. They are made of protein with a water-filled hole down the middle and to this extent they have similarities to ion channels. However, gap junctions provide a route for communication between two cells and are much bigger than ion channels. Molecules up to a relative molecular mass (molecular weight) of 1000 Da can pass through. The protein complex traversing the plasma membrane of one cell is called a **connexon** and when connexons in the walls of two adjacent cells are aligned, this forms a gap junction between the cells.

Connexons close if the intracellular $[Ca^{++}]$ rises. An example of when this happens is in cell death. Gap junctions exist in most tissues in the body with the exception of red blood cells and skeletal muscle cells. Because gap junctions allow the spread of a wave of 'electrical' activity through a sheet of tissue, they are sometimes referred to as '*electrical synapses*'.

Receptor-mediated events

A simple definition of a receptor is as follows:

> A receptor is a protein which specifically binds a chemical messenger and, as a result, produces a response within a cell.

Note that this definition does not make any stipulation about the location of these receptors. Although receptors for peptide hormones and neurotransmitters are mainly located on the outside (plasma) membrane of cells, those chemical messengers which can cross membranes because they are lipid-soluble have receptors which are intracellularly located. Examples of the latter category are steroid hormones, vitamin D, thyroid hormones and nitric oxide.

There are four classes of plasma membrane receptor:

▶ ligand-gated ion channels
▶ integrins linked to the cytoskeleton
▶ receptor-enzyme complexes
▶ G-protein coupled receptors.

These four types of receptor are now described in more detail.

Ligand-gated ion channels

In this case the chemical messenger (ligand) binds to a portion of the ion-channel protein. This results in either an opening or closing of the ion channel. An important example of this type of receptor is the 'nicotinic-type' receptor for the neurotransmitter acetylcholine (ACh). The term 'nicotinic-type' refers to the fact that the actions of ACh can be mimicked by the drug nicotine at this receptor. Nicotinic-type ACh receptors occur at the neuromuscular junction, the site of linkage between a motor nerve and a skeletal muscle. Nicotinic receptors also exist in the ganglia which form part of the chain of neurons in both the sympathetic and parasympathetic nervous systems (*see* page 117).

Integrins linked to the cytoskeleton

These are transmembrane receptors which link the extracellular matrix to events inside the cell. They are often referred to as **cell-adhesion molecules**. Integrin-linked receptors couple conformational changes in the matrix to, for example, events associated with blood clotting and to aspects of the immune response to produce cellular responses.

Receptor-enzyme complexes

A hormone-binding site on the outside of a cell is coupled to an enzyme complex on the inside of the cell. This is how, for example, some of the actions of insulin are mediated via an intracellular tyrosine kinase enzyme.

G-protein coupled receptors

This group of receptors is particularly important not only because of the physiological actions of the hormones that the receptors facilitate, but also because they are the target site for some common drugs.

The receptor in the plasma membrane is a protein which passes through the membrane seven times. It is therefore called a **seven transmembrane domain receptor**. The term **serpentine receptor** is also sometimes used. The binding site for the hormone is on the outside of the cell and on the inside the receptor protein is coupled to a **GTP binding protein**, also known as a 'G-protein' (*see* Figure 4.6).

Binding of a hormone on the outside of the cell results in activation of the G-protein and this, in turn, activates an enzyme to produce a '**second messenger**'. This concept means that a specific chemical is produced which triggers further reactions in

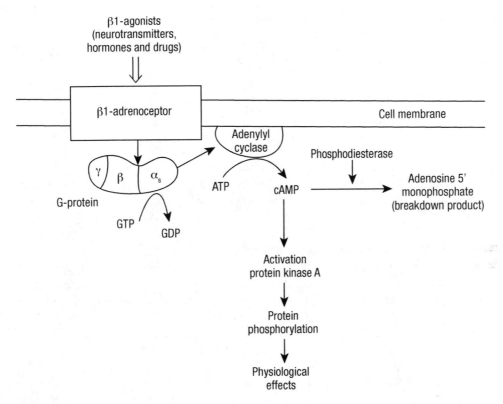

FIGURE 4.6 Example of a G-protein-coupled receptor, the effect of a β1-agonist on a β1-adrenoceptor

Source: Noble A *et al.*, op. cit.

the cell. Although the term 'first messenger' is never used, this would be equivalent to the hormone arriving at the cell – and the second messenger carries the information on and produces events inside the cell.

An example of a G-protein-coupled receptor is the β-adrenoceptor (*see* Figure 4.6) which mediates the response to hormones or drugs such as adrenaline (epinephrine). This hormone increases the force of cardiac muscle contraction (*see* page 131). The adrenaline binds to a seven-transmembrane domain receptor on the outside of the cell and, via a G-protein, activates the enzyme adenylyl cyclase. This enzyme is sometimes called adenyl cyclase or adenylate cyclase – all these names mean the same thing. The enzyme promotes the conversion of ATP to cyclic AMP, a second messenger. The cyclic AMP in turn activates a cascade of kinase enzymes which, via phosphorylation of proteins, eventually produces the increase in the force of cardiac contraction. The concentration of cyclic AMP in the cell is determined both by the rate of production but also by the action of the enzyme phosphodiesterase which promotes the breakdown of cyclic AMP.

The overall activity of this pathway can be manipulated pharmacologically in two key ways. Beta-adrenoceptor agonist drugs, such as adrenaline, isoprenaline, dobutamine and dopamine, can bind to the β-adrenoceptor and hence increase the activity of the whole pathway. This physiological effect can also be achieved by drugs such as caffeine, theophylline and milrinone which block phosphodiesterase, the enzyme which breaks down cyclic AMP. The effect of both these types of drug, the β-adrenoceptor agonists and the phosphodiesterase inhibitors, is therefore to increase the intracellular concentration of cyclic AMP.

The actions of the naturally occurring phosphodiesterase inhibitors theophylline and caffeine in tea and coffee and theobromine in chocolate are well known.

The 'inositol phosphate (phosphoinositide) pathway' is another important G-protein-coupled receptor mechanism. The second messengers produced in this case are inositol trisphosphate (IP_3) and diacyl glycerol (DAG). IP_3 promotes the release of calcium from intracellular stores and so increases the force of smooth muscle contraction (*see* page 120).

Intracellular receptors for steroid hormones

Steroids are lipids and hence can cross cell membranes. The receptor for these hormones is located either in the cytosol of the cell or on the nucleus. Activation of these receptors promotes gene transcription, and increases messenger RNA production and therefore increases specific protein synthesis. In the case of vitamin D, for example, some of the proteins synthesised are enzymes and calcium-binding proteins concerned with the absorption of calcium in the gastrointestinal tract.

Paracrine communication

This is an essentially local, short-distance communication mechanism between adjacent cell types. The paracrine hormone is released into the interstitial fluid surrounding the paracrine cell. It can then diffuse to affect nearby cells provided that they possess a receptor for the hormone. If we imagine a certain amount of hormone released at the centre of a sphere of cells, the concentration of hormone at the centre of the sphere will be high. However, as it diffuses outwards in all directions, the concentration of the hormone will progressively diminish until it is too low to generate a response from cells.

There are many examples of paracrine hormones. These include peptides which act as **growth factors**, such as platelet-derived growth factor (PDGF) and fibroblast growth factor (FGF). The endothelial cells which line blood vessels are an important source of paracrine hormones which affect the underlying smooth muscle layer to control the distribution of blood flow. These hormones include the peptide endothelin (vasoconstrictor), the prostaglandin prostacyclin (vasodilator) and nitric oxide (vasodilator). The paracrine effects of nitric oxide (NO) are mimicked clinically by the inclusion of NO in ventilator gases as part of the management strategy for neonatal pulmonary hypertension. Further mention of the physiological role of these paracrine hormones is included in Chapter 5, which is concerned with the cardiovascular system (*see* page 132).

Endocrine communication

The general characteristics of the endocrine system are that hormones are released into the interstitial fluid surrounding the endocrine cell and from there they leak into the circulatory system. It is a common misconception that endocrine hormones are secreted directly into the bloodstream. This is not quite correct.

Once in the circulatory system, an endocrine hormone can potentially be carried to any part of the body and can have an effect on any cell which carries an appropriate receptor. This is therefore a long-distance, often widespread but fairly slow, method of communication. Long-term, continuous regulation of aspects such as blood glucose concentration is accomplished.

Nervous communication

The mechanisms which determine the resting potential of a cell and the characteristics of action potentials have been dealt with earlier in this chapter under the heading 'Membrane potentials' (*see* page 102). We now consider the events leading to the triggering of action potentials and their subsequent transmission along nerve axons.

An individual nerve cell, particularly in the brain, may communicate with anything up to 150 000 other nerve cells via *synaptic connections*. Some aspects of synaptic function are dealt with below. Cell bodies of nerve cells have multiple projections called *dendrites*. Synaptic connections with other nerve cells occur mainly on the dendrites. The synaptic connections may be either excitatory (make the cell in question more likely to produce an action potential) or inhibitory (make the cell in question less likely to produce an action potential). Whether a synapse is excitatory or inhibitory is largely determined by the neurotransmitter and receptor type involved but the effects on the recipient postsynaptic cell will be as follows. An excitatory input, via release of neurotransmitter at a synapse, will lead to a small depolarisation of the cell called an *excitatory post-synaptic potential (EPSP)*. This takes the resting potential of the cell closer to the trigger (threshold) potential at which an action potential can be produced (*see* page 103). An inhibitory input via a synapse leads to a small hyperpolarisation of the cell and takes the resting potential further away from the trigger (threshold) potential; this is an *inhibitory post-synaptic potential (IPSP)*.

Thus, whether a nerve cell will generate an action potential often depends on the balance of inputs to the cell body from several other nerve cells, some of which are excitatory and some inhibitory. Only when the net effect of all these small changes in membrane potential takes the resting potential of a cell to the threshold will an action potential be produced. If an action potential does occur, it originates at the axon hillock, the join between the nerve cell body and the axon. The action potential at the axon hillock travels down the axon to cause release of neurotransmitter at a synapse onto another cell, either a nerve cell or another cell type such as skeletal muscle or a secretory cell. Nervous transmission can therefore be summarised under two headings:

▶ 'electrical transmission' down an axon
▶ 'chemical transmission' at a synapse.

'Electrical' transmission of action potentials

Nerve cells come in a range of sizes. Some cells in the brain are just a few micrometers in length whereas others are by far the biggest cells in the body. The cell body for nerves which supply the muscles in the big toe are in the lumbar region of the spinal cord and from there a motor axon projects down the leg and across the foot to the toe. In some adults, this means that nerve cells may be in excess of a metre long but even in neonates there are cells of the order of 20 cm long.

In a resting nerve cell, the inside of the cell has a net negative charge compared with the outside of the cell (*see* page 102). If an action potential is generated at the axon hillock, the inside of the cell at this point would acquire a net positive charge compared with outside the cell. Charged (positive) species inside the cell in the action potential region will be attracted towards the adjacent piece of resting nerve axon which still has a net negative charge. If the charge movement produced is sufficient to depolarise the resting piece of nerve as far as the threshold potential, then the voltage-gated sodium channels will open and an action potential will be produced. Thus, the action potential, or nerve impulse, has moved down the nerve and in turn the next segment of nerve axon will be activated in a similar way. The wave of depolarisation therefore spreads down the axon.

The speed of transmission of action potentials down a nerve varies hugely depending on the diameter of the nerve in question and on whether it is myelinated. The first generalisation is that large nerve fibres have a higher conduction velocity than do small nerves. Myelin is a phospholipid which wraps round some axons forming a sheath and it acts as an electrical insulation layer. Gaps in the myelin sheath, called **nodes of Ranvier**, mean that the process of transmission of nerve impulses, described above in a non-myelinated nerve, jumps from one node to the next. The local depolarisation events occur but an action potential can only be generated at the next non-insulated region, i.e. the next node of Ranvier. The second generalisation is that myelinated nerves conduct nerve impulses faster than do unmyelinated nerves. The physiological importance of myelination of nerve cells axon is sadly illustrated by the functional disorders which occur in auto-immune demyelinating diseases such as multiple sclerosis.

Conduction velocities in nerve cells vary from less than 0.1 m/sec in some small non-myelinated nerves to about 130 m/sec in some large myelinated nerves. The latter conduction velocity roughly equates to the speed of a Grand Prix racing car travelling flat out down the straight in a race. The use of the term 'electrical' transmission for nerves is not really appropriate. Electric current moves down a wire at a rate approaching the speed of light, approximately 186 000 miles (300 000 kilometres) per second.

'Chemical transmission' at a synapse

A synapse at the end of a nerve is a region where a chemical messenger (neurotransmitter) is released from a nerve ending into a gap (synaptic cleft) between the initial nerve ending and the tissue being supplied by the nerve. This might be another nerve but may be smooth or skeletal muscle, or a cell such as a secretory cell. The nerve cell before the synapse is referred to as the **pre-synaptic cell** and the cell after the synapse is the **post-synaptic cell**.

Neurotransmitters are synthesised in the nerve ending of the pre-synaptic cell and packaged into vesicles with the same wall structure as the plasma membrane of the cell. The best-known neurotransmitters are noradrenaline (norad) and acetylcholine (ACh). However, there are many other transmitters in specific areas of the body, especially in the brain. These include a group of amines, such as serotonin and dopamine; a group of amino acids, such as glutamate and glycine; and peptides, such as angiotensin II and vasoactive intestinal peptide (VIP). The latter group are among neurotransmitters that we think of as primarily serving other functions. Even ATP is a neurotransmitter in some circumstances. Sometimes a mixture containing more than one neurotransmitter may be released into a synapse. This is called a *co-transmission mechanism*.

The release of neurotransmitters into a synaptic cleft occurs by exocytosis (*see* page 100). When a wave of depolarisation (the action potential) spreads down a nerve it eventually reaches the nerve ending. Here a group of voltage-gated calcium channels open and Ca^{++} ions enter the nerve ending down their concentration gradient from the extracellular fluid. It is the rise in intracellular $[Ca^{++}]$ which triggers neurotransmitter exocytosis.

A considerable excess of neurotransmitter molecules is ejected into the synaptic cleft and only quite a small number actually hit a receptor on the post-synaptic cell and hence generate a physiological response. The remaining neurotransmitter molecules must be rapidly removed from the synaptic cleft as, otherwise, the tissue could not respond to a subsequent nerve stimulation. The methods available for neurotransmitter removal are:

▶ inactivation by enzymic breakdown, usually on the post-synaptic cell
▶ re-uptake into the pre-synaptic cell followed by re-packaging into transmitter vesicles ready for further release into the synaptic cleft. This is by far the most likely fate of the transmitter molecules in synapses in which noradrenaline is released.

The neurotransmitter which does reach a receptor on the post-synaptic cell may trigger an event in that cell usually either by opening ion-channel gates and thus altering the membrane potential or, sometimes, by interacting with a G-protein-coupled receptor (*see* page 106) leading to a cascade of intracellular protein phosphorylation events.

The process of synaptic transmission provides great potential for drug sites of action. These include the following.

▶ Drugs which modify the neurotransmitter synthesis pathway.
▶ Drugs which affect the release of neurotransmitter. This category includes drugs which bind to receptor sites on the pre-synaptic cell which are coupled to transmitter release mechanisms.
▶ Drugs which act as inhibitors of transmitter re-uptake mechanisms. The effect of such drugs is to increase the concentration of neurotransmitter in the synapse, thus increasing the effects of synaptic activation.
▶ Drugs which act as either agonists (mimic natural transmitter) or antagonists at the receptor on the post-synaptic cell.
▶ Drugs which block neurotransmitter inactivation enzymes on the post-synaptic cell. Again, these will potentiate the effects of synaptic activation.

Recent developments in our understanding of synaptic function include the recognition that NO is a neurotransmitter, but one which does not conform to the general pattern outlined above. It is not stored in vesicles and does not require entry of Ca^{++} ions to promote release which, for NO, can come from either the pre-synaptic or the post-synaptic cell. NO can therefore sometimes act as a retrograde transmitter – that is, from post-synaptic to pre-synaptic cell.

ACID-BASE BALANCE

Life is a battle against acidosis. Metabolic processes generate H^+ ions and these must be continually excreted so that an acceptable, slightly alkaline, pH is maintained in body fluids. Inability to achieve this leads to changes in the shape of proteins as a result of alterations in the charge distribution on proteins. The most critical proteins whose shape, and therefore function, must be maintained are probably ion channels in the heart. Activity of enzymes will also be affected. Failure to achieve adequate physiological control over H^+ ions therefore results in death. Some aspects of this opening paragraph on this topic need a little more explanation.

The range of normal pH in term infants (7.35 to 7.42), is very comparable to the widely quoted range for adults (7.35 to 7.45). In preterm infants, a slightly more acidic range (7.32 to 7.40) is acceptable. To put these figures into perspective, pH = 7.40 corresponds to $[H^+]$ = 40 nmoles/L (40×10^{-9} moles/L). A normal plasma $[Na^+]$ = 140 mmoles/L (140×10^{-3} moles/L). There are therefore 3.5 million Na^+ ions for every free H^+ ion in body fluids. However, it is relatively minor changes in $[H^+]$ which determine life and death. A minimum pH of 6.9, a level which could only be sustained for a limited period of time, is often quoted as a lethal level for adults. Neonates may be just a little more resilient to low pH, perhaps because of the relatively acidotic environment they have experienced *in utero*.

The definition of an acid is that it is a 'proton donor', i.e. something which generates extra H^+ ions in solution in water. Two types of acidic product are generated metabolically. Carbon dioxide (CO_2) is acidic because, when CO_2 dissolves in water, the following reaction takes place.

$$CO_2 + H_2O \leftrightarrow H_2CO_3 \leftrightarrow HCO_3^- + H^+$$

Failure to regulate CO_2 excretion adequately via the lungs leads to respiratory acidosis if excess CO_2 accumulates or to respiratory alkalosis if CO_2 depletion occurs.

The group of compounds which are generated metabolically also include acids such as lactic acid which accumulates in cases of tissue hypoxia; sulphuric acid from the oxidation of sulphur-containing amino acids (cysteine and methionine) in the diet, and products of metabolism such as the keto-acids generated in cases of poorly controlled diabetes. These acidic substances are excreted from the body via the kidneys. Alterations in these processes lead to metabolic acidosis or metabolic alkalosis.

Once acidic products of metabolism have been generated, the physiological problems can be grouped under two headings.

▸ Buffering of H^+ ions in order to minimise changes in blood pH during transport from site of production to site of excretion.

▸ Excretion of H^+ ions as CO_2 either via the lungs or via the kidneys.

Blood-buffering mechanisms

There are three main types of blood buffer:
) bicarbonate buffer
) protein buffers
) phosphate buffer.

The bicarbonate buffer mechanism is illustrated below.

$$CO_2 + H_2O \leftrightarrow H_2CO_3 \leftrightarrow H^+ + HCO_3^-$$

(Lungs) $\updownarrow$

$$NaHCO_3 \text{ (Kidneys)}$$

This is an important blood buffer for the following reasons.
) The concentrations of the main constituents can be regulated by the lungs (CO_2) and the kidneys (HCO_3^-).
) The concentrations of the constituents (CO_2 and HCO_3^-) are quite high and provide buffer capacity that is quantitatively effective.

Following addition of metabolic acid (H^+) to the bicarbonate buffer mixture, it binds to HCO_3^- and the bicarbonate buffer equation shown above is driven to the left. CO_2 is excreted via the lungs and the pCO_2 of blood is regulated by the respiratory system (*see* page 163). The bicarbonate that has been used up will be replaced by the kidneys.

Addition of more alkali in the form of hydroxyl ions (OH^-) to the bicarbonate buffer will drive the equation above to the right. Undissociated water molecules will be formed from H^+ ions and OH^- ions. The H^+ that has been used up will be replaced by the dissociation of more carbonic acid formed from extra CO_2 retention in the lungs.

The pH produced by the bicarbonate buffer mechanism is expressed by the Henderson-Hasselbalch equation.

$$pH = pKa + \log_{10} \frac{[HCO_3^-]}{[CO_2]}$$

pKa represents the pH at which the acid, in this case H_2CO_3, is 50% dissociated. It is a constant for any given buffer and for the bicarbonate buffer pKa = 6.1.

To illustrate how a physiological pH of 7.4 is obtained, the following figures are typical:

$$7.4 = 6.1 + \log_{10} \frac{[24]}{[1.2]}$$

In this case plasma $[HCO_3^-]$ = 24 mmoles/L.

The $[CO_2]$ is calculated from the pCO_2 and the solubility coefficient for CO_2 at 37 °C as follows:

$[CO_2] =$ $pCO_2 \times 0.223$ mmol/ L or $pCO_2 \times 0.03$ mmol/L
  (in kPa)   (in mmHg)
$[CO_2] =$ 5.3×0.223 mmol/ L or 40×0.03 mmol/L $= 1.2$ mmol/L

$[HCO_3^-]$ is regulated by the kidneys.

Note that it is the ratio of $\dfrac{[HCO_3^-]}{[CO_2]}$ which is important.

To achieve pH $= 7.4$

$$\log_{10} \frac{[HCO_3^-]}{[CO_2]} = 1.3$$

Thus $\dfrac{[HCO_3^-]}{[CO_2]} = 20$

As shown above, this is typically achieved with $[HCO_3^-] = 24$ mmol/L and $[CO_2] = 1.2$ mmol/L

If we imagine in a respiratory acidosis situation the pCO_2 of blood doubled to $pCO_2 = 10.6$ kPa or $pCO_2 = 80$ mmHg, in both cases, $[CO_2] = 2.4$ mmol/L.

If the kidney function altered so that the bicarbonate concentration also doubled, i.e.

$[HCO_3^-] = 48$ mmol/L, then the ratio $[HCO_3^-]/[CO_2] = 48/2.4 = 20$

the pH would therefore be 7.4 again. This is the basis for 'compensation'. In this case the kidneys are generating a metabolic alkalosis to compensate for a respiratory acidosis. The equivalent compensation for a respiratory alkalosis would be a renally generated metabolic acidosis.

Compensation also works the other way round. The response to a metabolic acidosis, for example diabetic keto-acidosis, would be hyperventilation to generate a compensatory respiratory alkalosis.

If, as a result of a compensatory change, the blood pH does not return all the way back to the normal range, then the primary change is said to be partially compensated; for example, a respiratory acidosis partially compensated by a metabolic alkalosis.

The Henderson-Hasselbalch equation is programmed into the software of acid-base analysis equipment. These machines can measure pH and pCO_2 using electrodes. The $[HCO_3^-]$ is therefore the only unknown in the equation and can be calculated. Acid-base machines do not directly measure $[HCO_3^-]$.

The amount of bicarbonate which would be required to replace the buffer base utilised by metabolic acids in an acid-base disorder is described as the 'base excess'. Thus, a normal base excess is in the range of −2 to +2 mmoles HCO_3^-/L. A metabolic alkalosis gives a positive base excess value and a metabolic acidosis gives a negative base excess value outside the normal range.

Protein buffering is quantitatively very important in blood and the protein in highest concentration is haemoglobin (Hb). In high-quality acid-base machines the [Hb] is measured as part of the full assessment of acid-base status. In lower-grade machines a normal [Hb] is assumed.

There are many side groups on proteins which can either absorb or give up H^+ as part of a buffering response.

Phosphate buffering relies on the following reaction – the conversion of the mono-hydrogen phosphate anion into the dihydrogen phosphate anion:

$$HPO_4^{2-} + H^+ \rightarrow H_2PO_4^-$$

The phosphate buffer is ineffective in blood because the plasma phosphate concentration is low, of the order of 1 mmol/L. This buffer system, however, becomes much more effective in urine because much of the filtered phosphate is retained in the kidney tubule whilst most of the filtered water is reabsorbed. The concentration of phosphate therefore rises steadily going down the nephron and it becomes an effective buffer.

Compensatory changes help to bring the blood pH back towards the normal range. The mechanisms involved in renal compensation for respiratory disorders are described in Chapter 6, on the renal system (*see* page 154). Correspondingly, the mechanisms which underlie the changes in respiratory function which compensate for primary metabolic acidosis or alkalosis are described under the heading 'Respiratory control mechanisms' in Chapter 7, on the respiratory system (*see* page 163)

In the interpretation of acid-base balance data, respiratory acidosis is shown by an increase in arterial pCO_2 and, correspondingly, respiratory alkalosis is shown by a decrease in pCO_2. Base excess value is negative for a metabolic acidosis and positive for a metabolic alkalosis.

Anion gap
Calculation of the anion gap (AG) can provide useful diagnostic information relating to the aetiology of a metabolic acidosis and also to the progress of treatment. The AG is the difference between the sum of the concentrations of the major cations in blood (sodium and potassium) and the major anions in blood (chloride and bicarbonate). That is:

$$AG = ([Na^+] + [K^+]) - ([Cl^-] + [HCO_3^-])$$

Inserting typical figures into this formula:

$$AG = (140 + 5) - (105 + 25) = 15\,mmol/L^*$$

---

* Note: Some authors omit potassium from the formula for calculating AG. The normal range for AG in this case is 4–5 mmol/L smaller.

On the basis of this simple formula, there are apparently more cations than anions in blood. A typical normal range for the AG is 10–18 mmol/L. In practice, there must be an equal number of positive and negative charges in blood so the AG represents the net amount of unmeasured anions and cations which are not included in the formula. Proteins at physiological pH carry a net negative charge. Albumin has the highest concentration of all the plasma proteins and this is the largest component of the unmeasured anions which make up the AG. It follows that what is accepted as a normal range for the AG must be adjusted downwards in the presence of hypoalbuminaemia. A host of other cations and anions, such as phosphate and sulphate, also contribute to the normal anion gap.

The concept of AG can be used to identify two groups of possible causes for a metabolic acidosis. In the first group the metabolic acidosis is accompanied by an increased anion gap. This is almost always due to an increase in the concentration of unmeasured anions. Examples of increased AG in these cases of metabolic acidosis include the accumulation of lactate anions in a lactic acidosis resulting from hypoxia or ischaemia, the formation of keto-acids such as β-hydroxybutyrate in a diabetic keto-acidosis and, in renal failure, a rise in phosphate and sulphate anions which are not being adequately excreted. In addition there are compounds which may be taken orally, such as aspirin, which provide an anion load and increase the AG. Finally, certain rare but important congenital metabolic disorders may lead to an AG because of enzyme defects which cause a build-up of acids which are not measured by routine electrolyte and blood-gas analysers. Examples of such disorders include abnormalities of the metabolism of: **amino acids** (e.g. methylmalonic aciduria, propionic acidaemia and maple syrup urine disease (MSUD); **fatty acids** (e.g. medium-chain Acyl-CoA dehydrogenase deficiency (MCADD)), and **carbohydrates** (e.g. glycogen storage disease) (*see also* Chapter 3).

'Normal anion gap acidosis'

However, there is a further group of metabolic acidosis patients with increased plasma [Cl⁻] ('hyperchloraemic metabolic acidosis') but a normal AG. This often occurs when there is increased loss of bicarbonate from the kidneys as the cause of the metabolic acidosis, such as occurs in proximal renal tubular acidosis ('type II renal tubular acidosis', including Fanconi syndrome), in which there is inadequate reabsorption of filtered bicarbonate in the proximal tubules. The reason that there is no AG is that the lost bicarbonate is replaced by an increase in reabsorbed chloride, leading to a raised plasma [Cl⁻] to maintain electroneutrality. Bicarbonate-losing states also occur as a result of gastrointestinal loss as diarrhoea, and failure of H⁺ excretion in the distal parts of the nephron ('type I renal tubular acidosis'). The latter mechanisms normally function such that every time an H⁺ ion is excreted into the urine, a bicarbonate ion is passed into the blood. The volume depletion associated with diarrhoea or diuresis activates renal retention of more Na⁺ and Cl⁻ via the renin-angiotensin system. Equal numbers of Na⁺ and Cl⁻ are reabsorbed in this way. Normal plasma [Na⁺] is about 140 mmol/L whereas normal plasma [Cl⁻] is only about 105 mmol/L. Retention of NaCl therefore leads to an increase in plasma [Cl⁻]. The extra Cl⁻ retained replaces the lost bicarbonate anion and so the AG is normal.

Stewart's 'strong ion theory'

A further perspective on these matters is to consider the 'strong ion difference' (SID). Strong ions are defined as those which are almost completely dissociated at physiological pH. The major strong cation in blood is Na^+ and the major strong anion is Cl^-. The other main 'strong' cations which can be measured include K^+, Ca^{++} and Mg^{++} while the main measured 'strong' anion is lactate. However, quantitatively it is Na^+ and Cl^- which are clinically important, the plasma concentrations of which are normally approximately 140 mmol/L and 105 mmol/L respectively. The relevant 'strong' ion difference in the normal state is, therefore, about 35 mmol/L.

Stewart's theory is based on the principle that, in order to maintain ionic electroneutrality, water will dissociate into its component ions if there is a change in ionic charge resulting from a change in concentration of strong ions:

$$H_2O \leftrightarrow H^+ + OH^-$$

So, as the **difference** between the concentrations of the 'strong ions' becomes less, there will be an increase of dissociation of water molecules, resulting in an increase in the concentration of hydrogen ions – i.e. an acidosis.

In clinical practice, it has been proposed that this may be an explanation for the acidosis which sometimes occurs in patients who are usually critically ill and who are receiving large amounts of intravenous fluids such as normal saline. Because the concentrations of Na^+ and Cl^- in normal saline are equal (153 mmol/L), there is no difference in ionic charge (or 'strong' ion difference). Therefore, if large volumes of normal saline are infused, the existing extracellular fluid, which had started perhaps with a 'strong' ion difference of 35 mmol/L (at least with respect to Na^+ and Cl^-), will be replaced by fluid which has no difference in ionic concentration. As a result, the 'strong' ion difference will become narrower, causing water to dissociate; this will result in an increased production of hydrogen ions and, therefore, an acidosis. There will be no AG, however, as there is no net increase in unmeasured anions. In this situation, it is not the chloride concentration which is driving the acidosis, but the difference between the sodium and chloride concentrations; indeed, the chloride concentration could be within the normal range.

AUTONOMIC NERVOUS SYSTEM

The autonomic nervous system (ANS) is part of the peripheral nervous system. Its functions are not under conscious control but they are regulated from the central nervous system (CNS). Many of the ANS functions involve regulation of smooth muscle but cardiac muscle and secretory tissues also come within the remit. Skeletal muscle contraction is not controlled by the ANS.

There are two major branches of the ANS:

‣ sympathetic nervous system (SNS)
‣ parasympathetic nervous system (PNS).

Various attempts have been made to define the difference between SNS and PNS on either a functional basis or a chemical basis. The functional definition, SNS speeds things up and PNS slows things down, applies to the heart but not to other organs such as the gastrointestinal tract. The chemical definition, sympathetic nerves release noradrenaline as a neurotransmitter and parasympathetic nerves release acetylcholine, also does not hold true throughout the body.

The only acceptable definition of SNS versus PNS has an anatomical basis. Sympathetic nerves emerge from the spinal cord in the segments between the first thoracic segment (T_1) and the second lumbar segment (L_2). The SNS is therefore 'thoracolumbar' in origin. The SNS nerves emerging from the spinal cord (pre-ganglionic nerves) are relatively short and form a synapse in a ganglion (a collection of synapses onto nerve cell bodies outside the central nervous system). The post-ganglionic nerves in the SNS are relatively long and run to the tissue being supplied.

Parasympathetic nerves emerge from the CNS in cranial segments III, VII, IX, and X and the sacral segments 2 to 4. The PNS is therefore described as 'craniosacral' in origin. The ganglia for the PNS are very close to, or even buried in, the tissue being supplied. Therefore, in contrast to the SNS, the pre-ganglionic nerves are relatively long and the post-ganglionic nerves are short.

Both branches of the ANS have both sensory functions (afferent nerves carrying information towards the CNS) and motor functions (efferent nerves carrying information away from the CNS towards tissues). Although the motor functions of the ANS receive most attention, for example regulating heart rate or controlling gastric acid excretion, the sensory nerves in the vagus trunk outnumber the motor nerves by about 10 to 1. This sensory function includes inputs to the CNS from stretch receptors monitoring distension of hollow organs such as the heart, blood vessels, stomach, bladder and airways of the lung. In addition, the vagus carries information about blood gases (pO_2, pCO_2, pH) and body chemistry (blood glucose). This sensory information enters the CNS at the level of the medulla.

Processing of sensory information from the periphery and organisation of the appropriate ANS motor outflow is primarily a function of medullary centres and the hypothalamus. Initial processing takes place in the medulla and information is then fed up to the hypothalamus. One of the functions of the hypothalamus is that it is the location of 'set-point' information. Just as with a domestic central heating system, which has a thermostat on the wall at which the desired room temperature can be set, many physiological control mechanisms function to regulate around a 'normal' set-point value. These parameters include, for example, body temperature and arterial blood pressure control. Taking the example of blood pressure control, the sensory information arriving in, and processed by, the medulla is relayed to the hypothalamus where it is effectively compared with the set-point. A signal is then sent back to the medulla so that the appropriate ANS motor response can be organised to keep blood pressure constant. These responses are described in Chapter 5 under the heading 'The baroreceptor reflex' (see page 134). When appropriate, these blood pressure control systems can be overridden to permit acute changes. Thus, acute increases in arterial blood pressure can occur in response to stress situations. These functions are organised by part of the limbic system of the brain. Blood pressure will return to normal when the cause of the stress disappears.

Autonomic control mechanisms become functional in the fetus for the regulation of parameters such as arterial blood pressure and heart rate changes in response to hypoxaemia or hypoglycaemia. However, it is at the time of birth that new demands are made on the ANS. Temperature regulation for the fetus is provided by the uterine environment but adaptive temperature control responses must become active at birth. Nutrition is provided directly and continuously via the placenta but functional parasympathetic control of gastrointestinal function is required in the neonate. Hunger, satiety and thirst centres in the hypothalamus must be involved to elicit appropriate feeding responses in the neonate.

The neurotransmitters mediating autonomic responses are not only of major physiological interest, they are also of practical therapeutic importance. At the ganglia for both SNS and PNS, the transmitter is acetylcholine (ACh) released on to nicotinic N_1-type receptors. Ganglion-blocking drugs, which do not have current clinical uses, therefore block the action of both branches of the ANS. Nicotinic N_2-type receptors are found at the neuromuscular junction in skeletal muscle. In both N_1 and N_2 receptors, the actions of the natural transmitter ACh can be mimicked by the plant compound nicotine and this is the origin of the name given to the receptors.

ACh is also the neurotransmitter released from post-ganglionic parasympathetic nerves but this time onto muscarinic-type receptors at which the actions of ACh can be mimicked by the fungal drug muscarine. Muscarinic antagonists, such as atropine, have important clinical uses.

For the SNS, the major neurotransmitter from the post-ganglionic nerve fibres is a mixture of mainly noradrenaline (norepinephrine) and some adrenaline (epinephrine), two catecholamines, although there are minor situations where other transmitters including ACh and peptides are used. The receptor types for catecholamines were classified as α and β subtypes in 1948 by the Swedish pharmacologist Ahlquist. Simply, at α-receptors, noradrenaline (norepinephrine) has a more potent effect than isoprenaline (isoproterenol). At β-receptors, the reverse classification is true. More recently, following the development of receptor antagonist drugs, sub-classifications of both α-receptors (α_1 and α_2) and β-receptors (β_1, β_2, β_3) have been established. Agonist drugs, such as dobutamine and dopamine, which mimic the effects of β_1-adrenoceptor stimulation by the naturally occurring catecholamines adrenaline and noradrenaline, have important clinical uses, particularly in the treatment of heart failure. Antagonist drugs for β-adrenoceptors such as propranolol, are important therapeutic agents in, for example, hypertension management. The effects of drugs such as adrenaline which stimulate α_1-adrenoceptors on vascular smooth muscle are important in raising arterial blood pressure in cardiovascular shock. Alpha-adrenoceptor antagonists (prazosin, doxazosin) have a limited use as antihypertensive agents.

Smooth muscle

Smooth muscle is found in the walls of hollow structures in the body. Many of the physiological functions mediated by the autonomic ANS involve control of smooth muscle. These include the regulation of blood flow distribution and blood pressure, bronchoconstriction and bronchodilation, gut motility and bladder emptying.

There are three broad types of muscle in the body:

▶ skeletal muscle
▶ cardiac muscle
▶ smooth muscle.

The contractile proteins, actin and myosin, are similar in all three types of muscle although the contractile mechanism (and its control) is different in smooth muscle compared with that in the other two types. Skeletal and cardiac muscle are both striated forms of muscle. This means that the microscopic appearance of the muscle has a regular pattern of stripes produced by the arrangement of the contractile proteins. Smooth muscle is not striated because the same regular arrangement of actin and myosin does not exist.

An increase in intracellular $[Ca^{++}]$ is essential to trigger contraction of all three types of muscle but the source of the Ca^{++} ions differs. In skeletal muscle, the Ca^{++} is released from intracellular stores, the sarcoplasmic reticulum, and returned to the intracellular stores during muscle relaxation. The calcium-binding protein, which plays an integral part in skeletal and cardiac muscle contraction mechanisms, is troponin. Calcium-channel blocking drugs do not have any effect on skeletal muscle because none of the Ca^{++} needed for the contractile process enters the cell through ion channels in the plasma membrane.

In cardiac muscle, entry of some of the calcium needed for contraction occurs through calcium channels. This initial rise in intracellular $[Ca^{++}]$ then triggers further release of Ca^{++} ions from intracellular stores. This is referred to as 'Ca^{++}-induced Ca^{++} release' (CICR) and it is the intracellular stores which are quantitatively most important in the overall rise in intracellular $[Ca^{++}]$. Cardiac muscle contraction is affected by appropriate calcium-channel blocking drugs. The contractile mechanism in cardiac muscle is essentially the same as in skeletal muscle. For further information about cardiac muscle contraction, see page 123.

In smooth muscle, much of the rise in intracellular $[Ca^{++}]$ needed to trigger contraction is provided by movement through calcium channels from the extracellular space. These calcium channels may be activated either as a result of smooth muscle depolarisation or following binding of a hormone or neurotransmitter to a receptor coupled to the calcium ion channel. CICR also occurs to further increase intracellular $[Ca^{++}]$. The calcium-binding protein, calmodulin, plays a key role in the activation of enzymes which promote myosin phosphorylation as a prelude to contraction of smooth muscle. This contractile mechanism is therefore markedly different from that in the other two types of muscle.

Calcium-channel blocking drugs reduce smooth muscle contraction and hence have a number of therapeutic roles, particularly in adult medicine. There are also some predictable smooth-muscle-mediated side effects, such as constipation.

REFERENCES

Abelow B. *Understanding Acid-Base.* Baltimore: Williams & Wilkins; 1998.

Marieb, E. *Essentials of Human Anatomy and Physiology.* 9th ed. San Francisco: Pearson; 2008.

Pocock G, Richards C. *Human Physiology.* 3rd ed. Oxford: Oxford University Press; 2006.

Tortora G, Derrickson B. *Principles of Anatomy and Physiology.* 12th ed. New York: Wiley; 2008.

Waller D, Renwick A, Hillier K. *Medical Pharmacology and Therapeutics.* 3rd ed. Edinburgh: Elsevier; 2009

CHAPTER 5

The cardiovascular system

Alan Noble

CONTENTS

ANATOMY OF THE FETAL AND NEONATAL CIRCULATIONS

Birth brings about a remarkable transition in the functioning of both the cardio-vascular and respiratory systems. There is a sudden change from the state where the respiratory, nutritive and excretory requirements of the fetus are provided by the placenta to a situation in the neonate where the lungs must suddenly become a viable gas exchange organ, and the circulatory system must support all the other characteristics of independent existence.

In the fetus, vascular resistance through the uninflated lung circuit is high. Pressure on the right side of the heart is greater than on the left and some of the blood which enters the right side of the heart is diverted through a hole in the atrial septum, the foramen ovale. The output from the right ventricle which does enter the pulmonary artery predominantly passes through a shunt, the ductus arteriosus, into the aorta and so again bypasses the lungs (*see* Figure 5.1). The distribution of the output from the left side of the heart includes a major low-resistance circuit, the placenta, and this contributes to the fact that pressure on the left side of the heart in the fetus is relatively low.

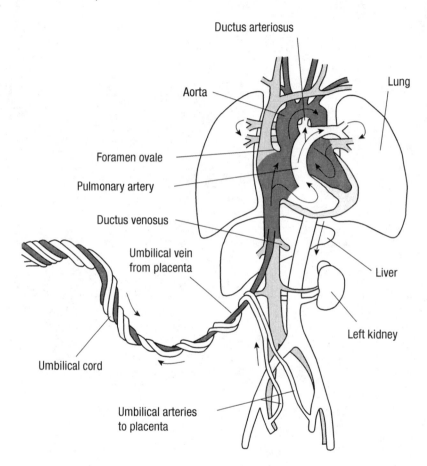

FIGURE 5.1 Fetal circulation

Source: Noble A, Johnson RA, Thomas A *et al*. *The Cardiovascular System*. Elsevier Health Sciences; 2005.

The lungs and their blood vessels expand at birth and this results in a fall in pulmonary vascular resistance. At the same time, the vascular resistance on the arterial side of the circulation is increased by clamping off the low-resistance placenta. The blood leaving the right side of the heart now preferentially flows through the lungs and returns to the left atrium. The atrial septal flap valve, the foramen ovale, closes once pressure in the left atrium exceeds that in the right atrium. This normally occurs within minutes of birth. Any residual flow through the foramen would not be from right to left, as in the fetus, but the altered pressure gradients would now dictate left-to-right flow.

The other short-circuit mechanism to bypass the lungs, the ductus arteriosus, connects the pulmonary artery with the aorta and in the fetus this is the route taken by about 90% of the blood entering the pulmonary artery. The fetus is in a relatively acidotic environment with a low pO_2. *In utero*, the ductus arteriosus remains patent because of the smooth muscle relaxant effect of locally synthesised prostaglandins. A rise in pH and pO_2, associated with the establishment of the lung function, inhibits the synthesis of prostaglandins and leads to smooth muscle contraction in the ductus arteriosus and hence to its closure. When necessary, this process can be speeded therapeutically by the use of the drug indomethacin, a prostaglandin synthesis inhibitor. Normally, the ductus arteriosus has closed within 24 hours of birth but in a significant proportion of neonates, a small left-to-right shunt through a partially patent ductus arteriosus may persist for days or even weeks. The effect of this is that some of the blood in the aorta does an extra circuit through the lungs.

CARDIAC MUSCLE

Some of the properties of cardiac muscle are described elsewhere (*see* page 120). The arrangement of the contractile proteins is shown in Figure 5.2.

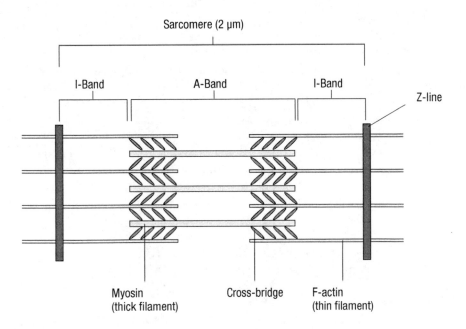

FIGURE 5.2 Arrangement of the actin (thin filament) and myosin (thick filament) fibres within the contractile unit of cardiac muscle, the sarcomere

Cross-bridges are formed between the myosin filament and the actin filament. This is the basis for contraction of skeletal and cardiac muscle.

Source: Noble A *et al.*, op. cit.

The contractile unit is the sarcomere. When stimulated, the actin filaments slide over the myosin filaments as a result of the breaking and reforming of cross-bridges between the filaments. The cross-bridges are formed from projections of the myosin filaments, the myosin head. This event is triggered by an increase in intracellular $[Ca^{++}]$ and involves the hydrolysis of an ATP molecule to alter the configuration of the myosin head. Cardiac muscle cells are repeatedly contracting and, as the ATP needed for contraction is derived aerobically from oxidative phosphorylation, the myocytes contain large numbers of mitochondria. Generation of ATP is actually limited by the contraction of the cardiac muscle because this crushes coronary blood vessels within the myocardium, particularly in the left side of the heart. This limits the delivery of the oxygen necessary for ATP synthesis in the cardiac muscle. In normal adults, this is frequently the predominant limiting factor on exercise performance. ATP is also needed for relaxation of cardiac muscle as the Ca^{++} must be pumped back into intracellular stores against a concentration gradient.

The neonatal myocardium undergoes important changes in the first month after birth. The myocytes become more cylindrical in shape and increase in number; i.e. they undergo hyperplasia. After the first month, the myocytes only increase in size – i.e. hypertrophy occurs, but hyperplasia ceases. This remains a characteristic of heart muscle for the rest of life. During cardiac muscle hypertrophy, extra sarcomeres can be added both in parallel and in series with existing sarcomeres. During the early neonatal period, there is an improvement in the ability of the cardiac muscle to contract and to generate force.

The term *compliance* refers to the ease with which a structure such as the heart or lungs can be inflated. It can be quantified as the change in volume of the structure per unit increase in pressure inside the structure. The compliance of the ventricles increases during the first few days after birth, probably due to alterations in the connective tissue in the heart wall. Compliance of the right ventricle increases more rapidly than in the left ventricle and this impacts on the mechanisms discussed below as preload effects on the heart.

Growth in the size of the myocardium in the neonatal period is not equal on the two sides of the heart. In the fetus the right side of the heart is the dominant pump. As the lungs are non-functional and are being bypassed via the foramen ovale and the ductus arteriosus, the right ventricle is the major pump for the systemic circulation. At birth, with the closure of the two bypass circulations, the right ventricle is now only perfusing the low-pressure pulmonary circulation and the left ventricle takes over the higher-pressure, higher-resistance systemic circulation. The size of the left ventricle myocardium therefore increases faster than that of the right ventricle.

CONTROL OF CARDIAC OUTPUT

The real driving force to propel blood round the body is actually arterial blood pressure. Although this is a function widely attributed to the heart, the major role of the heart is to top up the pressure in the aorta during systole, the ventricular contraction phase. The extra blood volume which enters the aorta during systole is accommodated by stretching the walls of the arteries. When the heart enters its refilling phase, diastole, the perfusion of tissues does not stop, it continues, driven by arterial blood pressure. This is maintained by the elastic recoil of the artery walls against the blood they contain. For this reason the arterial pulse pressure, the difference between systolic and diastolic pressures, provides an index of arterial wall stiffness. If arterial wall stiffness increases (compliance decreases), then the pulse pressure increases.

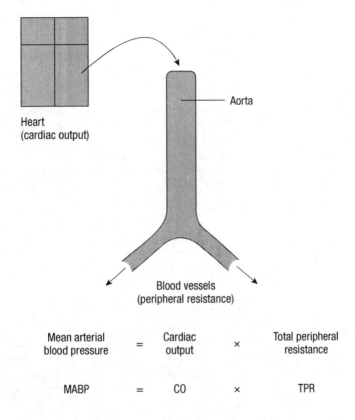

FIGURE 5.3 Simple model of the circulation to illustrate the factors determining arterial blood pressure

Source: Noble A *et al.*, op. cit.

Figure 5.3 shows a simple model of the circulation. Mean arterial blood pressure is determined by the product of the cardiac output and the peripheral resistance to flow. Mean arterial blood pressure is kept quite constant by the operation of the baroreceptor reflex. The baroreceptors are pressure-sensing devices and together with neural reflexes serve to adjust the cardiac output and peripheral resistance to keep mean arterial blood pressure constant on a moment-to-moment basis. The components of the baroreceptor reflex will now be dealt with individually, starting with the mechanisms which determine cardiac output.

Most of the general principles of circulatory control mechanisms in the neonate are broadly similar to those in the adult although there are quantitative differences which do not solely relate to body size. Even at rest, the neonate heart is functionally close to maximum performance and has little capacity to respond to an acute stress which might impose an increased workload on the heart.

Cardiac output = Heart rate × Stroke volume.

The factors determining cardiac output are as follows:
▶ heart rate regulation
▶ preload effects on the heart
▶ contractility effects on the heart
▶ afterload effects on the heart.

Preload, contractility and afterload are all parameters which determine the stroke volume of the heart.

Heart rate regulation

Cardiac excitation originates in the sino-atrial (SA) node in the right atrium of the heart, spreads through the atrial muscle to the atrioventricular (AV) node and then, after a short delay, progresses down the bundle of His to bring about depolarisation of the ventricular muscle (*see* Figure 5.4).

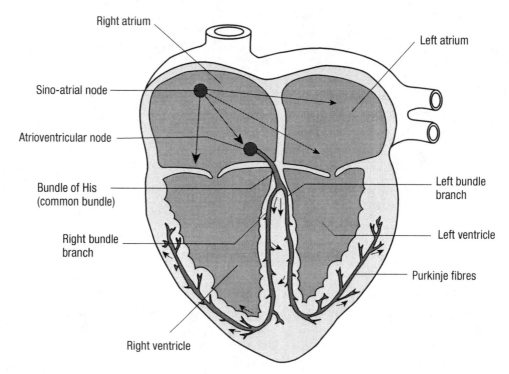

FIGURE 5.4 Conduction pathway in the normal heart

Excitation originates in the sino-atrial node, spreads through the atria and is then transmitted to the ventricles via the atrioventricular node. The bundle of His has right and left branches to carry the excitation to both ventricles

Source: Noble A *et al.*, op. cit.

This spread of depolarisation between the myocytes is aided by the widespread existence of gap junctions (*see* page 105) between the cells. As contraction of the heart is not dependent on stimulation by a nerve supply, this is called a myogenic mechanism. The individual parts of the heart muscle each have an intrinsic rhythm of their own but the rate of the intact heart is dominated by the part with the fastest intrinsic rhythm, the SA node. However, the sympathetic and parasympathetic nerves to the heart do modify heart rate.

The membrane potential at the SA node is illustrated in Figure 5.5.

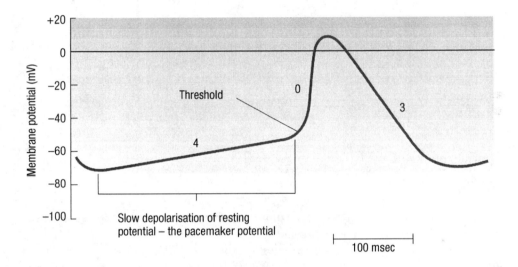

FIGURE 5.5 Sino-atrial node potential (pacemaker potential)

Increasing the slope of the slow depolarisation phase (phase 4) leads to earlier arrival at the threshold potential and therefore an increase in heart rate

Source: Noble A *et al.*, op. cit.

The resting potential (*see* page 102) in this pacemaker tissue is less negative than in other parts of the heart muscle because the cells are less permeable to K^+. A slow depolarisation occurs during the part labelled phase 4. The ionic mechanisms involved in this part of the action potential are complex but include a slow influx of Na^+ ions and Ca^{++} ions. When the threshold potential is reached, a population of calcium channels opens and the pacemaker cells depolarise (phase 0). Note that the involvement of Ca^{++} ions in the depolarisation is a different situation from the nerve action potentials (*see* page 103) and is also different from the ventricular muscle action potential shown in Figure 5.6.

In ventricular muscle, the depolarisation (the upsweep of the action potential: phase 0) is produced by an influx of Na^+ ions as in nerve action potentials. However, the ventricular muscle action potential is prolonged and lasts about 300 msec, compared to the 1–2 msec in a nerve (*see* page 104). The plateau phase (phase 2) is produced by an influx of Ca^{++} ions which triggers further release of Ca^{++} from intracellular stores (*see* page 120), resulting in contraction of the cardiac muscle.

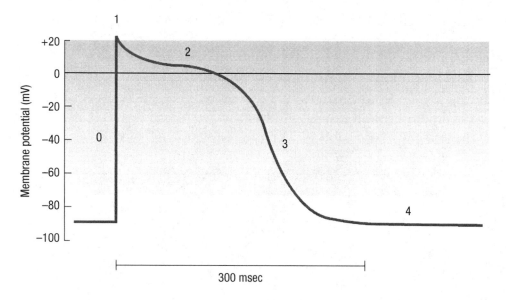

FIGURE 5.6 Ventricular muscle action potential

Source: Noble A *et al.*, op. cit.

Repolarisation of ventricular muscle (phase 3), as in nerves, is caused by an efflux of K^+ ions from the cells. These ionic events form the basis for the principles behind the actions of anti-dysrhythmic drugs. Different drug classes affect different components of the cardiac muscle action potential and hence provide an appropriate therapeutic response.

Aspects of the autonomic nervous system have been described previously (*see* page 117). The vagus nerve, cranial nerve X, slows the heart rate by releasing acetylcholine (ACh) onto muscarinic-type receptors on the SA node and AV node. The effect of vagus nerve stimulation is to slow the depolarisation shown as phase 4 on Figure 5.5. In addition, the muscarinic stimulation also results in hyperpolarisation of the SA node. As a consequence, the pacemaker potential takes longer to reach the threshold at which an action potential can be triggered. Heart rate is therefore slowed. This effect of ACh can be blocked by the drug atropine, a muscarinic antagonist, with a consequent increase in heart rate. This drug is used, for example, in the management of sinus bradycardia, a slow heart rate originating at the SA node.

The sympathetic nerves to the heart supply the SA node and AV node and also the cardiac muscle. The latter component can generate an increase in contractility of the heart (see below). Stimulation of the sympathetic nerve supply produces an increase in heart rate by release of noradrenaline (norepinephrine) on to β_1-adrenoceptors on the SA and AV nodes. These effects can be mimicked by agonists such as adrenaline and isoprenaline and can be blocked by β-adrenoceptor blocking drugs such as pro-pranolol. The effect on the pacemaker potential shown in Figure 5.5 is to increase the slope of phase 4 so that the threshold potential is reached more quickly and heart rate increases. The sympathetic nerve control of the newborn heart is not fully functional at birth and the production of noradrenaline is low during the first three weeks. Vagal control of heart rate is therefore dominant at this time.

The autonomic nervous system control of heart rate is mediated by the baroreceptor reflex (*see* below). Although general textbooks of physiology may quote values of 50–100 beats/min as a normal heart rate range in adults, this is not appropriate for children. A heart rate range of 100–160 might be more relevant for infants under 1 year old. Heart rate is relatively high in neonates and falls in the first 6 weeks after birth.

It has been suggested, partly on the basis of animal studies, that alterations in the autonomic control of the cardiovascular system may be abnormal in neonates who are small for gestational age. It has also been suggested that these abnormalities may persist throughout life and may be linked with adult disease patterns. There is strong epidemiological evidence of an inverse correlation between birth weight and subsequent increased risk of adult cardiovascular disease. This is known as the **Barker hypothesis**. Some studies which have tried to record altered autonomic function in neonates have failed to detect any changes.

Preload effects on the heart

The term *preload* refers to the net effect of a number of factors which determine the volume of blood contained in the ventricles of the heart at the end of diastole. If filling increases, then the cardiac muscle fibres are stretched and, within a limited physiological range, this leads to an increase in the force of ventricular muscle contraction. This is known as the **Frank-Starling law** of the heart.

The three major factors which influence ventricular filling are: first, blood volume; second, the rate at which blood returns to the heart from the periphery – the venous return; and third, the venous tone, which is the effect of the sympathetic nervous system maintaining the veins in a state of partial contraction. Two-thirds of the blood volume is contained in the veins and, without sympathetic venoconstriction, pooling of blood would occur in the lower part of the body, especially in an upright posture.

A simple explanation of the Frank-Starling law is that, after stretching the sarcomeres in the myocytes, it is possible to have a greater number of cross-bridges between the actin and myosin filaments (*see* Figure 5.2). This is possible because when the myocytes are not stretched, the actin filaments overlap and cross-bridges do not form in the overlap regions. The increased cross-bridge number means a greater force of contraction can be achieved. It is difficult, but not impossible, to measure muscle fibre length *in vivo*. However, under most circumstances the atrial pressure, the filling pressure of the ventricle, is an appropriate surrogate for end-diastolic volume or cardiac myocyte length. There are some specific circumstances, such as in the presence of atrioventricular valve stenosis, when atrial pressure is not appropriate to use.

In Figure 5.7, the two concepts of preload effects and contractility effects on the heart are illustrated. Considering either of the cardiac function curves shown on Figure 5.7, an increase in the end-diastolic volume (atrial pressure) means moving from left to right on the horizontal axis. This produces an increase in stroke volume of the heart (vertical axis). This is a change in response to altered preload on the heart. It is important to differentiate between the effects of changes in preload on

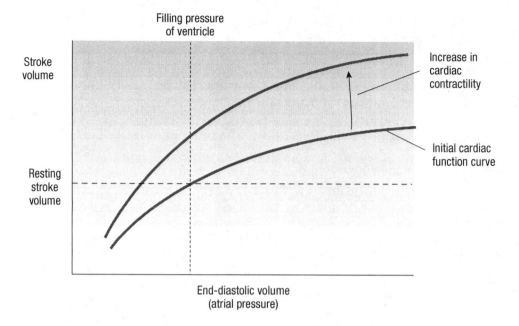

FIGURE 5.7 Cardiac function curves

Changes in preload on the heart are represented by changes from left to right on this diagram. Contractility changes are represented by upward or downward shifts in the position of the cardiac function curve

Source: Noble A *et al.*, op. cit.

the heart and contractility effects which are described below. This distinction is often poorly understood.

In neonates, the ventricles are less compliant than in older individuals. This means that the ventricles fill less easily. The Frank-Starling law does apply but the neonatal heart functions at the upper end of the range. In terms of the cardiac function curves shown in Figure 5.7, this means towards the plateau phase at the right-hand end of the curve. The neonatal heart operates at a higher filling pressure than adult hearts but has a relatively poor reserve capacity to increase stroke volume in response to alterations in preload. In neonates, as the right ventricle is more compliant than the left ventricle, adaptive responses of overall cardiac output are particularly determined by right ventricle function.

In mature individuals, the preload for the left ventricle is primarily the output of the right side of the heart. A failure of the left ventricle to respond adequately will lead to an increase in pressure through the pulmonary circuit. The consequent increase in preload on the left ventricle may result in a sufficient compensatory increase in left ventricular output. However, if this does not happen, the consequence may also be the development of pulmonary oedema.

The volume of the left ventricle increases at birth as the intraventricular pressure increases when the left ventricle assumes responsibility for perfusing the systemic circulation. This helps to provide an increase in cardiac output at birth via the Frank-Starling mechanism.

Contractility effects on the heart

It is possible to increase the stroke volume of the heart without increasing the end-diastolic volume or stretching the muscle fibres. An increase in 'contractility' leads to greater emptying of the ventricle during systole with a consequent reduction in end-systolic volume.

The effect of increasing contractility is shown graphically in Figure 5.7. The whole curve is displaced upwards and this means that at any given end-diastolic volume, illustrated by the vertical line labelled 'filling pressure of the ventricle', the stroke volume of the heart is increased. Physiologically, this can be achieved with an increase in intracellular $[Ca^{++}]$ produced by sympathetic nervous system stimulation and consequent activation of the β_1-adrenoceptor (*see* page 107) on the cardiac myocytes.

The increase in contractility produced by β-adrenoceptor stimulation can be mimicked by drugs such as dobutamine and dopamine which are described as positive inotropes. These drugs work through the production of cyclic AMP. Although such drugs are invaluable for short-term cardiac stimulation, they have been shown to have adverse effects in long-term use. Consequently, the drug digoxin which produces an increase in intracellular $[Ca^{++}]$ and a positive inotropic effect is still used for long-term administration. The mechanism of action is different; it does not lead to an increase in cyclic AMP as digoxin is a sodium pump (Na^+/K^+ ATPase) inhibitor. Digoxin was discovered in 1785 and was used for the treatment of congestive cardiac failure, then called the 'dropsy'.

There are many pathological mechanisms which can result in a decrease in cardiac contractility. These are often associated with intracellular acidosis. This may be a consequence of respiratory or metabolic acidosis or of hypoxia. The mechanisms by which acidosis reduces contractility are complex but the end result is decreased binding of Ca^{++} to troponin.

The initial increase in intracellular $[Ca^{++}]$ during cardiac muscle contraction results from opening of L-type Ca^{++} channels in the plasma membrane of the cell (*see* page 120). Blockers of these calcium ion channels, such as verapamil, therefore have a negative inotropic action on the heart.

Afterload effects on the heart

The aortic valve in the heart opens when the pressure in the left ventricle exceeds the pressure in the aorta. Ejection of blood from the ventricle will be opposed by any event which increases the resistance to outflow. This is called an ***afterload effect*** on the left ventricle. Afterload effects are often determined by aortic pressure but aortic valve stenosis will also impose an increased afterload on the left ventricle. Similarly, an increase in the afterload on the right ventricle will be produced by increased pulmonary artery pressure or pulmonary valve stenosis.

At birth, when the lungs start to function, the pulmonary vascular resistance suddenly decreases but, compared with the adult circulation, it still remains high for 6 to 8 weeks. The gradual reduction in pulmonary vascular resistance over this time is associated with remodelling of the smooth muscle layer in the pulmonary arterioles. The afterload on the left ventricle increases markedly at birth with the rise in arterial pressure.

THE PERIPHERAL CIRCULATION

The poor solubility of oxygen in water dictates the need for a very profuse circulatory system, about 60 000 miles (96 000 kilometres) of it in the textbook person (*see* page 96). There are two key roles that control mechanisms for the peripheral circulation must serve:

▶ Regulation of arterial blood pressure, the force which drives the perfusion of tissues of the body with blood.
▶ Providing an appropriate distribution of blood flow to all parts of the body in order to support the metabolic needs of tissues.

The key population of vessels for peripheral circulatory control are the arterioles. These vessels are located between the arteries and the capillary beds and they are often referred to as *resistance vessels*. This is because the arterioles constitute the greatest resistance to flow of any of the segments of the circulation. It also means that peripheral circulatory control is mediated by the control of arteriolar smooth muscle contraction. The arteriolar walls contain a significant amount of smooth muscle and, as with all blood vessels, they have a single layer of endothelial cells in contact with the blood. The contractile mechanisms for smooth muscle are discussed in Chapter 4, on page 120 . The factors influencing vascular smooth muscle contraction are as follows:

▶ endothelial factors
▶ local metabolites
▶ blood-borne hormones
▶ neural control mechanisms.

Endothelial factors

The endothelial layer produces a range of paracrine agents which alter the state of contraction of the underlying vascular smooth muscle.

Nitric oxide (NO)

NO is synthesised by NO synthase enzymes which use the amino acid L-arginine as a substrate. NO has a vasodilator action and it is produced continuously in blood-vessel walls. The main stimulus for production is the effect of shear stress on the endothelial cells, basically friction between flowing blood and the endothelium. If blood-flow velocity increases, this leads to more NO production and consequently vasodilation. This is a mechanism for adjusting the diameter of resistance blood vessels to fit the amount of blood flowing through them. NO production can also be stimulated by blood-borne agonists such as acetylcholine, bradykinin and thrombin. The use of NO in ventilator gas mixtures to induce smooth muscle relaxation as a part of the management protocols for neonatal pulmonary hypertension is well known.

There are, in fact, two forms of NO synthase enzyme. The vascular form described above is a constitutive enzyme because it is always present and continually producing NO. There is also an inducible form of the enzyme which is produced in cells exposed to chemical mediators, cytokines, produced as part of inflammatory responses. An example is in cases of septicaemic shock. Substantial amounts of NO are produced causing excessive vasodilation and a fall in arterial blood pressure.

Organic nitrates (nitrovasodilators) are drugs which may either spontaneously produce NO (e.g. sodium nitroprusside) or are enzymically degraded to produce NO (e.g. glyceryl trinitrate, isosorbide mononitrate or dinitrate). In addition to effects on the resistance vessels, these drugs also have effects on the capacitance vessels. These are the vessels which contain much of the blood volume, the veins. A major effect of nitrovasodilators is therefore to cause venous dilation and hence to reduce preload effects on the heart.

The endothelins

Endothelins are a group of peptides which were first discovered in 1988. They are produced by the endothelial cells and, in contrast to NO, are the most potent naturally occurring vasoconstrictor substances known. Endothelins are thought to play a role in normal blood pressure control and also to be involved in a range of cardiovascular and renal disease mechanisms.

The discovery of the endothelins provided an explanation for the way in which the Egyptian Queen Cleopatra died (in 30 BC). The venom of the Israeli burrowing asp, which bit Cleopatra, contains the peptide sarafatoxin which has the same effect as the endothelins. Coronary vasoconstriction was the probable cause of death.

Other vasoconstrictors produced by the endothelium include thromboxane A_2 and prostaglandin H_2. The endothelium therefore produces a cocktail of vasodilator and vasoconstrictor agents to contribute to local control of blood flow.

Local metabolites

Local metabolites enable the matching of blood flow to local metabolic conditions. The rationale for this is illustrated in Figure 5.8.

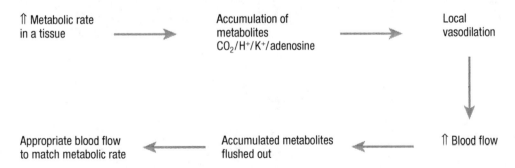

FIGURE 5.8 Pathway for metabolite regulation of peripheral blood flow

Source: Noble A *et al.*, op. cit.

A local increase in metabolic rate will lead to an accumulation of products such as H^+, CO_2, adenosine and lactic acid. These have a local relaxant effect on smooth muscle leading to a local increase in blood flow which flushes out the accumulated metabolites. The smooth muscle affected by metabolites is not just in the wall of arterioles but also, particularly, the precapillary sphincters. These are cuffs of smooth muscle at the entrance from the arterioles into capillary beds. The sphincters have no nerve supply and primarily respond to metabolite control. These mechanisms are the dominant factor determining distribution of blood flow.

In poorly perfused tissues, accumulation of metabolites may cause dilation of blood vessels and further compound the problems of stagnant flow. On the venous side of the circulation particularly, slow-flowing blood may result in rouleaux formation by red blood cells. This means that red cells become stuck together and stack up like a pile of plates. This increases the local resistance to blood flow and results in further deterioration in blood perfusion and in local oedema. This is part of the scenario of irreversible shock.

Blood-borne hormones

The renin-angiotensin system is described in Chapter 6 (*see* page 152). In addition to effects which are concerned with blood volume regulation, angiotensin II is a potent systemic pressor hormone. The renin system is functional in the fetus and activity increases at birth, thus helping to maintain arterial blood pressure.

Nerve supply to blood vessels

The characteristics of the autonomic nervous system are described on page 117. The dominant characteristics of the nerve supply to blood vessels are that it is sympathetic in origin and adrenergic – the main neurotransmitter is noradrenaline acting on α_1-adrenoceptors to cause vasoconstriction. Although there are examples of parts of circulatory control mechanisms in which individual parts of the neural control characteristics described above do not hold true, these are very specialised aspects of local circulatory control.

The major function of the sympathetic neural control mechanisms is the regulation of arterial blood pressure. This is described below.

Vascular control via the sympathetic nervous system starts to become functional early in gestation. However, at term birth it is still immature compared with that of the adult. Rapid development in function occurs after birth.

THE BARORECEPTOR REFLEX

The major components of the baroreceptor reflex are illustrated in Figure 5.9.

The major baroreceptors on the high-pressure, arterial side of the circulation are located at the carotid sinus and the aortic arch. The baroreceptors are modified nerve endings which are sensitive to stretch. They are buried in the wall of the blood vessels and, when arterial pressure rises, the vessels become inflated and the nerve endings are stretched. There is consequently an increase in the action potential number in the glossopharyngeal nerve (Cranial Nerve IX) because of stimulation of the carotid sinus and in the vagus nerve (Cranial Nerve X) because of stimulation of baroreceptors in the aortic arch. The increased activity passes along these cranial nerves into the medulla of the brain. Processing of this information in the medulla and hypothalamus leads to organisation of the autonomic outflow response (*see* page 118).

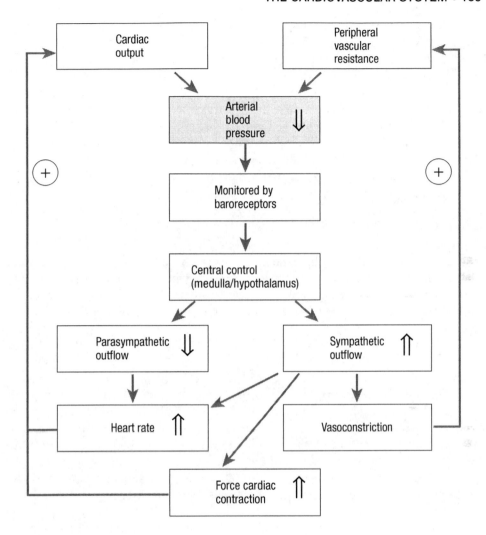

FIGURE 5.9 The baroreceptor reflex

The response to a fall in arterial blood pressure is an increase in both cardiac output and peripheral resistance that will restore blood pressure to the normal set-point.

Source: Noble A *et al.*, op. cit.

In Figure 5.9, the response to a fall in arterial blood pressure is illustrated. Heart rate is increased by a combination of inhibition of the vagus nerve supply to the heart and stimulation of the sympathetic nerve supply. There is an increase in the contractility of the heart muscle generated by the sympathetic nerve supply and, together, the heart rate and force of cardiac contraction changes lead to an increase in cardiac output. An increase in peripheral vasoconstriction occurs in response to sympathetic nerve activation. The combination of the increased cardiac output and the raised peripheral resistance brings the blood pressure back to the normal set-point. It is said that the timing of every heart beat throughout life is determined by the blood pressure at the carotid sinus.

In both the fetus and the newborn, the cardiovascular control mechanisms function to preferentially supply high-priority organs such as the brain and heart with oxygen. The baroreceptor reflex becomes functional in the fetus and is increasingly effective as gestational age increases. It appears that the parasympathetic nervous system plays the major role, via the vagus, in the regulation of the fetal heart rate in late gestation. Towards the end of gestation, and in the early neonate period, the baroreceptor reflex resets to a higher pressure range. This is necessary to accommodate the circulatory changes at birth when the left ventricle, rather than the right ventricle, becomes responsible for systemic vascular perfusion.

CAPILLARY FUNCTION

Capillary structure

The capillary circulation is where the major functions of the circulatory system take place. These are the exchange of oxygen and other nutrients into tissues and the removal of carbon dioxide and other cellular waste products. The regulation of this part of the circulation also plays a critical role in determining the distribution of water between compartments.

Capillary walls consist of a single layer of endothelial cells as illustrated in Figure 5.10.

This figure shows the most widespread type of capillary structure, called a *continuous capillary*. In *fenestrated-type capillaries*, which are much more permeable to water, there is a wider gap between adjacent endothelial cells with a thin membrane between the cells. This type of capillary structure is found in tissues which functionally have a high water flux across the capillary wall. This includes the glomerulus of the kidney and intestinal villi. A third type of capillary structure, called *discontinuous capillaries*, occurs in tissues such as the liver, bone marrow and spleen, where the tissue function requires the exchange of cells such as new and old red blood cells across capillary walls.

The structure illustrated in Figure 5.10 has a capillary lumen diameter of 3–8 μm. As red cells have a diameter of about 8 μm, the red cells have to deform to pass through many capillaries. Red cells are, in fact, very flexible and easily resume their normal shape when they exit from the 0.5–1.0 mm long passage through a capillary.

Some lipid-soluble molecules can diffuse through the lipid bilayer on either side of the endothelial cell wall. These include oxygen and carbon dioxide but also some drugs such as general anaesthetic agents. Small lipid insoluble ions and molecules cannot cross the lipid bilayer of cells so their movement across capillary walls is confined to the water-filled channels between cells. The glycocalyx is a layer of negatively charged macromolecules which coats the endothelial cells and lines the channels between cells. This has a major effect in determining how easily charged molecules and ions cross capillary walls.

Passage of larger molecules, such as proteins, is determined primarily by the type of capillary structure involved. Some continuous capillary structures are effectively impermeable to proteins but in tissues with discontinuous capillary structures significant amounts of plasma protein can leak into the interstitial space.

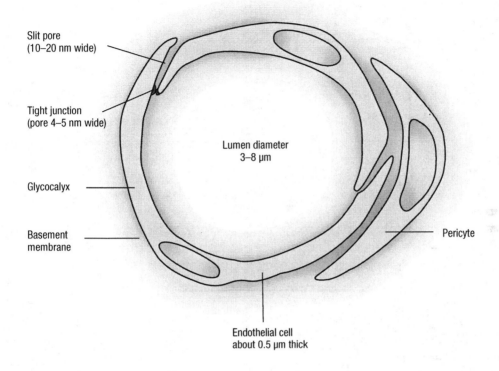

Slit pore
(10–20 nm wide)

Tight junction
(pore 4–5 nm wide)

Glycocalyx

Basement
membrane

Lumen diameter
3–8 µm

Pericyte

Endothelial cell
about 0.5 µm thick

FIGURE 5.10 Structure of a continuous capillary

Tight junctions between cells determine capillary permeability. Pericytes surround part of the capillary wall and provide support.

Source: Noble A *et al.*, op. cit.

Water movement across capillary walls

The distribution of water between compartments is described in Chapter 4 (*see* page 90). Movement of water between the capillary and the interstitial space depends on the balance between a gradient of hydrostatic pressure (capillary blood pressure – interstitial fluid pressure) and a gradient of colloid osmotic pressure (colloid osmotic pressure plasma – colloid osmotic pressure interstitial fluid). This is illustrated in Figure 5.11. These forces are discussed on page 90.

The model for movement of water across capillary walls was first described as the 'Starling hypothesis' in 1896. However, Starling did not recognise the role played by the lymphatics. Excess movement of water out of capillaries drains into the lymphatic system and is then returned to the circulation as described below.

The interstitial 'space' does not normally contain water which is free to move. The interstitial compartment contains macromolecules which immobilise the water to prevent its movement. An analogy might be the immobilisation of water between the fibres of a bath sponge. If the interstitial space is expanded and the macromolecules

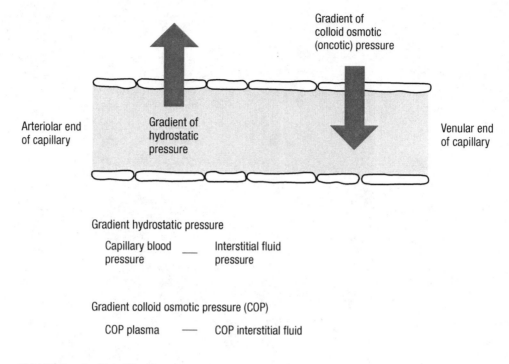

FIGURE 5.11 The 'Starling hypothesis' of capillary function

Source: Noble A *et al.*, op. cit.

are pushed further apart, they fail to immobilise the water and it becomes free to move under the effects of gravity. This is why oedema fluid accumulates in the dependent areas of the body.

Interstitial fluid pressure is in fact less than atmospheric pressure. This is why we can have the bodily shape we have rather than being spherical. Our skin is pressed back against underlying structures by atmospheric pressure.

The lymphatic system

Although the two sets of Starling forces almost balance, there is net outflow of water into the lymph capillaries. These are blind-ending tubes which, like vascular capillaries, consist of a single layer of endothelial cells. Lymph capillaries join together to form collecting lymphatics which have valves to prevent backflow. At intervals along the largest lymphatic vessels, there are lymph nodes. The functions of these structures are described below.

Most of the lymph flow re-enters the circulation in the left thoracic duct which enters the subclavian vein close to the left armpit. The lymph drainage for the right side of the thorax and head and the right arm enters a smaller lymph trunk which enters the right subclavian vein.

The functions of the lymphatic system can be summarised as follows:
▶ Tissue drainage system which helps to maintain an appropriate distribution of body water.

▶ Return of plasma proteins which have leaked out into the interstitial space back to the circulation.
▶ Absorption of digested fat, in the form of chylomicrons, from intestinal villi.
▶ Defence function at lymph nodes.

Lymph nodes are cavernous structures which contain phagocytic cells and lymphocytes. Lymph enters from large lymphatics and flows over the lymphoid follicles which have phagocytic cells with specific antigen recognition sites. Lymphocytes are not produced in lymph nodes; this occurs in primary lymphoid tissues, the bone marrow and thymus.

Mechanisms of oedema

Oedema is an accumulation of excess water in body fluid compartments. This often occurs in the interstitial fluid compartment following an imbalance in the Starling forces. The fundamental mechanisms which can result in oedema can therefore be summarised as follows:
▶ an increase in capillary blood pressure
▶ a decrease in colloid osmotic pressure
▶ blockage of the lymphatic drainage
▶ an increase in capillary wall permeability.

A common cause of oedema, due to an increase in capillary hydrostatic pressure, is right-sided heart failure. This generates a compensatory increase in preload to the heart in order to raise stroke volume. As this compensation increases the right atrial pressure, the pressure in all of the vessels feeding blood into the right atrium, including the capillaries, will also rise. Increased arterial pressure is not a direct cause of oedema. Hypertension results from excessive vasoconstriction in the arterioles, the vessels before the capillaries. Pressure in the capillaries after the high resistance is normal.

The major contributors to the colloid osmotic pressure of plasma are the plasma proteins, especially albumin (*see* page 94). All of the plasma proteins, with the exception of the immunoglobulins, are synthesised in the liver. Liver failure is therefore a cause of peripheral oedema. Malnutrition, when there is an inadequate intake of protein to provide for the synthesis of new plasma protein and renal disease, when there is loss of plasma protein in the urine, are further causes.

Lymphoedema is the name given to peripheral oedema caused by lymphatic insufficiency. This may be caused by blockage produced in many different ways including neoplasia and infection but congenital structural abnormalities are a potential cause in neonates.

Permeability changes in capillaries occur when inflammatory mediators such as histamine, bradykinin and serotonin increase the size of pores by causing contraction of the endothelial cells. This not only means that it is easier for water to move out of capillaries but may also mean that plasma proteins leak out as well. These changes occur as part of local inflammatory reactions and the consequence is localised tissue swelling. This occurs, for example, at the site of a local skin lesion.

REFERENCES

Blackburn S. *Maternal, Fetal and Neonatal Physiology.* 3rd ed. St Louis: Saunders; 2007.

Levick J. *Cardiovascular Physiology.* 5th ed. London: Arnold; 2009.

Levy M, Pappano A. *Cardiovascular Physiology.* 9th ed. St Louis: Saunders; 2007.

Noble A, Johnson R, Thomas A *et al. The Cardiovascular System.* Edinburgh: Churchill Livingstone; 2005.

Polin R, Fox W, Abman S. *Fetal and Neonatal Physiology.* 3rd ed. Philadelphia: Saunders; 2003.

CHAPTER 6

The renal system

Alan Noble

CONTENTS

INTRODUCTION

There are three fundamental processes involved in the production of urine:

▶ *Filtration* – driven by capillary blood pressure in the glomerulus.
▶ *Reabsorption* – almost all of the filtered water and dissolved solutes are reabsorbed during passage down the nephron.
▶ *Secretion* – the selective movement of substances from the blood into the proximal tubular fluid.

Each of these processes will now be considered individually.

GLOMERULAR FILTRATION
Structure of the filter

A human kidney has about one million glomeruli. Development of the kidneys starts early in gestation and the complete adult number of nephrons has formed by about 35 weeks. No further increase in nephron number occurs, only a change in the size and function of individual nephrons. By 9 to 10 weeks gestational age, urine formation starts and during the second half of pregnancy the fetal kidneys produce the urine which forms the major part of amniotic fluid.

Each glomerulus consists of a capillary network with an incoming afferent arteriole and an outgoing efferent arteriole. The glomerular capillary blood pressure provides the driving force for filtration and this is regulated by mechanisms which adjust the resistance to blood flow of the afferent and efferent arterioles. The efferent arteriole has a smaller diameter than the afferent arteriole and this helps to sustain a high pressure in the intervening capillary bed.

There are three main layers to the glomerular filter. The layer which is in contact with the blood is a fenestrated capillary endothelium. This is a very permeable layer which serves primarily to keep the red and white blood cells within the circulation. The main selective component of the filter for solutes in plasma is a double-thickness glomerular basement membrane. This is a non-cellular mesh of large negatively charged glycoprotein molecules such as collagen IV, laminin and fibronectin. These macromolecules are secreted by the two cell groups on either side of the basement membrane, the endothelial cells and the podocytes. These podocytes, via small projections called foot processes, provide support for the glomerular basement membrane and are contiguous with the epithelial cell layer which lines the kidney tubule. In between adjacent podocytes there are gaps called slit pores which also carry a negative charge. The main site of selectivity of the glomerular filter, on the basis of size, is the glomerular basement membrane. All three layers of the filter carry a net negative charge. Both size and charge are important determinants of the transit of solutes across the glomerular filter.

Mesangial cells are located between the capillary loops of the glomerulus. They have a dual phenotype in that they are contractile and therefore resemble smooth muscle cells (*see* page 120), and they are also phagocytic and bear some resemblance to macrophages. The role of mesangial cells is to adjust the surface area and permeability characteristics of the filter by their contractile properties and to remove debris from the filter by the phagocytic role.

Forces driving glomerular filtration

The forces determining filtration at the glomerulus are illustrated in Figure 6.1.
The three forces involved are the following.

▌ Glomerular capillary blood pressure, the prime driving force for filtration. In an adult kidney this is approximately 45 mmHg.

▌ Colloid osmotic pressure (oncotic pressure) of plasma (*see* page 94) which opposes filtration. This osmotic force is generated by the fact that there are proteins in plasma but, normally, very little protein in the filtrate. This gradient is equivalent to about 25 mmHg.

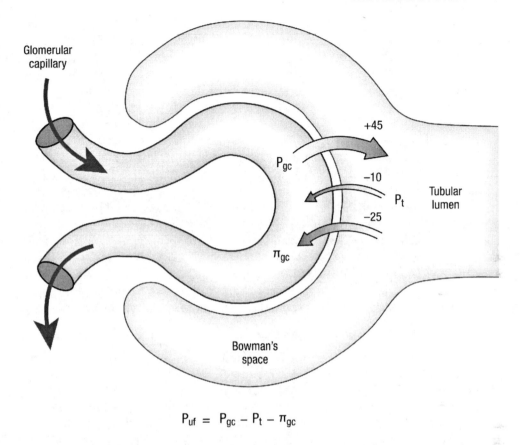

$$P_{uf} = P_{gc} - P_t - \pi_{gc}$$

FIGURE 6.1 Forces determining filtration rate at the glomerulus

P_{uf} is net filtration pressure; P_{gc} is glomerular capillary blood pressure; P_t is tubular pressure; π_{gc} is the colloid osmotic pressure (oncotic pressure) generated by the plasma proteins.

Source: Field M, Pollock C, Harris D. *The Renal System*. Elsevier Health Sciences; 2001.

▶ Tubular pressure is the pressure exerted by the fluid in the nephron. This is equivalent to about 10 mmHg and again opposes filtration.

The net filtration pressure, the difference between the force driving filtration and the two forces opposing it, is therefore only about 10 mmHg. Relatively small changes in any of the three component forces outlined above can result in significant changes in glomerular filtration rate (GFR). This is the volume of filtrate formed in the kidneys per unit time. It is usually expressed in units of mL/min or, less frequently, L/day. Appropriate figures for the textbook person are 125 mL/min or 180 L/day. The forces driving filtration are fundamental to understanding acute renal failure (*see* page 148), a situation in which GFR decreases.

Selectivity of the glomerular filter

The solutes which will pass through the glomerular filter are selected on the basis of size and charge. Molecules up to a relative molecular mass of 7000 Da pass through the normal filter unimpeded. These small items will include all of the ions, such as Na^+ and Cl^-, irrespective of charge, and small uncharged molecules such as urea and glucose. Most proteins carry a net negative charge at physiological pH. There is increasing size-related resistance to negatively charged proteins passing through the filter up to a total exclusion size of 70 000 Da. Albumin has a relative molecular mass (RMM) of 69 000 Da and about 0.02% of the albumin which enters the kidneys passes through the filter into the tubule.

Selectivity on the basis of charge means that positively charged or neutral proteins cross the filter more easily than negatively charged proteins. As noted previously, all the layers of the glomerular filter normally carry a negative charge and in this environment, negatively charged proteins are repelled. An illustration of this comes from the way the glomerulus handles haemoglobin if it has escaped from damaged red blood cells. Haemoglobin (RMM 68 000 Da) is a similar size to albumin but does not carry a substantial negative charge. Haemoglobin can pass through the glomerular filter much more easily than albumin, and can therefore appear in the urine.

Proteinuria

Albumin is relatively small as a plasma protein and it is the protein in the highest concentration in plasma. As noted above, about 0.02% of the albumin which passes through the kidney will enter the tubule. Nevertheless, quite large amounts of albumin, about 40 kg/day in a textbook adult, pass through the kidneys and so even a very small percentage entering the filtrate becomes significant. This protein is absorbed by endocytosis in the proximal tubule. Inside the epithelial cells the endocytotic vesicles join with lysosomes containing proteolytic enzymes. The absorbed proteins are broken down into their constituent amino acids and recycled via the circulation to protein synthesis sites.

Pathological damage to the glomerular filter may lead to changes in either the size selectivity or, sometimes, the charge selectivity on the filter. In this circumstance more albumin may escape through the filter and exceed the capacity of the proximal tubule cells to recycle the protein. As a result, albumin will appear in the urine and this is referred to as proteinuria.

Detection of proteinuria is often carried out using a dipstick test. These detect only albumin and not other proteins. They are also relatively insensitive. The early stages of some disease mechanisms, such as diabetes, may result in levels of albumin excretion which are below the threshold for dipstick tests but still of clinical interest. This is called microalbuminuria and is detectable only by laboratory-based tests.

Two other types of protein, which are not detectable with a dipstick test, may appear in urine samples. Tamm-Horsfall protein is secreted into the urine from tubular cells. The function of these proteins is obscure. In syndromes such as myeloma, there is over-production of small proteins which pass from blood through the glomerular filter and appear in the urine.

A modest level of albumin proteinuria is common in pregnancy but this does not necessarily indicate glomerular pathology or pre-eclampsia. The changes are normally reversible after delivery.

Regulation of renal blood flow and glomerular filtration rate

In a resting mature individual, renal blood flow (RBF) accounts for about 20% to 25% of resting cardiac output. This is a very high flow rate considering the small size and therefore limited metabolic activity of the kidneys. Within the kidney, much of the blood flow goes to the cortex of the kidney. The medulla of the kidney is relatively poorly supplied and so is mildly hypoxic and prone to ischaemic damage.

The term 'filtration fraction' refers to the glomerular filtration rate (GFR) expressed as a percentage of renal plasma flow (RPF). A typical value for filtration fraction is 20%. The remaining 80% of plasma which escapes the glomerular filter enters the efferent arteriole along with the red cells and subsequently passes to the vasa recta. These are capillary vessels which surround the kidney tubule and receive the water and solutes reabsorbed from the tubule.

Within normal physiological ranges, both RBF and GFR are kept quite constant over a range of arterial blood pressures from 70–200 mmHg. This is known as autoregulation. The prime mechanism for autoregulation depends on an intrinsic property of smooth muscle (*see* Chapter 4, page 120). When smooth muscle is stretched it responds by contracting. In the absence of autoregulation, if the pressure inside a blood vessel increased then the vessel wall would be stretched, the cross-sectional area of the vessel would expand and blood flow would increase. However, contraction of the vessel wall smooth muscle in response to stretch leads to a reduction in the vessel lumen and both the blood flow and GFR are kept constant.

A further component of the mechanism for the autoregulation of RBF and GFR is called tubuloglomerular feedback (TGF). A sensor in the distal nephron, at the macula densa, monitors [Na$^+$] and/or [Cl$^-$] passing down the tubule. If the NaCl passing the macula densa increases, then the GFR is down-regulated by release of local chemical mediators. In terms of the micro-anatomy, the macula densa is adjacent to the glomerular afferent arteriole and is therefore in an ideal position to take part in a local regulation mechanism. The GFR in individual glomeruli, termed *single nephron glomerular filtration rate* (SNGFR), is regulated in this way. There are still aspects of TGF which are poorly understood.

The overall importance of RBF and GFR autoregulation mechanisms is that fluctuations in arterial blood pressure do not lead to big changes in body fluid balance. Also, the delicate glomerular filter is protected from potential damage by large increases in blood flow.

Superimposed on the basic regulation of GFR there are mechanisms which regulate GFR by changing the resistance of the afferent and efferent arterioles to the glomeruli and hence altering glomerular capillary blood pressure.

These mechanisms can be summarised as follows:

▶ Constriction of the afferent arteriole will reduce GFR. This is mediated by the sympathetic nervous system (SNS) and by vasoconstrictor endothelins. Activation of the SNS is a particularly important determinant of GFR changes in circulatory shock. This mechanism involves the baroreceptor reflex (*see* Chapter 5, page 134).

❱ Dilation of the afferent arteriole will increase GFR. Active agents here include locally produced vasodilator prostaglandins, natriuretic peptides (*see* page 153) and nitric oxide. Non steroidal anti-inflammatory drugs (NSAID), such as aspirin, which block prostaglandin synthesis will therefore cause a reduction in GFR.

❱ Moderate constriction of the efferent arteriole will increase GFR and this is an effect of angiotensin II (*see* page 152) and natriuretic peptides. Intense constriction of the efferent arteriole would result in cessation of blood flow through the glomerulus and so GFR would fall.

❱ Dilation of the efferent arteriole would decrease GFR. This is not a physiologically important control mechanism but it is a side effect of drugs which block the renin-angiotensin system. These are mainly angiotensin-converting enzyme inhibitors (ACEI) and angiotensin receptor blockers (ARB) (*see* page 152).

Monitoring glomerular filtration

GFR can be measured using a clearance test. The definition of 'clearance' is the volume of plasma which is completely cleared of a marker substance per unit time. In order to assess GFR by a clearance test we need a marker substance circulating in plasma which is non-selectively filtered at the glomerulus; that is, filtrate [marker] is the same as plasma [marker]. Once it has been filtered, this marker is not reabsorbed during passage down the nephron and the marker remaining in plasma after passage through the glomerulus is not secreted into the tubule.

The following are then true:

Amount of marker filtered = Amount of marker excreted

Amount of marker filtered = GFR × [Plasma marker]

$$\text{Amount of marker excreted} = [\text{Urine marker}] \times \frac{\text{Urine volume}}{\text{Time}}$$

Therefore, with a small re-arrangement of these statements:

$$GFR = \frac{[\text{Urine marker}]}{[\text{Plasma marker}]} \times \frac{\text{Urine volume}}{\text{Time}}$$

This is called the clearance formula. Inulin is a polysaccharide compound which has the ideal characteristics as a marker for measuring GFR by a clearance method. It is not a naturally occurring compound in people and would need to be infused separately.

Creatinine

Creatinine is an endogenous compound which is normally released at a steady rate from skeletal muscle. It is a breakdown product from the metabolism of creatine phosphate, a compound held in skeletal muscle and used for the short-term rephosphorylation of ADP. Creatinine is not an ideal marker for measuring GFR because, although it is non-selectively filtered at the glomerulus, some secretion of creatinine into the tubule occurs in the proximal tubule. This means that using creatinine as a clearance marker would give about a 10% over-estimate of GFR. The major advantage of creatinine is that it is an endogenous non-toxic compound which is released at a steady rate into the circulation.

In practice, full clearance tests are very rarely performed clinically. However, using the same basic principles:

Creatinine produced = Creatinine filtered = GFR × Plasma [creatine]

As creatinine is released at a constant rate from muscles, there is an inverse relationship between GFR and plasma [creatinine]. Thus, for example, if GFR, halves and plasma [creatinine] doubles, then the same amount of creatinine is both filtered and excreted. Plasma creatinine measurements therefore provide an index of GFR: if GFR falls, then [creatinine] increases. This test is routinely used for the clinical monitoring of GFR.

Urea

Urea handling by the kidneys initially follows the same pattern as for creatinine, non-selective filtration. During passage down the nephron, about 40% of filtered urea is reabsorbed. Measurements of plasma [creatinine] and [urea] therefore tend to move in parallel in response to a change in GFR. However, two aspects may alter the urea-to-creatinine ratio. The first is increased protein turnover. Increased plasma [urea] will follow raised urea production as a result of a rise in dietary protein intake, a gastrointestinal bleed or major inflammatory events. These may all increase plasma urea-to-creatinine ratio. The second cause of selectively raised plasma [urea] is associated with increased anti-diuretic hormone (ADH) action (*see* page 150). Dehydration or hyperosmolar conditions commonly result in increased ADH secretion and, consequently, increased water and also increased urea reabsorption in the collecting duct of the nephron. Again, an increase in urea-to-creatinine ratio follows. This can be a useful diagnostic test.

Maternal, fetal and neonatal glomerular filtration rate

The GFR increases by 40–60% during pregnancy. The changes start to occur very early and are detectable 3 to 4 weeks post-conception. Peak changes are reached after 9–16 weeks. When this increase in GFR does not occur, this is sometimes associated with pregnancy loss. The mechanism of the increase in GFR is a rise in glomerular capillary blood pressure and a decrease in plasma colloid osmotic pressure as a result of haemodilution. Precise details of mechanisms are not very clear but several of the factors which regulate the tone of the afferent and efferent arterioles (*see* page 145) have been implicated. The GFR returns to non-pregnant levels by 3 months post-delivery.

RBF expressed per unit body surface area is low in absolute terms in both term and preterm infants. In adults, about 20–5% of resting cardiac output goes to the kidneys, but for a term infant this figure is only about 5%, increasing to 10% over the next few days. These figures reflect the high resistance to blood flow through the kidney at birth.

GFR is low in term neonates and very immature neonates have a particularly impaired GFR. This remains low initially until the full complement of nephrons has formed at about 35 weeks gestational age. Subsequent to this, a rapid increase in GFR allows premature infants to catch up with term babies.

In addition to potential deficits in the excretory functions of the kidney imposed by the slow development of full glomerular function, the limited renal function in both term and preterm infants may also alter the pharmacokinetics of drugs which are excreted by the kidney. Dosages of drugs used may need to be adjusted on this basis.

Acute renal failure

Acute renal failure is characterised by a decrease in GFR accompanied by a rise in plasma [creatinine] and [urea]. Changes in urine flow rate are not part of this definition. Oliguria or anuria may accompany acute renal failure but this is not necessarily the case and urine flow rate may remain unchanged. Acute renal failure has a short-term (hours/days) onset and is potentially reversible.

There are three basic types of acute renal failure:

▶ *Pre-renal failure* – a decrease in GFR as a result of a fall in glomerular capillary blood pressure. This often follows activation of the SNS and constriction of the afferent arteriole to the glomerulus. Inhibition of renal vasodilator prostaglandin synthesis by NSAID drugs is another cause.

▶ *Intrarenal failure* – a decrease in GFR as a result of structural changes in the glomerular filter (e.g. acute glomerulonephritis) or the kidney tubule. The tubular events are often the result of ischaemic or toxic insults to the early parts of the nephron which lead to acute tubular necrosis (ATN). In this case, necrotic tubular cells detach from their basement membrane and the cell debris accumulates in the tubule lumen. If the debris is eventually flushed out it may be seen as casts during microscopic inspection of a urine sample. Epithelial cell regeneration and a return of GFR to normal may occur after a week or more. Uncontrolled electrolyte loss can occur during this time.

▶ *Post-renal failure* – a consequence of outflow obstruction which leads to a rise in tubule pressure and therefore a reduction in the net filtration pressure (*see* Figure 6.1). Outflow obstruction can occur at any stage along the urinary tract including the renal pelvis, ureter, bladder and urethra.

Chronic renal disease (failure) is associated with permanent loss of nephrons and is not reversible. The time course is usually much longer than for acute renal failure.

REABSORPTION IN THE KIDNEY TUBULE

Most of the solutes and water in the glomerular filtrate are reabsorbed during passage down the nephron. Broadly, excretion of water and electrolytes is matched to physiological needs using hormonal control of carrier-mediated transport mechanisms (*see* page 97).

Proximal tubule

In the proximal tubule of mature individuals about 70% of filtered solutes such as Na^+, Cl^-, K^+, are reabsorbed together with about 90% of filtered bicarbonate and 100% of filtered glucose. Water reabsorption occurs because there is a transepithelial cell osmotic gradient generated by the solute absorption; the water follows the solutes. The fluid arriving at the end of the proximal tubule has the same osmotic strength as the filtrate entering the tubule. The term 'glomerulotubular balance' refers to the fact that the proximal tubule absorbs a constant proportion of the solute presented to it rather than a specific amount of solute. In neonates, the proximal tubule is still quite short and this limits the reabsorptive capacity of this segment of the nephron.

The drive to make tubular co-transport mechanisms work is usually provided by the $[Na^+]$ gradient between the filtrate and the inside of the epithelial cell (*see* page 98). The low intracellular $[Na^+]$ is maintained by the Na^+/K^+ ATPase (sodium pump) activity on the basolateral side of the cell. In preterm neonates decreased sodium pump activity may contribute to decreased proximal tubule function and lead to excessive sodium loss. In term newborns there is a rapid increase in sodium pump activity after birth. This, together with an increased sensitivity to aldosterone (*see* page 153), enhances the ability to regulate sodium balance.

Glucose is reabsorbed by sodium-glucose co-transporters (*see* page 98) in the proximal tubule and this is the only segment of the nephron where glucose reabsorption can occur. There is a limited number of the co-transporters in the proximal tubule and if the total amount of glucose in the glomerular filtrate exceeds the reabsorptive capacity of the proximal tubule, glycosuria will occur. The plasma [glucose] at which glycosuria just occurs is called the renal threshold and the maximum transport capacity is referred to as the T_M, (transport or tubular maximum). In preterm infants the T_M for glucose is lower than it is in term infants or in adults. This is due to a low number of glucose co-transporter proteins. However, most infants with a normal blood [glucose] are not glycosuric.

Role of the kidney in water balance
The loop of Henle and the collecting ducts

The ascending limb of the loop of Henle has an important role in the reabsorption of 20% to 25% of the filtered solute including Na^+, K^+ and Cl^-. Selective reabsorption of Mg^{++} and Ca^{++} also occurs in this segment of the nephron under the control of parathyroid hormone (PTH).

The major function of the transport mechanisms in the loop of Henle is to generate an osmotic gradient in the interstitial fluid outside the tubule between the cortex and medulla. In a mature kidney, the interstitial fluid in the cortex has an osmolarity which is similar to that of blood plasma, about 290 mosmoles/L. The interstitial fluid outside the bottom of the loop of Henle in the medulla typically has an osmolarity of about 600 mosmoles/L but under conditions requiring maximum water retention this can rise in mature individuals to 1200 mosmoles/L – about four times plasma osmolarity. There is a continuous gradient of interstitial osmolarity between the cortex and the inner medulla. This gradient is generated by a countercurrent mechanism which is driven by a $Na^+/K^+/2Cl^-$ co-transporter on the luminal surface of the thick ascending limb of the loop of Henle. This co-transporter is blocked by loop diuretics such as furosemide and bumetanide which are secreted into the tubular fluid in the proximal tubule. An important characteristic of the ascending limb of the loop of Henle is that it is impermeable to water. As Na^+ and Cl^- are transported out of this segment of the nephron, the fluid inside the tubule becomes more dilute. Accumulation of urea in the interstitium is also an important contributor to the osmotic gradient in the interstitium.

The importance of the interstitial osmotic gradient between cortex and medulla is that the collecting duct runs parallel to the loop of Henle and is therefore exposed to the same osmotic gradient. The collecting duct is intrinsically impermeable to water. If it is made permeable by the actions of a hormone, then water can move from the collecting duct down an osmotic gradient into the interstitial space. Water can then be taken away via the capillary blood vessels. If the hormonally induced increase in permeability reaches maximum levels, then the osmotic strength of urine produced will be the same as the osmolarity of interstitial fluid at the bottom of the loop of Henle. If the collecting duct is not made permeable to water then the osmolarity of urine produced will be the same as the fluid entering the collecting duct, typically down to about one-third of plasma osmolarity.

ADH

The hormone which alters collecting duct permeability is antidiuretic hormone (ADH). It is synthesised in the hypothalamus and passes down the inside of giant axons to be stored in the nerve endings in the posterior pituitary. The major physiological triggers for ADH secretion derive from osmoreceptors in the hypothalamus and from volume receptors located in the atria of the heart. Approximately two-thirds of the blood volume is held in the venous system and the volume receptors are modified nerve endings which relay information to the hypothalamus. An increase in plasma osmolarity or a decrease in blood volume will increase ADH secretion. This will increase collecting duct permeability and promote water reabsorption. Conversely, a decrease in osmolarity or an increase in blood volume will reduce water reabsorption by decreasing ADH secretion and lead to a diuresis.

The collecting duct epithelial cells contain pre-formed water channels called aquaporins. These channels can be inserted into both the luminal membrane and the basolateral membrane in order to increase the water permeability of the collecting duct.

Fetal urine production is an important source of amniotic fluid from about 18 weeks' gestation. However, the ability of the fetal kidney to produce concentrated urine is limited to 20% to 30% of adult capacity. Fetal urine is hypotonic, typically at about 200 mosmoles/L (plasma – 290 mosmoles/L) although it becomes less hypotonic with increasing gestational age. It must be remembered that sodium regulation is still under the control of the placenta at this stage. Although osmoreceptors and volume receptors control ADH secretion from about 26 weeks' gestation, the kidney has limited receptor sensitivity for ADH at this time.

Water regulation in the neonate

In newborn infants, although the basic principles of water regulation are similar to those in the adult, they only operate over a limited range. The ability to produce a dilute urine is similar to that in adults but the power to concentrate urine is less impressive. In preterm infants, urine concentrating ability is more limited than in term neonates but by 4 to 6 weeks after birth preterm infants have caught up in this respect. Almost every aspect of the mechanisms described above which lead to the production of a concentrated urine is impaired in preterm infants. This includes the osmotic gradient generation in the renal interstitium, the length of the loop of Henle, the actions of ADH, and the production of aquaporins. A further factor is that part of the solute in the interstitial space which produces the cortex-to-medulla osmotic gradient is urea. Increased reabsorption of urea occurs with water reabsorption under the influence of ADH. This increased interstitial [urea] is the basis for the increasing ability to generate a larger cortex-to-medulla interstitial gradient and hence form a highly concentrated urine sample in hyperosmolar or hypovolaemic states in adults. Neonates, of whatever gestational age, generate less urea because protein and amino acid sources are being preferentially used for growth.

Role of the kidney in sodium balance

The segment of the nephron between the ascending limb of the loop of Henle and the inner medullary segments of the collecting duct is the region where sodium excretion is regulated. Although this is often referred to as the distal tubule, this can be a bit misleading when considering the functions of this region of the nephron. The terms 'early diluting segment' and 'late diluting segment' are probably more appropriate.

In the early diluting segment, anatomically the early distal tubule, sodium is reabsorbed via a luminal Na^+/Cl^- co-transporter protein. This is not a site for significant hormonal control but it is the site of action of the thiazide diuretics such as hydrochlorthiazide.

In the late diluting segment, anatomically the late distal tubule and the early part of the collecting duct, hormonally controlled regulation of Na^+ and K^+ excretion occurs. There are three interrelated hormonal systems involved:

▶ renin-angiotensin system
▶ aldosterone
▶ natriuretic peptides.

The renin-angiotensin system

Renin is a hormone secreted, primarily by the kidneys, in response to a fall in arterial blood pressure or to a fall in blood volume. Part of the control of renin secretion is mediated by SNS activation as part of the baroreceptor reflex (*see* Chapter 5, page 134), but there are also intrarenal sensing mechanisms for intrarenal blood pressure and sodium excretion which alter renin secretion. The role of the renin system is to maintain blood pressure and blood volume by a combination of promoting Na^+ retention in the kidney and peripheral vasoconstriction.

Renin does not have direct actions of its own but is an enzyme which promotes the formation of angiotensin I from a protein substrate (angiotensinogen) (*see* Figure 6.2). Angiotensin I is physiologically inert but is cleaved by angiotensin-converting enzyme to make angiotensin II. There are two types of receptor for angiotensin II, the AT_1- and AT_2-receptors. The most important functions of the renin-angiotensin system, including the promotion of aldosterone synthesis and

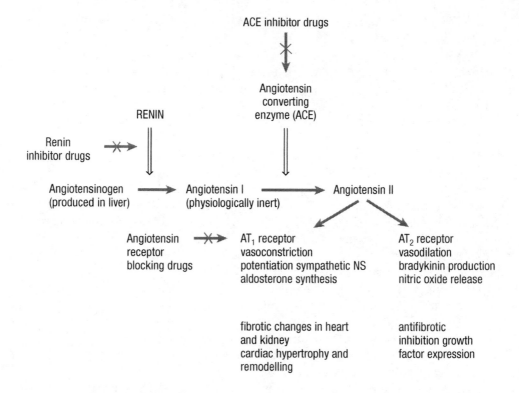

FIGURE 6.2 Renin-angiotensin system

The renin system produces a compensatory increase in cardiac preload in response to, for example, cardiac failure.

Source: Noble A, Johnson RA, Thomas A *et al. The Cardiovascular System*. Elsevier Health Sciences; 2005.

vasoconstriction, are mediated by the AT_1-type receptor. The roles of the AT_2-receptor are still being evaluated but it may be involved in promoting growth. The AT_2-receptor is expressed particularly in embryonic tissues but it is unclear what role it has.

Drugs which block the renin-angiotensin system are illustrated in Figure 6.2. Angiotensin-converting enzyme inhibitors block the formation of angiotensin II from angiotensin I. The generic names of all of these drugs end in –*pril* (e.g. ramipril). Inhibitors of the AT_1-receptor block the major physiological actions of angiotensin II. All of the names of this group of drugs end in –*sartan* (e.g. losartan). Renin enzyme inhibitor drugs (e.g. aliskiren) have not been used until recently. Blockers and selective agonists for the AT_2-receptor are available but have no current clinical uses. Beta-adrenoceptor-blocking drugs reduce sympathetically induced renin secretion. This is part of the antihypertensive action of this group of drugs.

There are important changes in the renin system during pregnancy with an increased concentration in plasma of all the components of the system but reduced sensitivity to the pressor actions of angiotensin II. This helps to maintain a normal blood pressure but still allows increased Na^+ and water retention in pregnancy. The increase in renin secretion does not come just from the kidneys – extrarenal sources such as the uterus and placenta also contribute.

The renin system is active from early in fetal development and a functional renin-angiotensin system is essential for normal development. In early intrauterine development the AT_2-type receptor predominates and is involved in growth promotion.

In neonates, the activity of the components of the renin-angiotensin system is inversely related to the gestational age with higher levels in preterm infants than in term babies. In newborn term infants, the plasma renin activity is still at 3 to 5 times adult levels and gradually declines in the weeks after birth. Hypertension in neonates is frequently related to factors which enhance the activity of the renin-angiotensin system.

Aldosterone

Aldosterone is secreted by the zona glomerulosa cells of the adrenal cortex. As it is a steroid hormone, increased secretion follows increased synthesis of aldosterone rather than the release of pre-formed stored hormone. The major controls on aldosterone synthesis are mediated by angiotensin II and increased $[K^+]$. The actions of aldosterone on the late diluting segment are to promote Na^+ retention and K^+ and H^+ excretion. As with other steroid hormones this occurs by promotion of protein synthesis. The proteins involved include a water-filled Na^+ channel which aids entry of Na^+ from tubular fluid into the epithelial cell and the Na^+/K^+ ATPase (sodium pump) which promotes movement of Na^+ out of the cell at the basolateral side. Production of a water-filled K^+ channel in the luminal membrane, the route by which K^+ ions enter the tubular fluid for subsequent excretion, is also promoted by aldosterone.

In term neonates the changes in aldosterone production broadly mirror the changes in the renin-angiotensin system described above. In very premature neonates the secretion of aldosterone is low compared with that in a term neonate and the tubule epithelial cells are less responsive to aldosterone.

Natriuretic peptides

The family of atrial natriuretic peptides are primarily involved in the regulation of blood volume. Atrial natriuretic peptide (ANP) was first isolated from cardiac muscle cells in the atria of the heart. An increase in blood volume in the venous system stretches the atria and provides the trigger for ANP release. The actions of ANP are to suppress the actions of aldosterone, to increase GFR and to have a peripheral vasodilator action. The resulting effect is an increase in sodium excretion. The natriuretic peptide family now includes brain natriuretic peptide (BNP), first isolated from the hypothalamus although the gene is not exclusively expressed there, and C-type peptide (CNP).

The circulatory changes at birth (*see* Chapter 5, page 121) with decreased pulmonary vascular resistance mean that there is an increase in the return of blood to the left atrium. ANP levels are increased for 2 or 3 days after birth, a time of post-birth diuresis.

Role of the kidney in acid-base balance

Fundamental aspects of acid-base balance are described earlier (*see* Chapter 4, page 112). The roles of the renal tubular mechanisms in this area can be summarised as follows:

▶ reabsorption of filtered bicarbonate, mainly in the proximal tubule
▶ acidification of the tubular fluid in the latter part of the collecting duct to achieve excretion of 'metabolic acid' (*see* page 112)
▶ generation of bicarbonate to support the bicarbonate buffer mechanism (*see* page 113).

Roles two and three on this list are tightly linked. Every time an H^+ ion is pumped into the urine, a new HCO_3^- ion is generated and this enters the bloodstream. The H^+ and HCO_3^- ions are generated inside the tubule epithelial cells from the combination of CO_2 and water, making carbonic acid (H_2CO_3), a reaction which is promoted by the intracellular enzyme carbonic anhydrase. Dissociation of the carbonic acid produces an H^+ ion which can be moved by an ATP-driven proton pump into the tubular fluid. In urine, the H^+ ions are buffered either by the phosphate buffer or by combination with ammonia (NH_3), produced by the tubular epithelial cells, to form ammonium ion (NH_4^+). An increase in $[CO_2]$ in the epithelial cells, as occurs in respiratory acidosis, will mean more H^+ is generated to excrete from the body in urine. This is the basis for renal compensation for a respiratory acidosis. The HCO_3^- ion, which is formed from carbonic acid along with the H^+ ion, enters the circulatory system.

Hyperventilation is a feature of the maternal changes which occur during pregnancy. The consequent respiratory alkalosis is compensated for by incomplete renal reabsorption of filtered HCO_3^-. The low $[CO_2]$ in body fluids will mean that less H^+ is generated in the epithelial cells for transport into the urine and so more H^+ is retained in the body. A compensatory metabolic acidosis therefore occurs in response to the hyperventilation-induced respiratory alkalosis.

In neonates, plasma $[HCO_3^-]$ and plasma pH are lower than in mature individuals. This is a consequence of a reduced ability to reabsorb filtered HCO_3^-. The more immature a baby is, the lower the plasma $[HCO_3^-]$ is likely to be. The ability to excrete an acid load increases with both gestational and post-natal age. Failure of the mechanisms described above leads to a 'renal tubular acidosis'.

TUBULAR SECRETION

Tubular secretion of organic compounds, particularly drugs, occurs in the proximal tubule. Many drugs circulate in blood in a protein-bound form and thus excretion via the kidneys would be limited by the characteristics of glomerular filtration.

The secretion mechanisms in the proximal tubule are broadly divided into two groups on the basis of the charge carried by the drugs they transport. Anionic drugs, which carry a net negative charge, include penicillins and furosemide. Cationic drugs, with a net positive charge, include quinidine and tetracycline. The renal handling of drugs will be affected by the pH of urine as this will alter the charge carried by molecules.

REFERENCES

Blackburn S. *Maternal, Fetal and Neonatal Physiology.* 3rd ed. St Louis: Saunders; 2007.

Field M, Pollock C, Harris D. *The Renal System.* Edinburgh: Churchill Livingstone; 2001.

Lissauer T, Fanaroff A. *Neonatology at a Glance.* Oxford: Blackwell; 2006.

Polin R, Fox W, Abman S. *Fetal and Neonatal Physiology.* 3rd ed. Philadelphia: Saunders; 2003.

Rennke H, Denker B. *Renal Pathophysiology.* 2nd ed. Philadelphia: Lippincott, Williams & Wilkins; 2007.

CHAPTER 7

The respiratory system

Alan Noble

CONTENTS

INTRODUCTION

The major functions of the respiratory system can be summarised as follows:

▶ Delivery of oxygen into the circulation for transport to the tissues in order to support oxidative metabolism. There are limitations on this process imposed by the relatively poor solubility of oxygen in water (*see* page 95).

▶ Excretion of carbon dioxide generated in tissues. Failure to achieve an adequate performance in this area results in potentially critical disturbances in acid-base balance (*see* page 112).

For the fetus, delivery of oxygen and removal of carbon dioxide are functions provided by the placenta. Although the fetus makes some breathing-like movements from as early as 10 weeks' gestation, the lungs are unventilated and still filled with fluid. Clamping the umbilical cord after birth separates the baby from the placenta. What triggers the first air breath is not well understood but it is thought that the rise in pCO_2 and fall in pO_2 as a result of the loss of placental function at birth are important.

CARRIAGE OF GASES IN BLOOD
Carriage of oxygen in blood

A consequence of the poor solubility of oxygen in water is that we have evolved with an oxygen-carrying pigment, haemoglobin. A haemoglobin (Hb) molecule has four sub-units, each of which can bind one oxygen molecule (O_2). Each sub-unit has a haem moiety surrounded by a peptide chain, globin. Haem is a porphyrin with an atom of iron in the Fe^{++} (ferrous) oxidation state at the centre of the porphyrin ring. The oxygen molecule (O_2) binds to the iron in an oxygenation (not an oxidation) reaction. If the iron atom in haem does become oxidised to the Fe^{+++} (ferric) oxidation state, it cannot carry oxygen and is called methaemoglobin. Small amounts of methaemoglobin are formed quite naturally and are reduced back to normal haemoglobin, with the iron in the Fe^{++} state, under the influence of a methaemoglobin reductase enzyme. Larger than normal amounts of methaemoglobin may be formed as a result of a genetically determined deficiency of the reductase enzyme. Exposure to some drugs such as nitrates and nitrites (as well as the gas nitric oxide) will also lead to excessive methaemoglobin formation. This is a potential cause of cyanosis (*see* page 162). Treatment is by the use of a physiologically acceptable reducing agent, methylene blue.

The structures of the globin peptide chains change from embryonic to fetal to adult configurations as development proceeds and this influences the affinity of haemoglobin to bind oxygen. Embryonic haemoglobin synthesis starts very early in gestation, at about 14 days. Fetal haemoglobin (HbF) is the predominant form from about 10–12 weeks of gestation. The main adult form of haemoglobin (HbA) starts to appear in relatively small amounts after only 6–8 weeks' gestation but increases rapidly after 16–18 weeks' gestation. HbF levels reach a peak at 30–32 weeks' gestation and subsequently the levels start to decline. At term, HbF represents 50% to 80% of total Hb. Almost all of the remaining 20% to 50% of Hb is in the main adult (HbA) form. The relative amounts of HbF and HbA present relate to post-conceptional age rather than post-birth age. Preterm infants therefore tend to have a higher percentage of HbF than term infants. Bilirubin is formed from the turnover of haem moieties from Hb. Increased turnover of red cells containing HbF and their replacement with cells containing HbA after birth is associated with post-natal jaundice.

Structurally, the difference between the forms of Hb relates to the globin chains. The main form of adult Hb has two α-chains and 2 β-chains. Although the main adult Hb normally predominates, about 5% to 10% of normal Hb exists with other structures. The most common of these is HbA_2 in which the β-chains are replaced by a different globin chain. There are a great many other genetically determined variations in globin chain structure, many of which are totally harmless and may never be identified in an individual. Others, which do produce symptoms, include the thalassaemias and sickle cell Hb. Variations in globin structure are the most numerous genetic variants of any protein in the body. Fetal Hb (HbF) has 2 α-chains and 2 γ-chains. Production of this form of Hb persists throughout life and remains at a level of 1% to 2% of total Hb.

The affinity of adult haemoglobin to bind oxygen is influenced by metabolic conditions within the red blood cell. This can be illustrated on an oxygen-haemoglobin dissociation curve (*see* Figure 7.1).

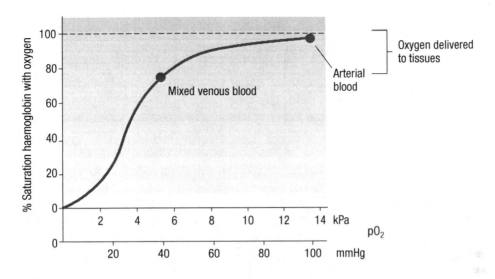

FIGURE 7.1 Oxygen-haemoglobin dissociation curve

Source: Noble A, Johnson RA, Thomas A *et al*. *The Cardiovascular System*. Elsevier Health Sciences; 2005.

The sigmoid curve describes the relationship between pO_2 and the percentage saturation of Hb with O_2. The most important factor which modifies the affinity of Hb to bind oxygen is 2,3 diphosphoglyceric acid (DPG). This is formed inside red cells and reduces the affinity of HbA to bind oxygen by binding to the β-chains of Hb thereby stabilising the deoxygenated form of haemoglobin. At first sight this seems to be an adverse effect but the pO_2 in the normal lung is high enough to almost saturate Hb with O_2 as shown by the flat top on the oxygen Hb dissociation curve. The presence of raised $[H^+]$ or [DPG] inside the red cell does not significantly affect the loading of oxygen to Hb in the lungs. An increase in $[H^+]$ also affects the shape of the haemoglobin molecule and reduces the affinity of Hb to bind oxygen. However, the effect of raised $[H^+]$ is to promote the release of O_2 from oxygenated Hb and increase the delivery of oxygen to the tissues. This is called the ***Bohr effect*** or ***Bohr shift***. Similarly, increased [DPG] promotes O_2 delivery into the tissues as, at any given pO_2 in the tissues, Hb is less saturated with O_2 in the presence of DPG than without it. The extra oxygen has escaped from binding to Hb and is delivered into the tissues. The effect of DPG is critical in ensuring that the placenta functions as a gas-exchange organ (*see* below).

Saturated Hb has four O_2 molecules bound to it, one on the haem of each of the four sub-units. The affinity of Hb to bind oxygen can be quantified as the P_{50} value. This is the partial pressure of oxygen at which the Hb is 50% saturated with oxygen. A typical P_{50} value for adult Hb is 3.5 kPa (26 mmHg). If the affinity of Hb to bind oxygen decreases under the influence of DPG or increased $[H^+]$, the dissociation curve shifts to the right, the P_{50} value increases and more oxygen is delivered into the tissues. Correspondingly, if the affinity of Hb to bind oxygen increases, the dissociation curve shifts to the left, the P_{50} value decreases and less oxygen is delivered into the tissues.

The [DPG] inside red cells at term birth is often similar to that of adults. The amount of DPG may fall in the first week after birth but levels are re-established in the next 2 to 3 weeks. Preterm infants may have reduced DPG levels and hence a lower P_{50} value. This will impair oxygen delivery into the tissues.

A key functional significance of structural difference between HbA and HbF is that DPG does not bind to HbF because it has γ-chains instead of β-chains. The differing shape of these peptide chains prohibits binding of DPG. The absence of an effect of DPG means that the HbF on the fetal side of the placenta has a stronger affinity to bind oxygen than the maternal HbA. This effect is magnified by an increase in maternal DPG production during pregnancy. The maternal Hb P_{50} value typically increases from 3.5 kPa to 4.0 kPa by term. These changes are important for the placenta to function adequately to deliver oxygen into the fetus.

Loading of oxygen into blood in the lungs occurs by diffusion, as illustrated in Figure 7.2.

This figure shows the interface between an alveolus and a pulmonary capillary. Blood returning to the lungs has a low pO_2 (typically $pO_2 = 5.3$ kPa) and, in a mature

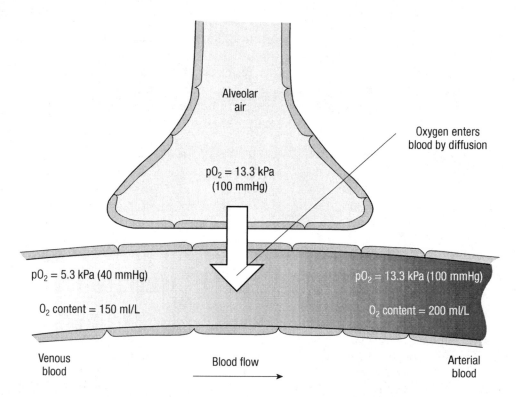

FIGURE 7.2 Loading of oxygen by diffusion from an alveolus into a pulmonary capillary

Source: Noble A *et al.*, op. cit.

lung, the alveolar $pO_2 = 13.3$ kPa (100 mmHg). Oxygen diffuses into the plasma and then across the red-cell membrane to bind to Hb. The transit time at rest for a red cell through a pulmonary capillary is about one second but, normally, complete equilibration takes place in only about a quarter of this time. The extra time available if necessary is one of the safety factors in lung function. Typical values for pCO_2 are, in venous blood $pCO_2 = 6.1$ kPa (46 mmHg), and in arterial blood leaving the lungs $pCO_2 = 5.3$ kPa (40 mmHg). The diffusive gradient to load O_2 into blood at the lungs (8 kPa) is therefore ten times greater than the diffusive gradient for unloading CO_2 (0.8 kPa). However, as CO_2 is about 20 times as soluble in water as O_2 it diffuses much more easily than O_2. These two factors, diffusive gradient and solubility, approximately cancel each other out so that, in the normal lung, exchange of the two gases occurs at an equivalent rate.

At the tissues, oxygen is utilised inside the mitochondria and there is a continuous diffusive gradient between the arterial blood entering a tissue ($pO_2 = 13.3$ kPa) and the inside of a mitochondrion ($pO_2 = 0.1$ kPa) (*see* Figure 7.3).

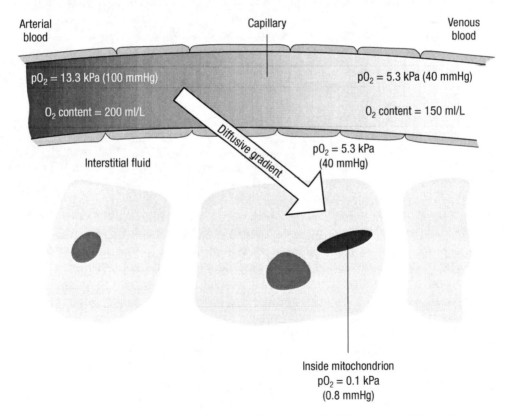

FIGURE 7.3 Delivery of oxygen down a diffusive gradient from arterial blood into a mitochondrion

Blood leaving the tissue, as venous blood, has equilibrated with the interstitial fluid just outside the blood vessel and so has the same pO_2.

Source: Noble A *et al.*, op. cit.

The interstitial fluid outside the cell is part of the way down the diffusive gradient with, typically, a $pO_2 = 5.3$ kPa (40 mmHg). The interstitial fluid is the last compartment that the blood equilibrates with before leaving the tissue as venous blood. Venous pO_2 for that tissue is therefore going to be the same as interstitial fluid pO_2. If a tissue becomes more metabolically active the oxygen will be consumed more quickly, the interstitial fluid pO_2 will therefore be lower and the venous pO_2 will also be lower as oxygen will diffuse more quickly into the mitochondrion.

Figures quoted for venous blood pO_2 usually represent mixed venous blood, the form in the right side of the heart which is an average for all the venous drainages for all tissues. The oxygen extraction is not the same for all tissues of the body. Heart muscle, for example, extracts about 75% of the oxygen in coronary artery blood even at rest. For the kidneys only about 10% of the renal artery oxygen content is used.

Hypoxaemia

Hypoxaemia is a term which specifically refers to low arterial pO_2. It does not necessarily directly relate to the oxygen content of blood because that is also determined by the haemoglobin content. Tissue hypoxia, poor oxygenation, may be a consequence of hypoxaemia or anaemia but poor perfusion of a tissue can also lead to tissue hypoxia. The limited amount of blood which does reach the tissue in this case could have a normal pO_2.

There are fundamentally five different mechanisms which can lead to hypoxaemia:

▶ *Low inspired pO_2*. In mature individuals this occurs at altitude. In the fetus poor delivery of oxygen from the placenta would be equivalent.

▶ *Underventilation of the lungs*. This, in an air-breathing individual, would mean that alveolar pO_2 is low, leading to low arterial pO_2. This form of hypoxaemia would be accompanied by raised arterial pCO_2.

▶ *Ventilation perfusion (V/Q) mismatch* (*see* below).

▶ *Extra-pulmonary shunt*. This means that some of the blood in the pulmonary artery does not go through gas exchange areas of the lung. This exists to a minor extent quite normally with the blood supply to structures such as the trachea. A more dramatic extra-pulmonary shunt would be a right-to-left shunt in the heart. The blood bypasses the alveoli. In a left-to-right shunt, some of the blood does an extra circuit through the lungs and so this is not a cause of hypoxaemia.

▶ *Alveolar to pulmonary capillary diffusion block*. This mechanism theoretically can exist in situations such as pulmonary oedema or fibrotic changes in the lung. It is difficult to envisage a situation in which diffusion of oxygen is significantly affected by a diffusion block but exchange of CO_2 is not. Hypoxaemia due to a V/Q mismatch is often wrongly attributed to a diffusion block mechanism.

Ventilation perfusion (V/Q) mismatch

The lung functions ideally as a gas exchange organ when the distribution of alveolar ventilation (V) and blood flow to alveoli (Q – standing for quantity of blood) are evenly matched. As most of the oxygen carried in blood is bound to Hb and, under normal functional conditions, the arterial blood is already 97–98% saturated with oxygen, a further increase in lung ventilation would have only a very minor effect on the amount of oxygen carried in arterial blood.

Let us consider a theoretical situation in which half of the lung is perfused but not ventilated and all the ventilation of the lung passes to the other half of the lung which is also perfused. Total ventilation and total perfusion of the lung are therefore both normal. Blood emerging from the over-ventilated side of the lung will only contain a small additional amount of oxygen because the blood is almost fully saturated with oxygen under normal ventilation conditions. Blood emerging from the unventilated part of the lung will have the same oxygen content and pO_2 as the venous blood entering that side of the lung. If we mix equal amounts of the over-ventilated and unventilated blood samples, we can work out an average value for the percentage saturation of the final blood sample with oxygen. Taking this percentage saturation back to an oxygen–Hb dissociation curve, we can read off the pO_2 expected from this blood sample. Because of the shape of the dissociation curve and because the relationship between percentage saturation and pO_2 is not linear, we find that the pO_2 of the blood in the pulmonary vein produced by mixing the blood from the under-ventilated and over-ventilated sides of the lung is much closer to that of the under-ventilated side of the lung than to that of the over-ventilated side. This is the basis for V/Q mismatch as a cause of hypoxaemia.

Although V/Q mismatch is a cause of hypoxaemia, it is not necessarily a cause of raised arterial pCO_2 (hypercapnia). There are two fundamental reasons for this. The first is that CO_2 carriage mechanisms in blood (see below) do not reach saturation levels and effectively the CO_2 dissociation curve, a graph of blood CO_2 content on the vertical axis and pCO_2 on the horizontal axis, is almost linear. The consequence of this is that in over-ventilated alveoli, extra CO_2 is unloaded into the alveoli. The second factor is that the main chemical drive to lung ventilation is CO_2 (see page 163). If arterial pCO_2 tends to rise as a result of V/Q mismatch, then overall lung ventilation will increase until the arterial pCO_2 returns to normal.

Uneven distribution of pulmonary blood flow is a common cause of V/Q mismatch hypoxaemia. In a normal individual this is a consequence of the effects of gravity on the lung. Both perfusion and ventilation of alveoli increase moving down the lung from the top to the basal parts of the lung. The gravity-induced effects on perfusion are more marked than the effects on ventilation. The upshot is that at the top of the lungs in an upright individual, the V/Q ratio is higher than ideal (too much ventilation for the blood flow) and at the base of the lungs the V/Q ratio is lower than is ideal (too little ventilation relative to the blood flow).

In areas of the lung which are under-ventilated and the pO_2 is low, another pulmonary safety factor becomes operative. In contrast to the rest of the body, hypoxia within regions of the lungs leads to pulmonary arteriolar vasoconstriction. This hypoxic vasoconstriction means that blood flow is diverted to other regions of the lung which are better ventilated.

Cyanosis

The term *cyanosis* refers to the blue colouration of the skin and mucous membranes produced by the presence of excessive amounts of deoxygenated Hb in arterial blood. Cyanosis can be classified into two types, as follows:

▶ *Central cyanosis*, generated by failure of the heart and lungs as a unit to ensure adequate oxygenation of arterial blood. This can be seen in warm, well-perfused areas such as the inside of the mouth.

▶ *Peripheral cyanosis* is visible in extremities such as fingers and ears and is produced by excessive extraction of the available oxygen from an impaired local blood flow. This may be caused by excessive vasoconstriction in response to, for example, a cold environment.

It is important to recognise the distinction between the terms cyanosis, hypoxia and anaemia. The affinity of Hb to bind oxygen increases progressively as the first, second and third oxygen molecules out of a total of four bind onto Hb. The effect of this is that, in a blood sample which is 50% saturated with O_2, half of the Hb molecules are fully saturated with four O_2 molecules bound, and half have no O_2 bound. There will only be trace amounts of intermediate forms between the fully saturated and unsaturated forms of Hb. Fifty per cent saturation does not mean that each Hb molecule has two O_2 molecules bound.

Cyanosis is produced when the amount of deoxygenated Hb exceeds a certain level. A common textbook definition for this 'certain level' is more than 5 g deoxygenated Hb per 100 mL blood but there is no internationally agreed standard definition. The anaemic patient with a total blood [Hb] of, for example, 7 g Hb per 100 mL blood can survive if all of the Hb is fully oxygenated in arterial blood. They may well have tissue hypoxia but could not be centrally cyanosed. There is insufficient total Hb available to support life if 5 g Hb per 100 mL blood is in the deoxygenated form. In contrast, the subject with [Hb] = 15 g per 100 mL blood could be centrally cyanosed and still have 10 g Hb per 100 mL blood which is fully saturated with oxygen.

Carriage of carbon dioxide in blood

Carbon dioxide is carried in the blood in three forms:

▶ *Dissolved CO_2*. The amount of CO_2 in solution at a given body temperature is directly proportional to the pCO_2. This is typically about 5% of arterial CO_2 carriage.

▶ *As bicarbonate (HCO_3^-)* formed inside the red cell, a reaction promoted by the enzyme carbonic anhydrase. The HCO_3^- diffuses out across the red-cell membrane in exchange for inward movement of Cl^- ions. This is called *the chloride shift*. Carriage of CO_2 as bicarbonate is quantitatively the dominant form of CO_2 carriage, typically about 90%.

▶ *As carbamino compounds*. This is a labile form of reaction between CO_2 and amine groups on proteins. This form of CO_2 is relatively easily given up when blood reaches the lungs. It accounts for only about 5% of CO_2 carriage normally but contributes about 27% of the CO_2 exhaled at the lungs.

Most of the CO_2 carried in blood continues to circulate. In a resting textbook adult, the following figures are appropriate. Arterial blood contains about 480 mL CO_2 per litre blood. During passage through the tissues, 40 mL CO_2 is added to each litre making a total of 520 mL CO_2 per litre blood. At the lungs, 40 mL CO_2 is unloaded from each litre, only about 8% of the total CO_2 carried. The recirculation of CO_2 is an important aspect of acid-base regulation (*see* page 112).

RESPIRATORY CONTROL MECHANISMS

Chemoreceptor function

The primary chemical controls on lung ventilation work by monitoring CO_2 as $[H^+]$ not [oxygen]. Blood in the pulmonary capillaries equilibrates with the pCO_2 in the alveoli. If tight regulation of acid-base balance is to be achieved, then the amount of CO_2 being generated metabolically and delivered into the alveoli must be diluted in an appropriate volume of alveolar gas to achieve an alveolar pCO_2 of close to 5 kPa (40 mmHg). An illustration of how this might be achieved in a textbook person is shown below. Equivalent calculations for a neonate would produce the same end result but correspondingly smaller volumes would be involved.

Typical textbook adult figures:

CO_2 production rate at rest $= 200$ mL/min
Alveolar ventilation rate at rest $= 4000$ mL/min

Assuming all of the CO_2 in the alveolus has come from the tissues, then 200/4000, i.e. one-twentieth of all the gas in the alveoli is CO_2.

If the atmospheric pressure, and therefore intra-alveolar pressure, is 100 kPa, then the alveolar pCO_2 is 5 kPa (one-twentieth of 100 kPa).

An appropriate alveolar ventilation rate is maintained to keep the arterial pCO_2 constant despite variations in CO_2 production, because blood leaving the lungs and becoming arterial blood is monitored via two sets of chemoreceptors.

▶ *Central chemoreceptors* located on the ventral surface of the medulla.
▶ *Peripheral chemoreceptors* located in the carotid and aortic bodies.

Central chemoreceptors

The central chemoreceptors do not directly monitor the $[CO_2]$ of the blood but actually the $[H^+]$ of the extracellular fluid surrounding the brain. CO_2 can diffuse out of cerebral capillaries and into the cerebro-spinal fluid (CSF). Here, CO_2 dissolved in water will form H^+ as shown below.

$$CO_2 + H_2O \leftrightarrow H_2CO_3 \leftrightarrow H^+ + HCO_3^-$$

The H^+ receptor on the brain actually detects $[H^+]$ changes in the CSF but effectively functions to monitor plasma $[CO_2]$. The cerebral capillaries are almost impermeable to H^+ and any other non lipid-soluble chemical. This concept is known as the blood-brain barrier. The changes in H^+ detected by the central chemoreceptor have therefore derived from changes in CO_2 in blood, not H^+ ions in blood. A further aspect which increases the sensitivity of the central chemoreceptor is that the protein concentration in CSF is very low, especially compared with plasma. In addition, there is no Hb in CSF. Proteins are effective buffers (*see* page 115). A given $[CO_2]$ will therefore generate a bigger change in $[H^+]$ in the CSF than the same amount of CO_2 in blood, because the H^+ ions are not so readily removed by binding to buffers. Information from the central chemoreceptor mechanism passes to the respiratory control centres in the brain (*see* below).

In term infants, the functioning of the central chemoreceptor mechanism is similar to that in adults but preterm infants may take four weeks to achieve this level of function. However, the ability of a term neonate to increase lung ventilation is already limited to only 3–4 times the baseline level compared with the up to twentyfold increases which are possible in adults. There is a resetting of the appropriate 'set-point' for pCO_2 in the first month of life. This may be attributable to the fact that fetal blood pCO_2 at about 6 kPa to 6.5 kPa is higher than the desired pCO_2 after the initial neonatal period (4.8 kPa to 6.1 kPa).

Peripheral chemoreceptors

The peripheral chemoreceptors, the aortic bodies and carotid bodies primarily respond to low pO_2 in arterial blood. They are also responsive to increases in pCO_2 and changes in pH but the main effect here is to make the chemoreceptors more sensitive to low pO_2. Under normal circumstances, pO_2 levels detected by the peripheral chemoreceptors have a very small role to play in overall respiratory control. However, hypoxaemia exerts an increasingly positive effect on lung ventilation as the pO_2 falls.

The fetus grows under relatively hypoxic conditions compared with the neonate. The fetal arterial pO_2 of about 3.3 kPa (25 mmHg) increases to about 9.3 kPa (70 mmHg) in the first few hours after birth. As the fetal peripheral chemoreceptors have adjusted to a low pO_2, they are not very responsive to changes in the relatively high arterial pO_2 in the neonatal period. A re-setting of the response occurs, however, and the peripheral chemoreceptors subsequently become increasingly sensitive to changes in arterial pO_2.

Brain centres controlling lung ventilation

The respiratory control area of the brain has three main components:
▶ *Medullary centre* which is where the basic rhythm is generated.
▶ *Apneustic centre* in the pons which is responsible for terminating inspiration.
▶ *Pneumotaxic centre* in the pons which is responsible for switching from inspiration to expiration.

The apneustic and pneumotaxic centres therefore modulate the activity of the medullary centre. The temptation to refer to these brain structures collectively as the 'respiratory centre' should be resisted as this name implies an anatomically and functionally discrete entity. This is misleading.

As noted above, in the medulla of the brainstem there are groups of neurons which generate a basic respiratory rhythm. There is still a great deal which is unknown concerning the precise location and the mechanism of action of these neural pathways. Superimposed on the activity of the basic rhythm generator there are inputs from various other structures, including the chemoreceptors already described, which generate an appropriate response to metabolic demands in situations such as exercise. Other inputs allow the moderations of respiratory control which facilitate speech and swallowing.

Muscle spindles in the intercostal muscles of the rib cage provide information concerning the volume of the thorax to the respiratory control neurons. There is relatively little contribution to the input of information from receptors in the diaphragm. Receptors in the large airways include stretch receptors and irritant receptors. The stretch receptors detect lung inflation and this input to the medulla helps to terminate inspiration. The irritant receptors in the mucosal lining of the airways are particularly sensitive to mechanical stimulation and will reflexly generate a cough response. This is typically seen in neonates over 35 weeks' gestation but not in younger infants.

Breathing must be inhibited during swallowing of food or drink. This is achieved by an upward movement of the soft palate accompanied by contraction of the upper pharyngeal muscles. The laryngeal muscles also contract, closing the glottis. Entry of food into the airways is therefore prevented and this is assisted by an expiration following swallowing. This helps to clear any particles of food which remain around the glottis. These responses are co-ordinated from the medulla and rely on sensory information deriving from the presence of food in the oropharynx.

PULMONARY MECHANICS
Lung ventilation
The mechanical work needed to achieve ventilation of the lungs has two components:
- ▶ *elastic forces* which have to be overcome in order to inflate the lungs
- ▶ *resistive forces* which are determined by the need to move air through the many-branched airways of the lung.

Neonates who have unusual difficulty with either of these components tend to adjust their respiratory rate to minimise the workload. Decreased lung elasticity, as in the respiratory distress syndrome (RDS), is associated with rapid shallow breathing, thus reducing the work done against the elastic elements of the alveoli by reducing the extent of their inflation. In cases where the airway resistance is increased, respiratory rate tends to be slower and deeper.

Movement of air into and out of the lung is generated by a combination of contraction of the diaphragm and contraction of the intercostal muscles of the rib cage. During forced breathing movements the accessory muscles of respiration, scalenes, sternocleidomastoids, neck and back muscles and upper respiratory tract muscles also come into use. This increases the volume of the thorax and generates a negative intrapleural pressure. In order to understand lung inflation, the mechanical properties of the lung and rib cage must be considered.

Within the thorax, the partially inflated lungs have a tendency to collapse inwards as a result of their elastic recoil. At the same time, under quiet breathing conditions, the chest wall has a tendency to recoil outwards. These two structures tending to recoil in opposite directions leave a negative pressure in the pleural 'cavity' between the lungs and the chest wall. The 'pleural cavity' is in reality a small volume of slimy fluid rather than a significant empty space. The role of the fluid is to lubricate between the visceral and parietal pleura which cover the lungs and line the inside of the chest wall.

The recoil properties of the neonate chest are rather different from those of mature individuals. In order to pass through the birth canal without fractures occurring, the chest wall must be quite flexible. The soft rib cage cartilage also aids the progress of future growth of the chest wall. The compliance of the chest, effectively the ease with which the chest can be inflated, is high. This means, firstly, that the generation of a negative pressure in the pleural cavity is relatively limited, but also that there is a tendency for the chest wall to collapse under the influence of any negative pleural pressure generated as part of inspiratory movements. The outward elastic recoil of the chest increases during the first two weeks of extra-uterine life but remains less than in an adult for a considerable period of time.

The high compliance characteristic of the neonatal chest wall is a limitation on the size of the tidal volume (TV) that can be generated as increasing TV requires a more negative-intrapleural pressure to be achieved. The other factor determining pleural pressure, the inward recoil of the lung, may also be compromised, especially in preterm infants who may have reduced lung compliance as a result of RDS. This necessitates more rigorous inspiratory muscle movement in order to expand the poorly compliant lungs.

At the end of a normal expiration, the volume of air in the lungs is called the functional residual capacity (FRC). If a pair of lungs was isolated from the chest and allowed to recoil down to a minimum volume, this is the residual volume (RV), the same as the volume of gas left inside the lungs after a maximum expiration. The volume of air beyond FRC that can be emptied from the lungs during a forced expiration is called the expiratory reserve volume (ERV). Starting from a maximum end-expiration position (RV) the total amount of air that can be taken into the lungs is the VC. When a maximum inspiration has been achieved, the volume of air contained in the lungs is the total lung capacity (TLC). The TLC therefore includes the maximum amount of air that can be moved in and out of the lungs, the VC, plus the air which remains in the lungs after a maximum expiration, the RV.

The relative, as well as the absolute, sizes of these gas volumes differ between term neonates and adults. TLC is typically 63 mL/kg body weight (BW) in infants and 82 mL/kg BW in adults. The RV in infants at 23 mL/kg BW, 37% of TLC, is greater than the 16 mL/kg BW, 20% of TLC which is typical in adults.

Viewed in isolation, the effect of expanding the volume of the thorax would be to make the intrapleural pressure more negative. The pressure inside the lungs at quiet end-expiration; that is, at FRC, would be the same as the atmospheric pressure. This is more positive than pleural pressure. During inspiration the lungs will be inflated until a new balance is reached between the increased elastic recoil of the inflated lung and the pressure gradient across the alveolar wall. The intra-alveolar pressure at end-inspiration is again the same as atmospheric pressure. The volume of air which enters the lung during a quiet inspiration is the TV.

Why should increasing the volume of the lung lead to an increase in elastic recoil? This is a property of any distensible (inflatable) structure. The law of Laplace for a given structure states that tension in the wall of the structure is proportional to the radius of the structure multiplied by the pressure gradient. Tension is the force which is tending to collapse the structure, i.e. the elastic recoil.

It is well known from childhood toys that it is impossible to produce air bubbles with pure water. This is because of the surface tension between the water molecules would immediately collapse a water bubble. If a detergent is introduced into the water it separates the water molecules, reduces the surface tension and therefore the elastic recoil of a bubble and allows a 'soap bubble' to be produced.

Within the lungs, surfactant plays the same role as the detergent in the soap-bubble game. Surfactant reduces the tendency of the alveoli to collapse at low lung volumes and also permits easier inflation of the lung. At low lung volumes surfactant molecules are in the form of a folded surface film. As the lung volume increases during inspiration the surfactant molecules become stretched and contribute to an increase in elastic recoil. This is important because quiet expiration is a passive process which relies on elastic recoil. Loss of elastic recoil of the alveoli, as in the adult smoking-related disorder emphysema, means that inflation of the lungs occurs easily but expiration is compromised. A change which helps to re-establish adequate elastic recoil in this situation is hyperinflation of the chest. Remember, from the law of Laplace tension in the wall of the alveoli is proportional to the pressure gradient multiplied by the radius. Increasing the volume of the chest therefore helps to increase tension in the wall of the alveoli and generate sufficient elastic recoil for expiration.

Alveoli will collapse if the pressure outside the alveoli is greater than the pressure inside. Despite the role of surfactant helping to keep them open, there is still a tendency for alveoli to collapse at low lung volumes. This occurs particularly at the base of the lungs. This is because the effect of gravity on the lungs means that the alveoli at the base of the lung are compressed by the lung tissue above them. This also has the effect of reducing the negative pressure in the 'pleural cavity' because the lung is pushed into this space. The 'closing volume' of the lungs is literally the lung volume at which alveolar closure occurs. In mature individuals below the age of about 40, closure of the alveoli occurs at lung volumes lower than FRC and so it is not a problem in normal quiet breathing. In children younger than 6 or adults older than 40, the closing volume may come above FRC due to low elastic recoil of the alveoli. This concept is important in relation to the protocols used for artificially ventilating neonates. Airways can be kept open by maintaining a positive airway pressure throughout the ventilator cycle.

Surfactant deficiency in the RDS in neonates is related to gestational age and the maturity of developing lungs. The effect is that the volume of air entering the lungs for a given alveolus to intrapleural space pressure gradient is markedly reduced. Any disease mechanism which leads to a decrease in surfactant synthesis, such as asphyxia or pulmonary oedema, will lead to problems both inflating and deflating the lungs.

Airway resistance

Resistance to air movement through the non-gas exchange airways is also a factor determining the mechanical effort needed to ensure successful inspiration and expiration. This is partly determined by airway diameter but also by whether gas flow follows a laminar or a turbulent flow pattern.

Airway resistance in a term infant is about 16 times greater than in an adult fundamentally because the airway diameter is much smaller. Resistance to fluid flow, including air flow, is not directly proportional to the radius of the tube but to the fourth power of the radius. This was worked out by the French physician Poiseuille in 1846. Small tubes therefore pose a disproportionately high resistance to air flow. Until a child is 5 years old the small peripheral airways contribute 50% of the total resistance to air movement. In an adult only 20% of the total resistance comes from this source. Bronchoconstriction which increases resistance can occur in response to a wide range of irritants.

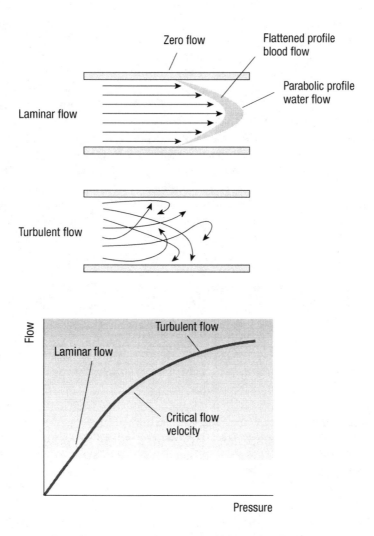

FIGURE 7.4 Laminar and turbulent flow shown here in relation to blood flow but the same principles apply to gas flow in airways

Source: Noble A *et al.*, op. cit.

Among the assumptions behind Poiseuille's law is that fluid (air) flow is laminar. In laminar flow, the particles in the gas flow parallel to the wall of the tube with the fastest moving molecules at the centre of the tube and, theoretically at least, the molecules next to the wall of the tube remaining stationary. Laminar flow, also called streamline flow, is essentially silent (*see* Figure 7.4). Air flow is directly proportional to the pressure gradient between two points.

When turbulent flow occurs, the molecules in the gas are not flowing parallel to the wall of the tube but in a much more random fashion with local vortices occurring. Turbulent flow is more likely to occur in large tubes than in small tubes and where the velocity of flow is high. Thus, turbulence may occur in large airways such as the bronchi and trachea. Turbulent flow is noisy flow which can be heard using a stethoscope to listen to the flow murmurs, known as wheezes.

REFERENCES

Blackburn S. *Maternal, Fetal and Neonatal Physiology.* 3rd ed. St Louis: Saunders; 2007.

Davies A, Moores C. *The Respiratory System.* Edinburgh: Churchill Livingstone; 2003.

Lissauer T, Fanaroff A. *Neonatology at a Glance.* Oxford: Blackwell; 2006.

Polin R, Fox W, Abman S. *Fetal and Neonatal Physiology.* 3rd ed. Philadelphia: Saunders; 2003.

Schwartzstein R, Parker M. *Respiratory Physiology.* Philadelphia: Lippincott, Williams & Wilkins; 2006.

CHAPTER 8

Bacterial and transplacental infection

Mark Anthony and James Gray

CONTENTS

INTRODUCTION

The perinatal period is the highest-risk period in life for acquiring a serious bacterial infection. In almost every measured aspect, babies' immune responses are less than those of children and adults, including macrophage and neutrophil killing, cytokine responses, and antibody production. Transplacental acquisition of antibody, and antibody and macrophages from colostrum all help to counter this relative immune deficit in term babies. Preterm babies, though, receive less protective maternal antibody and have greater immune immaturity. Skin and the normal bacterial flora help defend against pathogenic bacterial invasion, but the skin barrier is often breached by intravenous lines in premature babies, and the flora is frequently abnormal due to early antibiotic selective pressure and exposure to antibiotic-resistant bacteria resident in neonatal units. For all of these reasons, babies – and especially those born premature – are vulnerable to infection.

BACTERIAL STRUCTURE AND CLASSIFICATION

Bacteria are differentiated into two broad groups by Gram's stain, named after the eighteenth-century Dane, Hans Christian Gram. Bacteria are categorised by their ability to retain colour after crystal violet staining and acetone destaining. Bacteria that retain the stain have a thick outer peptidoglycan cell wall and are referred to as Gram-positive bacteria, whereas those that lose colour and take up a pink basic fuchsin counter-stain have a thinner cell wall and are referred to as Gram-negative. Bacteria can also be differentiated by their shape into cocci or bacilli. All of the common neonatal bacterial pathogens are either Gram-positive cocci or Gram-negative bacilli, with the exception of *L. monocytogenes*, which is a Gram-positive bacillus (*see* Table 8.1).

TABLE 8.1 Common Gram-positive and Gram-negative neonatal bacterial pathogens

	Classification	Bacterial species	Commonly used antibiotics
	Gram-positive cocci causing chorioamnionitis	*Streptococcus agalactiae* (group B streptococcus)	Benzylpenicillin Cefotaxime*
	Gram-positive cocci causing late-onset sepsis	*Staphylococcus epidermidis* (coagulase negative staphylococcus) *Staphylococcus aureus* (coagulase positive staphylococcus)	Vancomycin/ Teicoplanin Flucloxacillin
		Enterococcus spp.	Vancomycin/ Teicoplanin
		Streptococcus agalactiae	Benzylpenicillin Cefotaxime*
	Gram-positive bacilli causing fetal/early-onset neonatal sepsis	*Listeria monocytogenes*	Ampicillin**
	Gram-negative bacilli causing chorioamnionitis	*Escherichia coli*	Gentamicin Cefotaxime***
	Gram-negative bacilli causing late-onset sepsis	*Escherichia coli* *Pseudomonas aeruginosa* *Klebsiella pneumoniae* *Serratia marcescens* *Enterobacter cloacae*	Gentamicin Cefotaxime*** Meropenem****

Notes:
* Cefotaxime used when meningitis is suspected or proven.
** *Listeria monocytogenes* is not sensitive to cephalosporins.
*** Cefotaxime is used with an aminoglycoside to give 'double Gram-negative cover' or when meningitis is suspected or proven.
**** Meropenem is used when an organism is resistant to aminoglycosides and/or cephalosporins.

The distinction between Gram-positive cocci and Gram-negative bacilli is an important one because Gram staining assists with early identification of the organism, and because different antibiotics are effective against these two broad categories of bacteria. Thus, Gram-stain information can direct initial antibiotic choice.

The cell walls of Gram-positive and Gram-negative bacteria differ in the quantity and cellular location of the cell wall peptidoglycan (*see* Figure 8.1). In Gram-positive bacteria, a thick layer of peptidoglycan lies outside of a single bacterial cell membrane. In this location, the enzymes that create the petidoglycan are vulnerable to attack by β-lactam and glycopeptide antibiotics. Gram-negative bacteria, in contrast, have a thin peptidoglycan cell wall that is sandwiched between inner and outer membranes. In this location the peptidoglycan matrix is hidden from immediate access by cell-wall-acting antibiotics, which must first cross the outer membrane to exert their action.

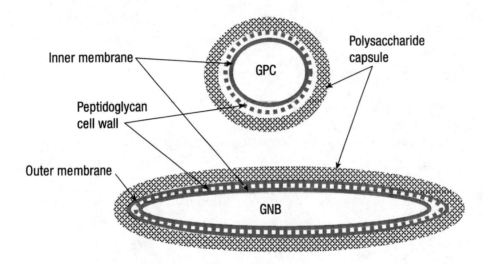

FIGURE 8.1 Bacterial cell wall composition

Streptococci explained

Streptococcal colonies when cultured on sheep blood agar produce either no haemolysis (γ-haemolytic; e.g. enterococci), green partial haemolysis resulting from the action of peroxides (α-haemolytic; e.g. *S. viridans*), or a clear zone of complete haemolysis caused by haemolysins (β-haemolytic; e.g. *S. agalactiae* or *S. pyogenes*). Rebecca Lancefield classified β-haemolytic streptococci in 1933 by antibody reactivity with cell-wall antigens (*see* Table 8.2), to give Lancefield groups A, B, C, etc. Group B streptococci (*S. agalactiae*) are further subdivided by serological responses to the polysaccharide capsule, into serotypes Ia–VIII. Microbiology laboratories will report the identity of an infecting streptococcal species firstly as Gram-positive chains visualised by microscopy, then as α-, β- or non-haemolytic. Subsequently, where appropriate, the laboratory will determine the Lancefield group and/or species, and finally it will report the antibiotic resistance profile. A β-haemolytic streptococcus causing newborn sepsis could be either *S. pyogenes* (GAS) or *S. agalactiae* (GBS); but, in this era it is likely to be GBS rather than GAS, as newborn disease and puerperal fever caused by the latter is now rare (*see* Box 8.11).

TABLE 8.2 Streptococcal classification explained

Species	Lancefield group*	Serotype**	Haemolysis
S. pyogenes	Group A (GAS)	–	β
S. agalactiae	Group B (GBS)	Ia–VIII	β
Enterococcus spp.	Group D	–	variable
Viridans streptococci	–	–	α
S. pneumoniae	–	–	α

Notes:
* Lancefield group is defined by serological responses to cell-wall antigens.
** Serotype of GBS is defined by serological responses to the capsular polysaccharide.

Diseases caused by different streptococci

▶ GAS – historical cause of puerperal fever
▶ GBS and occasionally viridans streptococci – cause ascending infection, chorioamnionitis, and early-onset sepsis
▶ Enterococci – cause late-onset sepsis, for instance via central venous lines

---

BOX 8.1 PUERPERAL FEVER

Puerperal fever is caused by locally invasive *S. pyogenes* (GAS) in which the mother develops a streptococcal tissue infection and then septicaemia, and the newborn can become secondarily infected. The pathological process is different from ascending infection caused by *S. agalactiae* (GBS).

Ignaz Semmelweiss in 1844, at the Vienna General Hospital, noted that puerperal fever, also called childbed fever, was responsible for maternal perinatal deaths. The mortality reached 16% of all women in labour in the ward training doctors, whereas the mortality was only 2% in the ward training midwifery students. Student doctors were undertaking autopsies in the morning on women who had died of puerperal fever, and then examining mothers in labour in the afternoon, and since the students were not washing their hands, GAS was passed each day to otherwise healthy women.

Semmelweiss was the first to propose hand washing with chlorinated lime to control the spread of healthcare-associated infections. Hand-washing still needs reinforcing today, over 150 years later; and lack of hand washing is responsible for the spread of virulent and multi-resistant organisms in hospitals.

Genes and genomes

Genome sequencing is the process in which the DNA code of every gene in an organism is identified, thus providing a blue-print of the genes and the proteins that are necessary for the organism to live. The larger the genome, the more adaptable is the organism (*see* Box 8.2). Gram-negative bacteria, for instance, have large genomes and can survive and multiply for long periods in the environment; whereas many Gram-positive bacteria are highly adapted to and need the environment of an animal host, for instance *S. agalactiae*. Genome-sequencing technology will ultimately lead to the development of new antibiotics and vaccines; and in the future, during outbreaks, strains will be tracked by genome sequencing of each isolate.

BOX 8.2 BACTERIA, GENES AND GENOMES

Bacterial species	Genome size*	Number of genes	Lifestyle
S. agalactiae	2.21 Mb	2094	Commensal of animals and man
S. aureus	2.83 Mb	2623	Commensal of animals and man
E. coli K12	4.63 Mb	4289	Commensal of animals and man, able to survive in the environment
K. pneumoniae	5.92 Mb	5814	Commensal of animals and man
P. aeruginosa	6.26 Mb	5565	Soil organism found in a wide variety of habitats, and part of the normal human flora

*1 Mb = 1 000 000 base pairs

Bacteria usually have a single circular chromosome, containing 2000+ genes. In general, the more genes within a chromosome, the more adaptable is the organism to living in different environments. Bacteria with smaller genomes tend to encode fewer enzymes and nutrient transporters and have less metabolic flexibility – for instance, *S. agalactiae* is highly adapted to living only within an animal host and not in the outside environment. *P. aeruginosa*, in comparison, has a large genome, lots of metabolic capability, and can live almost anywhere where there is moisture.

Bacteria may carry antibiotic resistance genes on plasmids, transposons and integrated phages – all are forms of mobile elements that can spread themselves between bacteria.

A **plasmid** is a transferable circle of DNA, usually much smaller than the genome itself, and sometimes contains genes for bacterial conjugation (the process by which plasmids are transferred from one bacterial species to another).

Transposons and phages are other forms of mobile genetic elements that can jump between bacterial species, and which often carry advantages genes such as those encoding antibiotic resistance.

ANTIBIOTIC STRUCTURE AND MECHANISMS OF ACTION

Three classes of antibiotic are predominantly used in neonatal intensive care settings: β-lactams, glycopeptides and aminoglycosides. The first class, β-lactam antibiotics, include benzylpenicillin and flucloxacillin (penicillins), cefotaxime (a cephalosporin)

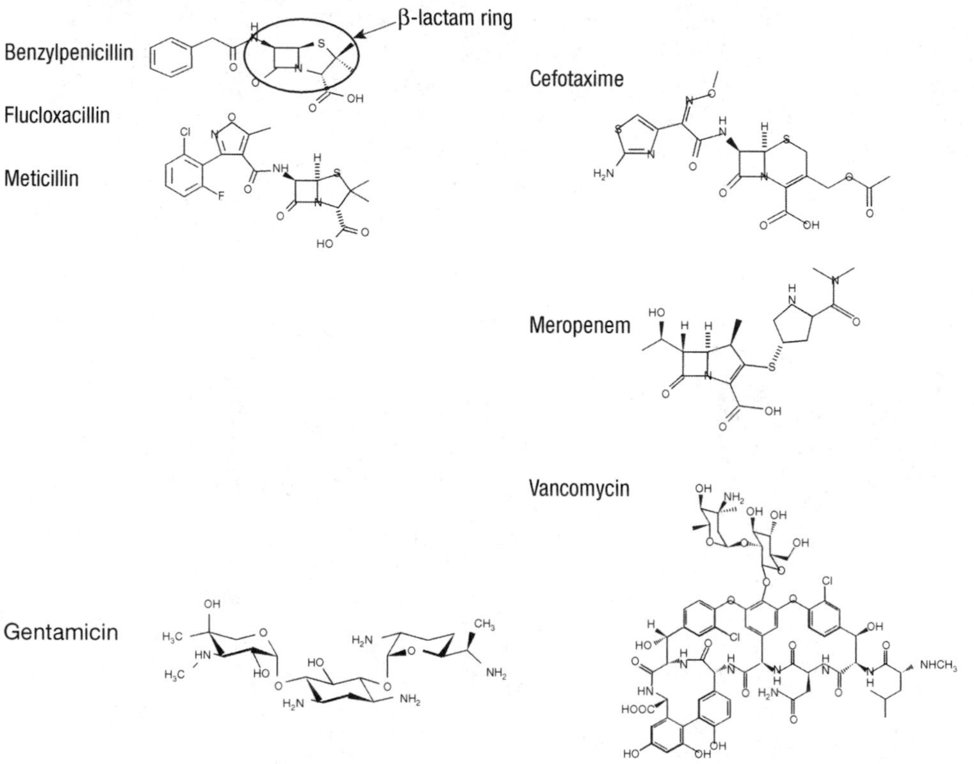

FIGURE 8.2 Antibiotic structures

and meropenem (a carbapenem – *see* Figure 8.2). Although structurally very different, they all share a common feature, a β-lactam ring that is an analogue of D-alanine-D-alanine, the dipeptide that is the building block of petidoglycan. The β-lactam ring binds to and inhibits the transpeptidase enzymes (also called penicillin-binding proteins) that are necessary for forming cross-links between peptidoglycan molecules. Disruption of the cell wall in this way causes bacterial lysis. Hence, β-lactam antibiotics are usually bactericidal (causing cell death). Group B streptococcus is universally sensitive to benzylpenicillin, and hence this antibiotic remains a good choice for first-line treatment of early-onset sepsis.

Vancomycin (*see* Figure 8.2) and teicoplanin also act on the peptidoglycan cell wall. For various reasons, including inability to reach the peptidoglycan layer in Gram-negative bacteria, glycopeptides are only active against Gram-positive bacteria.

Gentamicin (*see* Figure 8.2), tobramycin, and amikacin are aminoglycoside antibiotics that work by impeding the 30S subunit of bacterial ribosomes, thereby preventing protein synthesis. Aminoglycoside-exposed bacteria do not die immediately; lack of new protein production prevents bacterial replication and eventually leads to bacterial death. Aminoglycosides are effective against many Gram-negative bacteria, and against some Gram-positive bacteria, notably having a synergistic action with flucloxacillin against *S. aureus*. By contrast, streptococci and enterococci are resistant to aminoglycosides, resulting from poor uptake of the antibiotic.

However, when combined with a cell-wall-active antibiotic, aminoglycosides can have some synergistic bactericidal effect against these bacteria.

BACTERIAL RESISTANCE

Many bacteria, especially Gram-negatives, are resistant to penicillins because they produce β-lactamases – enzymes that break the β-lactam ring. Commonly encountered β-lactamases may act on penicillins (penicillinases) and cephalosporins (cephalosporinases). Flucloxacillin was developed because its additional side-chain protects it from the action of the S. aureus b-lactamase.

Meticillin-resistant S. aureus (MRSA) and meticillin-resistant coagulase-negative staphylococci are resistant to virtually all b-lactams because of alteration of the target site in the cell wall to which the antibiotics bind. Meticillin was a precursor to the development of flucloxacillin, and is no longer commercially available (see Figure 8.2).

Cefotaxime and meropenem (see Figure 8.2) are not susceptible to penicillinases, and are therefore useful antibiotics for treatment of both Gram-positive and Gram-negative bacteria. Meropenem has an extremely wide spectrum of action, so good that it abolishes the normal bacterial flora and predisposes to Candida infection, as do cephalosporins. Cefotaxime resistance can be mediated by alternative b-lactamses, the cephalosporinases, and meropenem resistance can also occur by metalloenzymes that hydrolyse all β-lactams. Carbapenem-resistant isolates are currently rare in most developed countries. β-lactamases are encoded by genes that can reside on plasmids, transposons or integrated phages (see Box 8.2), and most are transferable between bacterial strains and species.

Some Gram-negative bacteria are aminoglycoside resistant, due either to transferable resistance genes encoding enzymes that break down the antibiotic, or to poor uptake, or mutation of the ribosomal targets so that the aminoglycoside cannot bind.

ANTIBIOTIC CHOICE IN NEONATAL UNITS

The use of broad-spectrum first-line antibiotics (e.g. ampicillin and cefotaxime) on a neonatal unit encourages more antibiotic-resistant flora on babies compared with using narrow-spectrum antibiotics (see Figure 8.3). For this reason, most neonatal units use relatively narrow-spectrum antibiotics wherever possible. For instance, benzylpenicillin and gentamicin are given for initial therapy of suspected early-onset sepsis, aimed at treating S. agalactiae and E. coli infections. Not all neonatal units do this, however. Some units use cefotaxime for first-line empiric antibiotic therapy because of ease of administration, and to avoid toxicity of aminoglycosides and the need for monitoring levels. Flucloxacillin and gentamicin are often used for suspected late-onset sepsis, directed at S. aureus and Gram-negative bacteria. Glycopeptides, vancomycin or teicoplanin, are used to replace flucloxacillin when long-line infection is suspected, to treat coagulase negative staphylococcal and enterococcal infections. A third-generation cephalosporin (e.g. cefotaxime) is often added to the empiric regimen when meningitis is suspected or proven.

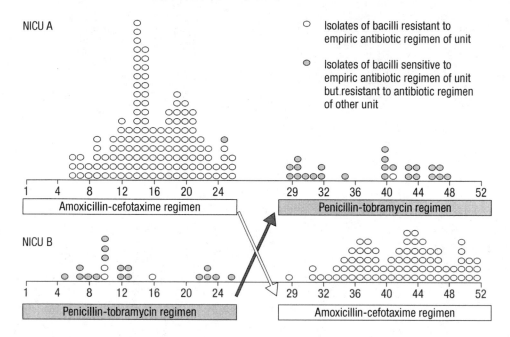

FIGURE 8.3 Broad-spectrum antibiotics encourage multi-resistant bacterial flora on neonatal units

In a Dutch cross-over study, the resistance profile of colonising Gram-negative bacteria was determined over a period of one year. Neonatal unit A used amoxicillin and cefotaxime for six months, and neonatal unit B used penicillin and tobramycin, and then the units switched their regimens. When a unit used the broad-spectrum combination of ampicillin and cefotaxime their babies were more frequently colonised with Gram-negative bacteria and these isolates were almost all resistant to the broad-spectrum antibiotics used. When the narrow-spectrum antibiotics, penicillin and tobramycin, were given, the babies were infrequently colonised with Gram-negative bacilli and when they were they were usually sensitive to these antibiotics.[1]

ROUTES OF INFECTION

Routes of infection are transplacental, ascending, and post-partum. The organisms that most commonly cause neonatal infection (*see* Table 8.1) are described to highlight the pathogenic mechanisms. Ascending and post-partum infections are usually caused by bacteria, whereas transplacental infections are usually caused by viruses and parasites. *Listeria monocytogenes* is an exception. Post-partum viral infections are not the subject of this chapter.

Bacterial infection in the neonatal period can be categorised as either early-onset or late-onset sepsis, and the cut-off between the two categories is variously defined as anywhere between 48 hours and a week old. A more useful definition is a pathogenic one. Early-onset sepsis originates *in utero* (typically once the membranes have ruptured) and disease is usually clinically obvious soon after birth or within the first 24–48 hours; whereas bacteria causing late-onset sepsis are usually acquired after birth.

EARLY-ONSET SEPSIS
Mode of acquisition of infection

Almost all early-onset infections are caused by bacteria that have ascended into the amniotic fluid from the vaginal flora. We know that this is the route of infection because in newborn infected twins, the first twin to be born is always infected whereas the second twin may or may not be (*see* Box 8.3). Chorioamnionitis is the initial event and the baby becomes secondarily infected, first with pneumonia, because the lungs are in direct contiguity with amniotic fluid. Depending on the duration and the density of pneumonia, the organism then seeds into the bloodstream and from there to the blood-brain barrier and into the cerebro-spinal fluid to cause meningitis. All babies with early-onset bacterial sepsis therefore have pneumonia, but they may not have bacteraemia or septicaemia, and meningitis is relatively rare.

Amniotic fluid obtained by amniocentesis at > 30 weeks gestation from women with apparently intact membranes contains bacteria in a small percentage of samples, implying that low-grade seeding of the amniotic fluid with bacteria occasionally occurs. The vast majority of bacteria cannot survive in amniotic fluid; amniotic fluid *in vitro* has strong anti-bacterial properties, and does not support the growth of many bacterial species, the exceptions being *Escherichia coli, Streptococcus agalactiae*, and occasionally other streptococci.

BOX 8.3 EARLY-ONSET SEPSIS

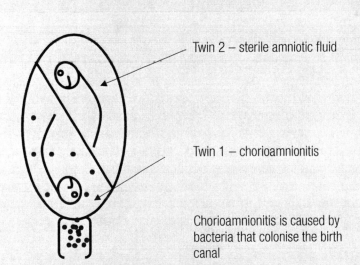

Twin 2 – sterile amniotic fluid

Twin 1 – chorioamnionitis

Chorioamnionitis is caused by bacteria that colonise the birth canal

Invasion of the amniotic fluid by bacteria from the birth canal leads to chorioamnionitis. The fetus is secondarily infected, and develops pneumonia and the newborn baby has respiratory signs of early-onset sepsis. For every seven babies with *S. agalactiae* (GBS) pneumonia, only one will have a positive blood culture, and very few will have meningitis.

Group B streptococcal infection

S. agalactiae (group B streptococcus; GBS) chorioamnionitis only occurs in women who are colonised with the organism, and the risk of chorioamnionitis in carriers is increased markedly by prolonged rupture of membranes > 18 hours. *S. agalactiae, in vitro*, can reach a density of 10^8 to 10^9 bacteria/mL of amniotic fluid in much less time than 18 hours. *S. agalactiae* can also invade amniotic membranes *in vitro*, hence it is likely that chorioamnionitis *in vivo* can be established even without prior rupture of membranes, and that *S. agalactiae* is one cause of premature rupture of membranes and preterm labour.

The proven *S. agalactiae* infection rate in the UK is 0.5 cases/1000 births, whereas the 'probable' infection rate is 3.6 cases/1000 births or 1:280 births. These rates may be an underestimate of the potential magnitude of the problem because at the time when these UK prospective observational studies were done, many obstetricians were giving intrapartum antibiotic prophylaxis to attempt to prevent early-onset *S. agalactiae* sepsis. 'Probable' infection is carefully defined as likely infection in babies from whom *S. agalactiae* is recovered from surface swabs taken at birth, and who have respiratory distress and radiographic changes of pneumonia. Thus, for every seven babies with *S. agalactiae* pneumonia only one has detectable bacteraemia. The proven infection rate enormously underestimates the burden of *S. agalactiae* disease – for instance, the UK has a birth rate of ~650 000 babies/year, which equates to only ~300 proven infections/year. However, the probable 'real' infection rate is seven times higher, equating to 2300 infections/year in the UK, or, in an average sized maternity unit of 5000 deliveries, 18 infections per year.

Other bacterial causes of early-onset sepsis

E. coli is a less frequent cause of early-onset sepsis, and occasionally infection is caused by other streptococci, such as α-haemolytic *S. viridans*. The limited range of pathogens causing early-onset sepsis means that it is mostly appropriate to use narrow-spectrum benzylpenicillin and an aminoglycoside for first-line treatment. Anaerobic bacteria occasionally also cause chorioamnionitis, often as part of mixed-organism infections, but the pathogenic potential of the anaerobes is low, and the bacteria are usually sensitive to penicillin. *Gardnerella vaginalis* is a Gram-variable bacterium that is associated with vaginosis, and which is occasionally isolated from surface swabs of babies with signs of early-onset pneumonia. It is more likely to be a marker organism of difficult-to-culture anaerobes, rather than being a neonatal pathogen per se. *Listeria monocytogenes* is discussed later in the chapter.

LATE-ONSET SEPSIS

Infections occurring after the first day or two of life have a different pathogenesis to early-onset sepsis. These infections are acquired *ex-utero*, and fall into two groups – commensals with low virulence that have gained iatrogenic access to normally sterile sites (such as coagulase-negative staphylococcal central venous line infection), or invasive bacteria with real pathogenic potential, such as serotype III *S. agalactiae* infections.

Low-virulence commensals

Staphylococci (both *S. aureus* and coagulase-negative staphylococcus), enterococci, and Gram-negative bacteria gain access to sterile sites, blood or lungs, usually by tracking along plastic or lodging on plastic and establishing a foothold.

Bacteria in the mouth may gain access to and cause infection in the normally sterile respiratory tract of ventilated babies. Oropharyngeal surveillance cultures can inform antibiotic choice for ventilation-associated pneumonia, prior to endotracheal cultures becoming available. Such surveillance cultures, however, do not give clues to the likely identity of bacteria causing late-onset sepsis in the absence of pneumonia.

Central venous lines are the usual source of late-onset sepsis on neonatal units, and the culpable organisms are skin commensals, staphylococci, or intestinal organisms such as enterococci and Gram-negative bacilli. Some of these infections will occur from loss of sterility at connection ports, and others will arise from bacteria seeding into the bloodstream from the intestine, and forming microcolonies on *in situ* plastic.

Pathogenic bacteria

Bacteria causing late-onset sepsis include *S. agalactiae*, *S. aureus* causing skin infections and then seeding elsewhere if untreated, and those organisms that cause urinary tract infections.

A specific sub-group of *S. agalactiae* cause late-onset infection; most isolates are capsular serotype III and/or multilocus sequence type ST-17 strains. Disease is different from early-onset *S. agalactiae* sepsis in that there does not have to be pneumonia; blood spread is usually low-grade bacteraemia rather than septicaemia, and the presenting feature is focal *S. agalactiae* infection, such as septic arthritis or meningitis. Serotype III/ST-17 strains almost certainly have a genetic propensity for causing invasive disease. Hence, these strains are likely to be intestinal commensals for a period of time, much the same as for the other *S. agalactiae* serotypes, but at some point in time the serotype III/ST-17 strains are able to breach the mucosal barrier and establish bacteraemia. Early-onset *S. agalactiae* sepsis may be seen as a chance event in which any serotype of *S. agalactiae* finds itself in the normally sterile amniotic fluid; the organism has sufficient defence mechanisms to protect itself against host innate immunity; it establishes chorioamnionitis, and the fetus is incidentally affected. In contrast, in late-onset *S. agalactiae* infection, disease propensity is related to the organism's ability to cause disease.

When *S. agalactiae* disease occurs in the few days after birth, the route of infection is likely to have been of the 'early-onset' type if the baby has pneumonia, and of the 'late-onset' type if the baby has focal disease without pneumonia. The distinction between early- and late-onset *S. agalactiae* sepsis is important because severe illness or death in early-onset sepsis is potentially preventable by the administration of intrapartum antibiotic prophylaxis by the obstetrician or as a result of the neonatologist identifying respiratory distress and treating the newborn baby early.

Late-onset sepsis is not preventable by intrapartum antibiotic administration, and the signs of impending illness are more subtle and don't necessarily include signs of pneumonia.

TRANSPLACENTAL INFECTIONS

Parasites, viruses and one bacterium may be acquired by a fetus. The organisms include *Toxoplasma gondii*; rubella; members of the *Herpesviridae* – cytomegalovirus (CMV), herpesvirus (HSV), and varicella-zoster (chickenpox virus – VZV); and *Listeria monocytogenes*. Maternal primary infection leads to parasitaemia, viraemia or bacteraemia and the organism spreads via the placenta to infect the fetus, usually causing damage that can be seen on placental histology after birth. Depending on the stage of fetal development, the damage to the baby can be anything from asymptomatic to profound.

Toxoplasma gondii

Toxoplasma gondii is a protozoan parasite whose definitive host is the cat. Other mammals and man are secondary hosts. It is only in cat-family members that the parasite has its sexual cycle, in which the organism replicates in the intestine and eggs are shed in their millions in faeces. In other mammals and man the organism is acquired either through eating undercooked meat or vegetables contaminated with parasite eggs. Toxoplasmosis in an immune pregnant woman is usually asymptomatic or causes only subclinical illness. However, the fetus is at risk of severe damage, with CNS and eye involvement caused by the parasite invading and destroying neuronal and retinal cells, leading to microcephaly or hydrocephalus with brain destruction and/or chorioretinitis. Mid-trimester, weeks 20–4, is the period of greatest risk to the fetus – before 20 weeks' gestation the risk of acquisition is low, and after 30 weeks, fetal immunity is sufficiently mature to control the infection without CNS damage.

Cytomegalovirus (CMV)

Fetal disease and neuronal damage occur following early-gestation acquisition of CMV, and can result from maternal primary infection or from secondary reactivation of maternal CMV. The fetal liver, lungs, intestine and brain may be damaged with conjugated hyperbilirubinaemia, pneumonitis, intestinal inflammation and neuronal damage. CMV has an especial propensity for causing sensorineural hearing loss. Reactivation of maternal CMV is less likely to cause severe fetal disease, presumably because there is some degree of protective maternal immunity. Some studies with small numbers of patients given ganciclovir intravenously for six weeks, commencing in the neonatal period, have suggested a lower rate of hearing loss in the treated babies. If hearing is improved in the treated group, this may be a surrogate marker of better global neurodevelopmental outcome. However, the evidence that treatment is effective is far from definitive, with the studies undertaken so far being flawed by lack of follow-up. For this reason, national ganciclovir treatment guidelines do not yet exist.

Varicella-zoster virus (VZV)

Chickenpox in pregnancy can be life-threatening for the mother, and transplacental spread establishes chickenpox in the fetus. The fetus may recover with no lasting effects, or dermatomal reactivation throughout the remainder of pregnancy can lead to circumferential scarring, limb deformity or even limb loss.

Maternal chickenpox in the peripartum period can lead to infection in the newborn baby. In keeping with other transplacental infections, the newborn baby can have liver involvement and pneumonitis. The mortality is reported as up to 30%, but this figure likely reflects publication bias. When a fetus is exposed to maternal chickenpox just prior to delivery, disease can be severe as there is no transplacental transfer of maternal protective anti-varicella antibody. In this situation, varicella-zoster immunoglobulin protects against severe disease evolving after the incubation period of 10–21 days.

Listeria monocytogenes

Listeria is a Gram-positive bacillus that lives in soil and contaminates crops. It is acquired through ingestion of contaminated food, particularly soft cheeses and undercooked meats. The organism grows well at fridge temperatures of 4–8 °C. Following maternal infection, transplacental spread occurs to the fetus. The placenta and newborn baby may be covered in miliary granulomata (granuloma infantiseptica). Most cases are associated with maternal symptomatic 'flu-like illness, indicating that bacteraemia in the mother is necessary. Amoxycillin or ampicillin are the most effective antibiotics when tested *in vitro* against *Listeria*, but *in vivo* benzylpenicillin may be as effective. As this fact is difficult to prove, on the rare occasion that a baby has a proven *Listeria* infection it is prudent to administer amoxycillin or ampicillin.

SUMMARY

Bacteria can be divided into two broad groups by the Gram stain. Gram-positive cocci include *Streptococcus spp.* and *Staphylococcus spp.* and are sensitive to β-lactam and glycopeptide antibiotics. Gram-negative bacteria include *E. coli*, *P. aeruginosa*, etc., and are sensitive to aminoglycosides, cephalosporins, and the higher order β-lactams such as meropenem. Neonatal units generally aim to have empiric antibiotic regimens that promote the narrowest-spectrum antibiotic use, as broad-spectrum antibiotics lead to babies being colonised with Gram-negative flora that is resistant to the antibiotics. Early-onset sepsis commences with ascending infection, and leads to chorioamnionitis, then pneumonia in the fetus, then septicaemia +/− meningitis. Empirical treatment with penicillin and an aminoglycoside covers the two main causative organisms, *S. agalactiae* (group B streptococcus) and *E. coli*. Late-onset sepsis is caused either by low-grade commensals obtaining access to normally sterile sites (e.g. tracking along plastic endotracheal tubes to the lung or along central venous lines to the bloodstream), or by organisms that are hyper-virulent and which have a propensity to cause disease (e.g. serotype III/ST-17 *S. agalactiae*). Late-onset sepsis that is seen on neonatal units is predominantly caused by low-grade commensals from the skin (e.g. coagulase-negative staphylococci) or from the intestine (e.g. enterococci or Gram-negative bacilli). Empiric initial treatment for suspected late-onset sepsis should be with narrow-spectrum antibiotics – for instance, flucloxacillin or a glycopeptide, and an aminoglycoside; and broad-spectrum antibiotics (e.g. cefotaxime or meropenem) should be reserved for the treatment of known antibiotic-resistant Gram-negative bacilli, and only occasionally used when a baby is deteriorating on initial narrow-spectrum agents. Newborn babies may acquire infections *in utero*, and predominantly these infections are parasites (*Toxoplasma*) or viruses (rubella and the *Herpesviridae* family members).

KEY POINTS FOR PRACTICE

▶ Bacteria causing neonatal infections can be divided into two broad groups by the Gram stain.

▶ Gram-positive bacteria include *Streptococcus spp.* and *Staphylococcus spp.* and are sensitive to β-lactam and glycopeptide antibiotics.

▶ Gram-negative bacteria include *Escherichia coli*, and *Pseudomonas*, *Klebsiella* and *Serratia* species, and are sensitive to aminoglycosides, cephalosporins, and the higher-order β-lactams such as meropenem.

▶ Neonatal units should aim to have narrow-spectrum empiric antibiotic regimens, as broad-spectrum antibiotics lead to colonisation with resistant Gram-negative flora.

▶ The sequence of systemic infection in early-onset sepsis is ascending: chori-oamnionitis, then pneumonia in the fetus, then septicaemia +/– meningitis.

▶ Empiric treatment with penicillin and an aminoglycoside covers the two main causative organisms of early-onset sepsis – *S. agalactiae* (group B streptococcus) and *E. coli*.

▶ Late-onset sepsis is caused either by low-grade commensals obtaining access to normally sterile sites (e.g. tracking along plastic endotracheal tubes to the lung or along central venous lines to the bloodstream), or by organisms that are hyper-virulent and which have a propensity to cause disease (e.g. serotype III/ST-17 *S. agalactiae*).

▶ Late-onset sepsis that is seen on neonatal units is predominantly caused by low-grade commensals from the skin (e.g. coagulase-negative staphylococci) or more virulent organisms from the intestine (e.g. enterococci or Gram-negative bacilli).

▶ Narrow-spectrum antibiotics are best for the empiric treatment of suspected late-onset sepsis – for instance, flucloxacillin or a glycopeptide combined with an aminoglycoside.

▶ Broad-spectrum antibiotics (e.g. cefotaxime or meropenem) are mostly reserved for the treatment of known antibiotic-resistant Gram-negative bacilli, or used when a baby is deteriorating on initial narrow-spectrum agents.

▶ Newborn babies may have acquired infections *in utero*. Predominantly these infections are parasites or viruses.

REFERENCE

1 De Man P, Verhoeven BAN, Verburgh HA, *et al.* An antibiotic policy to prevent emergence of resistant bacilli. *Lancet.* 2000; **355**: 973–8.

FURTHER READING

Rennie JM. *Robertson's Textbook of Neonatology.* 4th ed. Amsterdam: Elsevier; 2005.
Isaacs D, Moxon ER. *Handbook of Neonatal Infections: a practical guide.* 2nd ed. London: Balliere Tindall; 1999.

CHAPTER 9

Pharmacokinetics

Keith Hillier

CONTENTS

DRUG MOVEMENT THROUGH THE BODY

General considerations

Pharmacokinetics studies the way that the body handles drugs; essential pharmacokinetic knowledge of a drug includes information about the proportion of an administered dose that is *absorbed* into the bloodstream, its *distribution* to the tissues – including the site(s) where it acts – and its *elimination* from the body. Pharmacokinetics also studies the time taken for these processes to occur. Before a drug reaches the commercial market, detailed quantitative studies of its *absorption*, *distribution* and *elimination* profile provide characteristic benchmark figures for a drug's half-life, volume of distribution and clearance (*see* below).

The databases of dose quantities and dose intervals that are listed in formularies such as the *British National Formulary* have been derived from pre-marketing

extracellular fluid

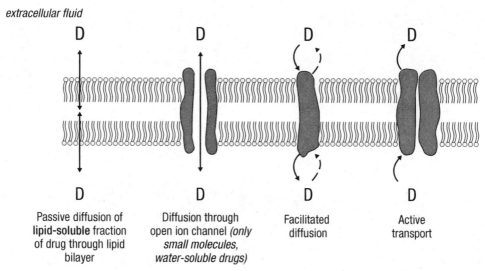

Passive diffusion of **lipid-soluble** fraction of drug through lipid bilayer

Diffusion through open ion channel *(only small molecules, water-soluble drugs)*

Facilitated diffusion

Active transport

cytosol

FIGURE 9.1 Mechanisms by which drugs can cross lipid membrane barriers

Passive diffusion of a drug in its lipid-soluble form only occurs from an area of high drug concentration on one side of the membrane to an area of lower drug concentration on the other side and will continue until concentrations are balanced. *Facilitated diffusion* is similar to passive diffusion but the rate of drug transport is enhanced by carrier mechanisms, such that it is greater than would be predicted by concentration differences alone. *Active transport* occurs against a concentration gradient and requires the use of energy-consuming transport processes.

pharmacokinetic studies and it is generally taken at face value that they provide safe and effective blood concentrations in the **majority of adults**. Pharmacokinetic studies also provide practical information about:

▶ why different routes of administration may require different doses
▶ the time interval between doses during chronic treatment
▶ the dosage modifications that are required in diseases such as hepatic and renal disease
▶ dosage calculations for the very young and the elderly.

Although there is a variety of pharmacokinetic information about the majority of commonly used drugs in adults, this is much less true of drug administration in neonates, particularly preterm neonates.

The **principles** that determine how a drug is handled in the bodies of neonates, infants and children are similar to those that determine how this occurs in adults but there is a host of differences in the physical and biochemical make-up of the young that might alter the amount of an individual drug that is absorbed, the way it is distributed around the body and the way that it is safely metabolised and excreted. Quantitative values for half-life, volume of distribution and clearance may differ from the adult values, making simple extrapolation of dosage regimens inaccurate. Because of the variability in the pharmacokinetics of different drug groups there is no general rule that simply relates adult dosage regimes to those for the young. There also remains a lack of knowledge in some areas about how pharmacokinetic parameters change in relation to the time lines of the different stages of infant development.[1]

From the time that a drug is administered until its elimination in urine, faeces or breath, its passage around the body requires that it dissolves in and passes through many membrane barriers that essentially consist of two layers of phospholipids that also contain proteins. For example, an enterally administered drug needs to cross gastric and small-intestinal membranes into the hepatic portal circulation and then pass through the liver, where it may be partially metabolised before it reaches the general circulation; further barriers exist as it passes out of the circulation into cells where it exerts its biological action and into cells (generally the liver and kidneys) where it can be made safe and eliminated from the body. The essential structure of a lipid membrane and the ways that a drug can move through it are shown in Figure 9.1.

Passive diffusion

This is the mechanism by which many drugs cross lipid membranes; this process involves the drug passing from a site of high concentration on one side of the lipid membrane to a site of lower drug concentration on the other side of the membrane. The drug will move down the concentration gradient at a rate proportional to the concentration difference until equilibrium occurs. For the drug to pass through the lipid membrane it must be soluble in lipids (e.g. diazepam). Most drugs can chemically co-exist in two forms – either lipid-soluble or water-soluble. The relative proportion of each form depends upon the pH of the body fluid that the drug is dissolved in and whether the drug is a weak acid or a weak base. In general terms, if a drug is a weak acid the proportion that is lipid-soluble rises as the bodily fluid in which it is dissolved becomes more acidic (*see* Figure 9.2).

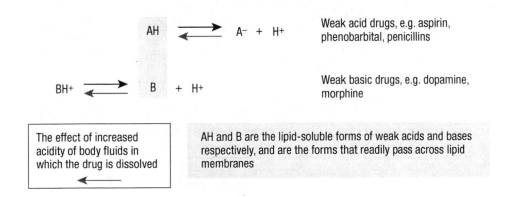

FIGURE 9.2 The effect of pH on the proportion of an acidic or basic drug that is present in lipid-soluble form

For drugs to cross membranes by passive diffusion, they must be in a lipid-soluble form without charge (i.e. AH for acids or B for bases). The pH of the body fluid in which the drug is dissolved will partially determine the proportion of total drug that is in the lipid-soluble form.

An example is aspirin, which is a weak acid. At the pH (1–2) of the adult stomach, a larger proportion of the drug is lipid-soluble and it is readily absorbed across the gastric mucosa. Once in the general circulation (pH 7) a much smaller proportion is in the lipid-soluble form and it is overall less able to pass from the circulation into tissues. However, when it is secreted into the renal tubular fluid (typically pH 4–6) the proportion in a lipid-soluble form will again rise, although not to the same proportion found in the gastric acid and this fraction can be reabsorbed back into the circulation, thus maintaining plasma concentrations (*see* Figure 9.3).

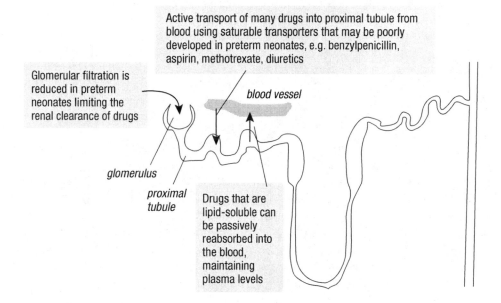

Active transport of many drugs into proximal tubule from blood using saturable transporters that may be poorly developed in preterm neonates, e.g. benzylpenicillin, aspirin, methotrexate, diuretics

Glomerular filtration is reduced in preterm neonates limiting the renal clearance of drugs

blood vessel

glomerulus

proximal tubule

Drugs that are lipid-soluble can be passively reabsorbed into the blood, maintaining plasma levels

FIGURE 9.3 The role of the kidney in drug excretion

The mature and optimally functioning kidney is important both for the elimination of drugs but also the biological activity of some drugs such as diuretics. Glomerular filtration rate and the proximal tubule secretory enzyme systems are immature in the neonate, particularly before term.

Facilitated diffusion

This involves a drug passing across a membrane down a concentration gradient; facilitated diffusion is, however, faster than would be predicted from the concentration difference alone across the membrane because families of carrier mechanisms which are widely distributed but are particularly important in the kidney enhance diffusion of the drug; these carrier proteins may be less well developed in neonates (*see* below, under 'Distribution of drugs').

Active transportation

Active transportation of drugs utilises fairly non-specific transport proteins which are found in the membranes of most cell types and can, for example, transport many drugs into and out of cells (*see* below, under 'Distribution of drugs'). Transport can take place against the concentration gradient and can be blocked by other drugs.

Dysfunction of these transporters can partially explain resistance that develops to some drugs; if a particular transporter is underactive a drug may not be taken into cells or if a transporter (such as P-glycoprotein) is overactive, the drug may be rapidly transported out of cells and away from its site of action. In both situations the concentration of drug in the cell may not reach that required for biological activity.

Transport through ion pores or channels
Only small molecules such as lithium or iodide can pass directly through membrane pores down a concentration gradient (see Figure 9.1).

ABSORPTION
Most enterally administered drugs need to be lipid-soluble to pass into the general circulation. In preterm neonates the pH of gastric contents is reported to be very variable but can be as high as pH 6–8 due possibly to duodenogastric reflux.[2] The pH falls to adult values over several months although some studies suggest the fall is quicker than this. Weakly acid drugs, such as aspirin and phenobarbital, cross membranes less well at a higher pH and will therefore be less well absorbed through the stomach; conversely, weakly basic drugs such as dopamine, erythromycin and morphine will be better absorbed.

The most active site of absorption for most enterally administered drugs is the small intestine. Gastric emptying is highly variable in neonates and is influenced by the frequency and composition of food intake, reaching adult patterns up to nine months to a year after birth; therefore the absorption of drugs through the duodenum will be less predictable than in adults.[3] It is advantageous for some drugs not to be absorbed when administered orally; for example, laxatives such as bulking and osmotic laxatives are not lipid-soluble under any bodily conditions and remain in the intestine, thereby reducing systemic side effects.

DISTRIBUTION OF DRUGS
Many drugs, after absorption into the systemic circulation, are widely distributed, metabolised and eliminated. These three processes are happening at the same time, although not at the same rate, and it is helpful to discuss them separately.

Protein binding
Drug distribution from the bloodstream into tissues can be delayed if it is extensively bound to plasma proteins (see Table 9.1).

TABLE 9.1 Drugs that are extensively bound to plasma proteins and may show interactions

Bound to albumin	Bound to a_1-acid glycoprotein
Digitoxin	Propranolol
Furosemide	Quinidine
Ibuprofen	Tricyclic antidepressants

(continued)

Bound to albumin	Bound to a_1-acid glycoprotein
Indomethacin	Lidocaine
Phenytoin	
Salicylates	
Sulphonamides	
Thiazides	
Tolbutamide	
Warfarin	

Protein binding is important for the transport of drugs in plasma and the fraction that is protein-bound will not cross membranes, including the blood-brain barrier, to reach drug receptors and produce a biological effect. The protein-bound drug does, however, provide a depot of potentially active drug as it can be rapidly released from its protein-binding site as the free concentration in the plasma falls. Protein binding is a saturable process, however, and drugs such as warfarin that are extensively protein-bound can occupy more than 90% of the available plasma protein-binding sites. Administration of another drug (such as aspirin) that is also highly protein-bound can result in competition for the limited number of binding sites and displaces warfarin from its protein binding; the increase in free warfarin may potentially cause a bleeding problem. In neonates the affinity of the plasma proteins, plasma albumin and a_1-acid glycoprotein for drugs is reduced and total levels of the latter protein are lower. Adult values are not acquired until about one year of age, and the potential for protein binding of drugs is therefore reduced. However, there is the possibility of competition between binding of endogenous substances and drugs; bilirubin which is extensively reversibly bound to albumin reduces the number of protein-binding sites available for extensively bound drugs such as ampicillin and phenytoin, and some drugs such as sulphonamides can displace bilirubin from albumin, thereby exacerbating neonatal jaundice.

The blood-brain barrier

Many drugs need to enter the CNS for their biological actions. However, there are particular barriers that limit the access of some drugs. Passage across capillaries into the CNS is more difficult relative to other capillaries as the former have tighter overlapping junctions, which restrict diffusion, and their basement membranes are lined with glial cells (astrocytes) that further limit drug entry; these additional barriers are called the blood-brain barrier (BBB). The BBB also possesses an enzymic dimension. P glycoprotein and organic acid transporters (*see* below) are important in transporting drugs and neurotransmitters out of the brain. An intact BBB prevents bilirubin crossing into the brain and causing kernicterus. In neonates, the BBB is not fully developed until about 6 months of age; therefore a range of drugs and bilirubin can access the CNS more readily than in older children and adults.

Entry of highly lipid-soluble drugs into the CNS does occur readily, as shown by the ability of anaesthetics such as thiopental to induce anaesthesia in seconds. Other drugs can gain entry by crossing the BBB using special transport processes; levodopa for the treatment of Parkinson's disease gains entry to the CNS in this way. The permeability of the BBB can increase in pathological situations such as inflammation, hypertension and oedema. Benzylpenicillin does not readily penetrate the healthy CNS but when the meninges are inflamed due to meningitis, access is increased and this is important in the treatment of bacterial meningitis.

Volume of distribution

'Standard' doses of administered drugs that are both safe and effective have been worked out from clinical trials before a drug is released onto the market. In trials it is clearly possible to take frequent sequential samples of plasma and other blood cells and urine but you cannot readily measure drug concentrations directly in tissues and cells outside the bloodstream except in special circumstances. Therefore safety and dose regimen data are derived by administering a series of doses and assessing the plasma concentration of the drug and matching these concentrations to the biological and toxic effects of the drug. Some drugs are so toxic (e.g. digoxin, theophylline) that the difference between the safe plasma concentration and the concentration producing toxicity – **the therapeutic index** – may be a factor of two or less. From these studies a value called the **volume of distribution (Vd)** has been derived for each drug and this is used to calculate the amount of a single dose of a drug to administer to achieve a desired concentration in plasma. The principle of Vd is that when different drugs are given they can move out of the plasma and into the tissues at different rates and to different extents. The formula relating the dose that needs to be administered with the concentration in plasma and Vd is:

Dose administered = Concentration in plasma × Vd

If drug A has a Vd of 8 L/kg body weight, whereas drug B has a Vd of 16 L/kg body weight, in order to achieve the same concentration of each drug in plasma, twice the dose of drug B would be required relative to drug A.

The **volume of distribution** of a drug is usually given as L/kg body weight and in the main has been derived from studies in adults. *However, it is incorrect to assume that this 'constant' derived in adults would apply to neonates when simply calculated according to the babies' weights.* In particular, in preterm neonates compared with older children and adults, Vd would tend be larger due to a greater proportion of the body weight that is water and fat and a higher body surface area to weight ratio.

ELIMINATION

Most but not all biologically active drugs are metabolised by the liver and excreted in the urine and bile. There are usually two phases of metabolism (the detail of which will not be covered here) but the overall products of metabolism generally have no or less biological activity than the active parent drug and are more water-soluble, which means they are readily excreted. In some limited cases, metabolism can occur in tissues other than liver, such as plasma (e.g. suxamethonium), and for some drugs the product of metabolism does have biological activity or toxicity (e.g. the benzodiazepine diazepam is metabolised to temazepam and oxazepam; paracetamol is partially metabolised to a toxic product).

Metabolism and clearance of drugs

Metabolism and clearance of drugs can be affected by:
▶ disease of the liver
▶ decline in renal function
▶ genetic polymorphisms (abnormal less active forms) of metabolising enzymes
▶ co-administration of drugs that inhibit or activate liver-metabolising enzymes.

Liver metabolism

A *family* of liver enzymes metabolises and makes safe the majority of drugs before they can be excreted from the body. Although in pregnancy the liver of the mother is the prime organ of metabolism of drugs, some metabolising enzymes can be detected in the liver early in fetal life where they are involved in the metabolism of endogenous products. They are known as cytochrome P450 (CYP) enzymes, and the CYP3A4 enzyme subfamily is involved in the metabolism of about 50% of all drugs used while CYP2D6 is involved in metabolism of about 30% of drugs.[4,5] Table 9.2 shows a limited selection of different enzymes and examples of the drugs they metabolise.

TABLE 9.2 Examples of the array of liver enzymes and the drugs they metabolise, and drugs that can inhibit or enhance enzyme activity

Isoenzyme	Selected examples of drugs metabolised	Inhibitors (examples)	Inducers (examples)
CYP1A2	Caffeine, paracetamol, theophylline,	Cimetidine, clarithromycin, erythromycin, grapefruit juice, isoniazid, ketoconazole	Omeprazole, cigarette smoke
CYP2B6	Cyclophosphamide, efavirenz ifosfamide	Fluoxetine, paroxetine	Carbamazepine, phenobarbital, phenytoin, rifampicin
CYP2C9	Glibenclamide, ibuprofen, losartan, tolbutamide, warfarin	Amiodarone, cimetidine, fluconazole, fluoxetine, ketoconazole, omeprazole, valproic acid	Carbamazepine, dexamethasone, phenobarabital, rifampicin
CYP2C19	Omeprazole	Cimetidine, fluvoxamine, omeprazole	Carbamazepine, rifampicin
CYP2D6	Amitriptyline, bisoprolol, codeine, many SSRIs, metoprolol, ondansetron, propranolol	Amiodarone, cimetidine, fluoxetine, haloperidol, methadone, quinidine	Carbamazepine, phenobarabital, phenytoin, rifampicin
CYP2E	Ethanol, paracetamol,	Disulfiram, isoniazid	Ethanol

(continued)

Isoenzyme	Selected examples of drugs metabolised	Inhibitors (examples)	Inducers (examples)
CYP3A4	Numerous drugs of different classes, e.g, amiodarone, carbamazepine, cisapride, clonazepam, diltiazem, diazepam, erythromycin, felodipine, fluconazole, lidocaine, midazolam, nifedipine, saquinavir, tamoxifen, terfenadine, verapamil, etc.	Cimetidine, clarithromycin, clotrimazole, erythromycin, fluconazole, grapefruit juice, ketoconazole, saquinavir	Carbamazepine, dexamethasone, phenobarabital, phenytoin, rifampicin

Although some CYP enzymes are detectable early in fetal life, *in general* compared with adults liver metabolism is lower in the neonate, particularly in the preterm neonate. Total CYP enzyme levels reach adult levels by about one year of age but individual CYP isoenzymes mature at varying rates and therefore the ability to metabolise different drugs is variable (*see* Table 9.3).

TABLE 9.3 The effect of some parameters on drug handling in neonates

Variation in pharmacokinetic parameter in neonates compared with adults	Comment
Increased gastric pH	Decrease in absorption of weak acids but enhanced absorption of weakly basic drugs (*see* Figure 9.2)
Delayed and erratic gastric emptying	Reduced absorption of drugs that occurs when the drug reaches the small intestine where the majority of absorption occurs
Reduced plasma protein binding	Greater proportion of drug in plasma not bound to plasma protein and potential for toxicity (*see* Table 9.1)
Larger ratio of body water to body weight	Larger volume of distribution of drug
Immature liver enzymes	Reduced metabolism resulting in higher systemic drug concentrations
Immature transport enzymes in renal proximal tubule	Enhanced plasma levels of some drugs, e.g. benzylpenicillin but reduced access of some drugs to their sites of action, e.g. diuretics acting on renal tubular wall receptor sites
Decreased glomerular filtration rate	Decreased ability to excrete some drugs, in some cases may increase the possibility of toxicity
Immature blood-brain barrier in preterm neonates	May allow greater access of some drugs to CNS

In a subset of individuals there is a genetic polymorphism in some CYP enzymes resulting in slow metabolising ability. For example 5–10% of Caucasians have low levels of CYP2D6 and therefore excrete drugs metabolised by this enzyme only slowly (*see* Table 9.2). An increasingly important aspect of CYP enzymes and their drug-metabolising abilities is the fact that some drugs will inhibit the metabolising ability of enzymes (*see* Table 9.2). A major example of this is cimetidine, which will inhibit several CYP subtypes; an example of the clinical relevance of this is that co-administration of cimetidine with warfarin will significantly inhibit CYP2C9 and cause an increase in serum warfarin levels and anticoagulant actions.

Renal clearance of drugs

Renal clearance of drugs involves filtration and secretion but also reabsorption (*see* Figure 9.3). The efficient functioning of the kidney is important in that it is involved in the elimination of a number of water-soluble drugs and metabolites of drugs that have been made inactive and water-soluble by drug metabolism and conjugation in the liver.[6]

Drugs and metabolites are delivered to the renal tubules in the following two ways:

▶ Filtration through the glomerulus, which is dependent upon the glomerular filtration rate.

▶ Some drugs are secreted into the proximal tubule from the circulation via active transporters in the membranes of the walls of the proximal tubule.

A drug in active parent form or as a metabolite that is in the proximal tubule will be excreted into the bladder if it is in its ionised form but if lipid-soluble, it can be reabsorbed back across the tubule into the circulation. The pH of the renal tubular fluid is important in determining whether the drug is in its lipid or water-soluble form. The clinical relevance of this can be illustrated with the example of a weak acid such as aspirin. If an individual is overdosed with aspirin, large amounts of salicylate will be secreted into the proximal tubule; if the tubular fluid is acid (pH 4–6) a significant proportion will be lipid-soluble and will be reabsorbed maintaining plasma levels and prolonging toxicity (*see* Figure 9.3). If the tubular fluid is made alkaline (achieved by administering oral or intravenous bicarbonate) most of the aspirin in the proximal tubule will be in its water-soluble form (*see* Figure 9.2) and it will not be reabsorbed.

The basolateral and apical membranes of the proximal tubule contain families of transport enzymes that are very important for the secretion of drugs and endogenous substances into the proximal tubule and therefore elimination from the body.

An example of these enzymes is a particular **O**rganic **A**cid **T**ransporter (OAT1) which transports drugs such as penicillin from the circulation across the proximal tubule. The efficiency of the transporter is the main reason in adults that benzylpenicillin is rapidly excreted in the urine with a half-life of only 30 minutes. In preterm neonates these transporters may be immature and the half-life of penicillin can be much longer. In preterm neonates only 24–74% of penicillin G is excreted in the urine in 12 hours.

Rapid excretion in adults is mainly by proximal tubule active transport into the lumen but in preterm neonates it is mainly by GFR, suggesting that the tubular mechanisms are immature.[7] The fact that benzylpenicillin is rapidly secreted into the proximal tubule by transporters can be exploited as administration of probenicid, which blocks the transporter, substantially increases the half-life of benzylpenicillin in the circulation.

Some drugs, such as thiazide and furosemide diuretics, exert their diuretic action on receptors on the apical surface of the renal tubules and mainly reach their site of action by secretion via the organic acid transporter. However, the transporters have a limited capacity and can be saturated; for example, aspirin and diuretics use the same transporter and if aspirin is co-administered it reduces the secretion of diuretics into the tubules and they are therefore rendered less effective.

Competition for the transporter can also make drugs more toxic. Both methotrexate and aspirin use the organic acid transporter and if they are co-administered, higher and prolonged plasma concentrations of methotrexate will occur, resulting in potential toxicity.

In neonates GFR is also lower than in adults and elimination of drugs may be relatively restricted. An archetypal example where this is important is the highly toxic drug gentamicin, which is eliminated from the body unchanged by the kidney. Ototoxicity and renal toxicity can result if doses are not adjusted if there is a decline in renal function.[8]

CONCLUSION

The administration of drugs to neonates can in some cases be inappropriate if dose regimens are calculated using adult guidelines. However, there is no overarching guidance for drugs about procedures to be followed, except that each drug and neonate should be assessed individually.

REFERENCES

1 Yaffe SJ, Aranda JV, editors. *Neonatal and Pediatric Pharmacology: therapeutic principles in practice*. Philadelphia: Lippincott, Williams and Wilkins; 2004.
2 López-Alonso M, Moya MJ, Antonio J, *et al*. Twenty-four-hour esophageal impedance-pH monitoring in healthy preterm neonates: rate and characteristics of acid, weakly acidic, and weakly alkaline gastroesophageal reflux. *Pediatrics*. 2006; **118**(2): e299–308.
3 Kaufmann RE. Drug action and therapy in the infant and child. In: Yaffe SJ, Aranda JV, op. cit.
4 Johnson TN, Thomson M. Intestinal metabolism and transport of drugs in children: the effects of age and disease. *J Pediatr Gastoenterol Nutr*. 2008; **47**: 3–10.
5 Alcorn J, McNamara PJ. Ontogeny of hepatic and renal systemic clearance pathways in infants *Clin Pharmacokinet*. 2002; **41**(12): 959–8.
6 van den Anker JN. Renal function and excretion of drugs in the newborn. In: Yaffe SJ, Aranda JV, op. cit.
7 Metsvaht T, Oselin K, Ilmoja M-L, *et al*. Pharmacokinetics of penicillin G in very-low-birth-weight neonates. *Antimicrob Agents Chemother*. 2007; **51**(6): 1995–2000.
8 Tetelbaum M, Finkelstein Y, Nava-Ocampo A, *et al*. Back to basics: understanding drugs in children: pharmacokinetic maturation. *Pediatr Rev*. 2005; **26**(9): 321–8.

CHAPTER 10

Nutrition

Intan Faizura Yeop

CONTENTS

INTRODUCTION

Developments in neonatal nutrition have contributed significantly to improving morbidity and mortality outcomes in premature infants. It plays an important role in achieving one of the main aims of neonatal care – that is, growth and development.

ACCUMULATIVE DEFICIT

Over the years, the approach to nutritional management has changed. Currently, efforts are made to reduce or eliminate the effect of **accumulative deficit**. Premature infants have very little reserve capacity, and what is considered to be a small deficit can actually be significant. The accumulative effect of small deficits gradually builds up to a large deficit and the need for catch-up growth. On the other hand, rapid weight gain in infancy has been associated with later adult complications. With adequate nutrition and steady weight gain from birth the need for catch-up growth is minimised or avoided.

AGGRESSIVE NUTRITION

The principle of **aggressive nutrition** in premature infants involves the continuous nutritional supply with minimal interruptions from birth. The supply should be sufficient to enable adequate growth and development. Infants in neonatal units often experience periods of illness that may lead to disruption of their nutrient flow. The disruption may be necessary as the gut is not able to contain, digest or absorb foodstuff.

CAUSES OF NUTRITIONAL COMPROMISE

Neonatal patients can pose a challenge from a nutritional perspective. It is not always possible to predict which infants will have added complications during their course of admission. However, by identifying those at particular risk and ensuring good nutrient delivery from birth, i.e. aggressive nutrition safely managed, the risk of complications can be reduced, recovery from complications aided, nutritional deficit minimised and overall outcome improved. Some of the factors which are associated with nutritional compromise are shown in Table 10.1.

TABLE 10.1 Factors predisposing to nutritional compromise

Maternal factors	Intra-uterine factors	Neonatal factors	Environmental factors
• Chronic disease, e.g. diabetes mellitus, depression, hypertension • Substance abuse • Underweight, low BMI	• Placental insufficiency • Multiple pregnancy	• Anatomical abnormalities, e.g. cleft lip/palate • Abdominal abnormalities, e.g. gastroschisis • Prematurity • IUGR • Polycythaemia • Sepsis	• Social circumstances

Maternal and antenatal factors
Metabolic programming

Sufficient supply of nutrients is important for fetal well-being as well as later adult health. The Barker hypothesis postulates that infants born small are at increased risk of cardiovascular diseases as adults.[1] This is thought to be due to permanent alterations in fetal metabolism, known as 'programming', partly as a result of insufficient supply of nutrients at critical times in pregnancy. There is recent evidence to suggest that this occurs partly through gene–nutrient interactions such as alteration of the fetal epigenome through DNA methylation and histone modifications.[2,3]

Maternal nutrition and health
BEFORE PREGNANCY
Maternal weight, health and nutrition at the time of conception are thought to have an impact on the health and growth of the fetus.[4-6] In addition to weight and height, body composition provides an indication of the mother's metabolic capacity and ability to support the growth and development of her fetus.[7] There is also some evidence suggesting that mothers with a greater lean body mass have higher rates of protein turnover, and that this is associated with greater birth length.[8]

DURING PREGNANCY
A Cochrane Review of balanced protein/energy supplementation in pregnancy reported that supplementation was associated with a gain of only 37 grams in birth weight, which was not statistically significant.[9] Epidemiological studies of women in the south of England have not shown any conclusive positive correlation between maternal diet and birth weight.[10,11] However, a strong relationship between antenatal maternal nutrition and infant birth weight was demonstrated in epidemiological studies of women during the Dutch famine of World War II.[12,13,14]

The role of the placenta in fetal health
Growth occurs at its fastest soon after conception, initially as cell division and later as a combination of cell division, cell hypertrophy and differentiation. The placenta provides the fetal environment and supports growth. Consisting of a fetal portion – the chorion – and maternal portion – the decidua basalis – it is where exchange of gases, metabolic products, antibodies and hormones between fetal and maternal circulation take place. It is also an endocrine gland, producing steroid and peptide hormones as well as prostaglandins.[15]

In pregnancy, physiological and metabolic adaptations occur to increase the availability of substrates such as glucose and LDL cholesterol to the fetus. Fetal growth is a result of a complex interaction between the mother, fetus and placenta through the production and metabolism of hormones. Placental hormones alter maternal metabolism, facilitate transfer of substrates and promote fetal growth and development. Adequate utero-placental blood flow is necessary for all of these interactions to occur. In the presence of maternal under-nutrition, fetal growth restriction occurs as a result of reduced glucose, which is the main substrate, as well as fetal insulin and IGF-1. Placental dysfunction can result in growth restriction and has been associated with increased infant morbidity.[16]

From conception to birth, fetal growth and development are reliant on maternal health and nutrition as well as a healthy, functioning placenta. In assessing an infant from a nutritional perspective, it is important to consider maternal, placental and intra-uterine factors.

NUTRITIONAL REQUIREMENTS IN THE NEONATAL PERIOD
Energy requirements
For adequate weight gain, a minimum of 90 kcal/kg/day is required, with some infants needing up to 160 kcal/kg/day.[17] This is to meet the requirements for basal metabolic rate (BMR), diet-induced thermogenesis (DIT), physical activity, and

growth. BMR, which is the amount of energy required for the maintenance of the body's vital processes, can increase with inflammation, pyrexia and chronic diseases. It can also decrease in the event of energy deficit. DIT represents the energy required for the digestion and absorption of food and synthesis of tissue.[18] The rapid growth and organ maturation which occurs after birth requires a significant supply of energy and is, therefore, affected in the event of energy insufficiency and deficiency.

The approximate requirements for a stable term infant growing at 10 g/kg of weight gain per day are set out in Table 10.2.

TABLE 10.2 Energy requirement[19]

Requirement	Energy
Resting energy expenditure (REE) to maintain essential body functions	50 kcal/kg
Occasional cold stress	+ 10 kcal/kg
Minimal activity	+ 5 kcal/kg
Faecal loss	+ 15 kcal/kg
Growth	+ 45 kcal/g
Total requirement	125 kcal/kg/day

Neonatal energy requirements vary, depending on:
▶ gestational age
▶ post-natal age
▶ weight
▶ increased respiratory effort against artificial ventilation or to maintain adequate gas exchange
▶ stressful procedures such as line insertions and radiological imaging
▶ hypothermia or heat loss, to which premature infants are susceptible due to their higher surface area to weight ratio and lower energy reserves
▶ acute illness, such as sepsis or chronic ill health, e.g. chronic lung disease
▶ surgery, which is reported to transiently increase energy requirements in neonates[20]
▶ route of nutrient delivery.[21]

Bearing in mind maternal, placental and intra-uterine factors, the infant's current nutritional needs require consideration of the above factors as part of a nutritional assessment and management plan. This is to ensure that adequate calories and nutrients are delivered safely and effectively.

Macro- and micronutrient requirements
Infants who are enterally fed are likely to receive a balanced intake of nutrients from breast milk or infant formula. Specially formulated milk products are available for premature and low-birth weight infants. However, if enteral feeding is not possible, more thought is required to ensure that adequate macro- and micronutrients are received.

Protein

The energy consumed by an infant is directed towards maintaining bodily functions, growth, and organ maturation and development. Growth and organ development require adequate protein intake in the form of essential, non-essential and conditionally essential amino acids (*see* Table 10.3). To maintain nitrogen balance, an adequate intake of essential amino acids is required, as protein synthesis depends on the availability of rate-limiting amino acids. The aim in infants is to achieve a positive nitrogen balance and prevent catabolism. Amino acid supply should be started on the first day after birth, with a recommended minimum of 1.5 g/kg/day to prevent a negative nitrogen balance. Higher intakes of up to 4 g/kg/day may be necessary for protein deposition in premature infants. In infants receiving parenteral nutrients, less is required due to intestinal bypass.[21]

TABLE 10.3 Essential, non-essential and conditionally essential amino acids[21]

Essential	Non-essential	Conditionally essential
Histidine	Alanine	Arginine
Isoleucine	Aspartic acid	Cysteine
Leucine	Asparagine	Glycine
Lysine	Glutamic acid	Proline
Methlonlne	Glutamlne	Tyroslne
Phenylalanine	Serine	
Threonine		
Tryptophan		
Valine		

Carbohydrate

Utilising the amino acids available requires an energy supply of 30–40 kcal per 1 g amino acids.[21] Non-protein calories should consist of 60–75% carbohydrates and 25–40% lipid.[22,23] Glucose is the main metabolic fuel. Carbohydrate, in the form of glucose, should be started after birth, and gradually increased. Endogenous glucose production varies depending on age. The rate of glucose production is 11.5 g/kg/day (or 8 mg/kg/min) in premature infants, and is highest during the post-natal period, decreasing gradually with age.[24,25] Exogenous glucose delivered in excess of the rate of glucose oxidation, which is a maximum of 6–8 mg/kg/min in premature infants and 12 mg/kg/min in term surgical infants,[26] causes increased lipogenesis and fat tissue deposition. Administration of glucose should not exceed 18 g/kg/day in infants, and lower rates should be considered if the infant is critically ill.[22] In excess, glucose can give rise to complications such as hyperglycaemia, glycosuria, liver steatosis, enhanced production of VLDL triglycerides, increased risk of infections, impaired protein metabolism, and increased infection-related mortality; and increased carbon dioxide production and minute ventilation can occur.

TABLE 10.4 Recommended glucose supply (g/kg/day)[22]

Weight	Day 1	Day 2	Day 3	Day 4
Up to 3 kg	10	14	16	18
3–10 kg	8	12	14	16–18

Fat

The fat content in human breast milk varies with gestation and feeding phase, with an average of 3–4 g/100 mL.[17] In milk formulae designed for premature infants, the fat content varies but is generally higher than in breast milk. This is of potential benefit to premature infants as they have lower fat stores compared with term infants. Infants receiving breast milk benefit from long-chain polyunsaturated fatty acids, such as docosahexaenoic acid and arachidonic acid, present in breast milk, and these have been reported to enhance visual and cognitive development. However, premature infants on exclusive expressed breast milk may require additional calories for adequate weight gain as the content of fat may gradually decline. For infants who are parenterally fed, fat is delivered as a lipid emulsion, available as long-chain triglycerides (LCT) or a combination of medium-chain triglycerides (MCT) and LCT-based emulsions. Compared with LCT emulsions, MCT/LCT emulsions have been reported to lead to higher net fat oxidation, reduced liver derangement, improved white-cell function and reduced adverse effects on respiratory gas exchange.[23,27–30] However, there is insufficient evidence to support its preferential use in neonates.[23] It provides high energy in a low-osmolarity and low-volume solution, along with essential fatty acids and fat-soluble vitamins. Its oxidation is dependent on total energy intake and expenditure, as well as carbohydrate intake. Lipid infusion could be started after birth, and should be started by Day 3. A maximum of 3–4 g/kg/day is recommended in infants,[23] as fat oxidation reaches its peak at that rate.[31] To prevent essential fatty acid deficiency, a minimum of 0.25 g/kg/day of linoleic acid should also be given to premature infants.[23] The infusion rate should not exceed the capacity for lipid clearance. This should be monitored closely in premature infants, especially if they are ill, as adjustments of lipid infusion may be required to prevent complications such as hypercholesterolaemia, cholestasis, respiratory failure and thrombocytopenia.

Minerals

Equally important is the adequate supply of micronutrients to prevent deficiency states. As the majority of micronutrient accretion occurs in the third trimester, supplementation is recommended for long-term parenteral nutrition (PN) (more than 3 weeks) in premature infants, with close monitoring due to the risk of toxicity.[32] Iron, in excess, could impair immune function and stimulate bacterial overgrowth, thereby increasing the risk of infections.[33]

Electrolytes

Infants receiving PN should also be provided with sodium, potassium, chloride, calcium, phosphate and magnesium. Sodium, potassium and chloride supplementation is initially closely linked to fluid management and in extremely preterm infants sodium intake is restricted during the first few days. Adequate sodium is required for body mass accretion, and a higher requirement exists in premature infants. There is also a high requirement of potassium, which can be lost from the intestinal tract, thus requiring further supplementation or replacement.

Calcium and phosphate are required for skeletal development, and their retention is proportional to growth. Supplementation with 1.3–3 mmol/kg/day of calcium and 1–2.3 mmol/kg/day of phosphorus is also recommended, with a Ca:P ratio of 1.3–1.7. Magnesium is also important for bone mineralisation and growth, and should be supplemented in PN (5 mg or 0.2 mmol/kg/day).[32]

Trace elements

Trace elements should be supplied in PN.[32] Chromium, copper, iodine, manganese, molybdenum, selenium and zinc are essential micronutrients with several functions.

TABLE 10.5 Recommended supplementation of trace elements[32,34,35]

Trace elements	Requirements (μg/kg/day)	Importance
Chromium (Cr)	0.2	• Processing carbohydrates and fats • A constituent of the glucose tolerance factor (GTF), thus works synergistically with insulin in promoting cellular glucose uptake • High Cr levels compete with iron for transferring • Cr contaminates PN, thus supplementation is considered unnecessary
Copper (Cu)	20	• Important component in many enzymes • Regular monitoring if on long-term PN
Iodine (I)	1 μg/day	• Essential part of thyroid hormones
Manganese (Mn)	1 (maximum)	• Important component of many enzymes • In high levels, contribute to cholestasis and hepatic dysfunction. • Reported reversible high-intensity areas in basal ganglia, brainstem, thalamus and cerebellum with toxic levels of Mn.
Molybdenum (Mo)	1	• Important for many enzymes involved in DNA metabolism • In high levels, may interfere with Cu metabolism
Selenium (Se)	2–3	• Anti-oxidant, protective against oxidative damage
Zinc (Zn)	450–500	• An activator of certain enzymes, important role in energy metabolism and immune function • High cutaneous or gastrointestinal losses require additional supplementation • Essential for tissue accretion

Vitamins

Premature infants established on enteral feeds are often supplemented with multivitamins. Infants receiving PN should receive lipid- and water-soluble vitamins. The ideal doses for infants are not known but a guide is available based on expert opinions (*see* Table 10.6). Low-birth weight infants have low fat stores and, as a result, low body stores of fat-soluble vitamins and high risk of deficiencies. The delivery of lipid-soluble vitamins requires consideration as vitamin A is photosensitive and can be degraded in intensive sunlight.[36] Water-soluble vitamins are not stored (except for vitamin B12), but excreted by the kidneys. As a consequence, there is a need for regular supplementation and the risk of toxicity is low.

TABLE 10.6 Recommended vitamin supplementation for preterm infants[36]

Vitamins	Recommended supplementation (dose per kg weight per day)	Importance
Vitamin A (μg) (Fat soluble)	150–300	● Immune function ● Differentiation and maintenance of epithelial cells
Vitamin D (μg) (Fat soluble)	0.8	● Calcium and phosphorus homeostasis
Vitamin E (mg) (Fat soluble)	2.8–3.5	● Anti-oxidant, free-radical scavenger
Vitamin K (μg) (Fat soluble)	10	● Regulation of coagulation factors
Ascorbic acid (Vitamin C) (mg)	15–25	● Co-factor in hydroxylation reactions ● Anti-oxidant ● Catabolism of tyrosin
Thiamine (Vitamin B1) (mg)	0.35–0.50	● Carbohydrate metabolism ● Lipid synthesis
Riboflavin (Vitamin B2) (mg)	0.15–10.20	● Energy metabolism
Niacin (Vitamin B3) (mg)	4.0–6.8	● Essential for synthesis of co-factors involved in energy metabolism
Pantothenic acid (Vitamin B5) (mg)	1–2	● Precursor for coenzyme A, involved in energy metabolism
Pyridoxine (Vitamin B6) (mg)	0.15–10.20	● Protein and carbohydrate metabolism ● Immune and neurologic functions
Biotin (Vitamin B7) (μg)	5–8	● Metabolism of proteins and fat ● Role in citric acid cycle and carbon dioxide transfer
Folic acid (Vitamin B9) (μg)	56	● Biosynthesis of pruines and pyrimidines ● Metabolism of certain amino acids
Cobalamin (Vitamin B12) (μg)	0.3	● DNA nucleotides synthesis

MONITORING OF PARENTERAL NUTRITION

Parenterally delivered nutrition, although of great benefit, is not without its complications including:

▶ line-related infection
▶ reduced availability of venous access
▶ intestinal disuse atrophy
▶ bacterial overgrowth
▶ PN-related liver disease.

PN related liver disease

Cholestasis occurs in 40–60% of infants on long-term PN. Most are moderate in severity and reversible with alterations or discontinuation of PN. Infants at particular risk of PN-related liver disease are:

▶ premature or low birth weight
▶ those with a short length of bowel with absent ileo-caecal valve
▶ a lack of enteral feeding
▶ recurrent sepsis
▶ excess lipid and/or glucose concentration in PN
▶ protein malnutrition or excess.

This common complication can be minimised or avoided by:

▶ continuing with the maximum enteral feeds tolerated
▶ stopping or reducing lipid infusion e.g. alternate-day lipid infusion. Consider the possibility of lipid toxicity in the prescence of thrombocytopaenia and high liver transaminases
▶ meticulous line handling to prevent line sepsis
▶ consider the possibility of bacterial overgrowth
▶ consider ursodeoxycholic acid.

In persistent cholestasis, the possibility of biliary obstruction, infection and drug toxicity should be considered, investigated and addressed.

It is important to monitor for these complications, especially with long-term (i.e. more than 3 weeks) PN. Regular measurements of plasma electrolytes, renal function and bone profile are required to ensure adequate amounts of relevant nutrients are prescribed in appropriate volumes of fluid. Urinary sodium levels are more sensitive to sodium depletion than are plasma concentrations and can therefore be useful for PN management. Serum bilirubin and triglyceride levels should be monitored with increments of lipid and carbohydrate to ensure that the rates of oxidation are not exceeded. Monitoring of liver transaminases can be used as a guide to reduce and/or avoid the complication of PN-related liver disease. Trace-element concentrations should be interpreted with caution, especially in stressful situations such as infections. Zinc levels decline in stressful situations and serum concentrations may not be a good indicator of inadequate supply. Once the patient is stable on a regimen, monitoring can be then relaxed.

TABLE 10.7 Monitoring of parenteral nutrition

Timing	Monitoring
3–4 times a week	Electrolytes, renal function
Twice weekly	• Albumin/TP
	• GGT/ALT
	• ALP/AST
	• Bilirubin
	• Ca, Mg, PO_4
	• Urinary electrolytes
Weekly	Triglycerides (unless rising)
After 3 weeks, then monthly	• Fat-soluble vitamins
	• Trace elements (with CRP)

There have been many advances in the development of infant formula feeds, especially for premature infants. This has resulted in improved nutrient delivery in enterally fed infants. Despite these, regular monitoring of weight gain and growth is required to ensure that the infants are receiving sufficient calories. Infants receiving breast milk could have added fortifier to increase caloric intake, but cautious addition may be required due to the high osmolar load.

In many premature infants, full enteral feeds are not possible due to instability and/or immature gut function. PN therefore enables nutritional support until enteral feeds are possible, but regular monitoring is needed to avoid possible complications. It is also important to persist in trying to restart enteral feeds and trophic feeds should always be considered. Trophic feeding is the provision of minimal volume of feeds, preferably breast milk, that have been reported to stimulate the gastrointestinal system, promoting gut hormone secretions, enzyme activities, gut motility and the acquisition of favourable gut flora. Such feeds also improve enteral feed tolerance and hasten the process of establishing enteral feeds.

GROWTH PARAMETERS

Good growth and weight gain are measures of successful neonatal care. The current practice of plotting serial measurements on a growth chart is a useful exercise to monitor growth and for future reference. It also provides an opportunity to assess current status regularly and to reassess nutritional management.

Growth charts in use are based on the UK90 reference, which is the most representative of British children today.[37] However, it makes no allowances for multiple births,[38,39] breastfed or formula-fed infants,[40,41] nor for neonatal weight loss in the first week of life.[42] In addition, growth percentile lines for premature infants are based on expected weight gain and growth of the fetus, not of the post-natal premature infant.[43] The differences in nutrient supply and environment between fetus and premature infants of the same gestational age raise the question of the validity and suitability of these growth standards. However, they remain a useful tool in assessing the trend of growth and weight gain in premature infants.

Weight

Infant weight at birth can reflect the nutritional supply and fetal well-being during pregnancy. In the post-natal period, serial weight gains of 10–15 g/kg/day may indicate adequate growth but in isolation give an incomplete assessment. Weight as a measurement of true mass in premature infants can be inaccurate due to attachments such as cannulas, lines and wires, as well as excessive fluid. Also, a weight gain of more than 10–15 g/kg/day may suggest fluid retention, but in the presence of oedema, serial weights could be useful in monitoring fluid loss or accumulation. On the other hand, a large weight gain may represent catch-up growth in infants who have been nutrient deficient. Although body weight for age can provide an indication of nutritional state, its use is limited without proportions or percentages of body compositions of fat and non-fat tissues.[44]

Occipitofrontal circumference

Head circumferences are useful measures of growth in infants but an accurate measurement at birth can be difficult to obtain due to overlapping sutures, caput, and moulding from delivery. In addition, conditions such as hydrocephalus, hypoxic ischaemic encephalopathy, intracranial haemorrhages and central nervous system malformations may complicate head circumference measurements. After the first week or two, serial measurements of head circumferences can give a good indication of head growth, which can have implications for later development.[45]

Length

Length is not always measured at birth in premature infants. This may be due to the technical difficulties of measuring a premature infant, usually flexed in an incubator, and the minimal-handling approach to managing these infants. However, a length would add another dimension. Serial lengths could give an indication of growth. Lengths for age and comparison of weight and length percentiles could give an indication of the proportion, e.g. long and thin or short and fat. Its incorporation in ponderal index (PI = [weight (kg)/length^3 (cm)] × 100) is thought to be a useful measurement in disproportionate intra-uterine growth.[44,46] At present, there are no percentile charts for premature infant lengths and this does not encourage routine measurements of infant lengths.

Body composition

Information on body composition could provide a useful indication of reserve capacity and an estimate of tissue deposition.[47,48] The estimation of body composition by means of skin fold thickness, mid-arm circumference and arm area measurements in the UK appears to be limited to specialist centres and research settings, and can be subject to inaccuracies.[49,50,51] Decreased skin fold thickness is suggestive of protein deficiency, and excessive thickness, of obesity. Muscle mass can be calculated by subtracting skin fold measurement from mid-upper arm circumference,[52] although these measurements may be challenging in the premature infant.

Estimation of body composition such as serial measurements of muscle and adipose tissues could be useful indicators of effectiveness of nutrient delivery. The proportion of adipose tissue would be of particular interest, including brown fat.

Brown fat contains a unique protein, known as thermogenin, which enables the release of large amounts of heat, without ATP utilisation, as part of the non-shivering thermogenesis process.[53,54] It accounts for approximately 5% of body mass in a term neonate and is distributed along the upper half of the spine,[55] but is smaller in size and percentage in premature neonates.[56] It is more abundant in twins than in singletons,[57] and its deposition in later pregnancy is sensitive to maternal nutrition.[58] It gradually disappears during childhood years, as the mitochondrial content disappears.[55]

Serial measurements of growth parameters are an important part of neonatal management. Despite the limitations, they remain useful, providing an indication of successful management and guiding further nutritional management. Children have smaller reserves and a greater need for energy, for their growth and development, than do adults. The rapidly developing brain needs nutrients, and can be significantly affected if supply is inadequate.[59] Poor post-natal growth has been associated with poor developmental outcomes.[60,61] However, rapid growth in infancy has been associated with long-term cardiovascular and metabolic diseases as well as adult obesity, as discussed earlier.

RAPID WEIGHT GAIN AND THE RISK OF OBESITY AND THE METABOLIC SYNDROME

Achieving the right balance of nutrient delivery in neonatal care is not always easy, and complications are sometimes unavoidable. However, by aiming for consistent adequate nutrient flow from as early as possible following birth, steady weight gain and growth are achievable. This would avoid the need for catch-up growth, which is of particular benefit, as there is evidence to support the increased risk of adult obesity and the metabolic syndrome in infants with rapid weight gain in the first six months of life. The development of insulin resistance and hypertension in later life has also been reported with rapid weight gain in early childhood. Thus, consistent appropriate weight gain and growth from early life are important in reducing these risks.

REFERENCES

1 Barker DJ, Osmond C, Simmonds SJ, *et al.* The relation of small head circumference and thinness at birth to death from cardiovascular disease in adult life. *BMJ.* 1993; **306**: 422–6.
2 Duttaroy AK. *Evolution, Epigenetics, and Maternal Nutrition.* Available at: www.mukto-mona.com/Special_Event_/Darwin_day/evolution_asim120206.htm (accessed 14 April 2009).
3 Dolinoy DC, Weidman JR, Waterland RA, *et al.* Maternal genistein alters coat color and protects Avy mouse offspring from obesity by modifying the fetal epigenome. *Environ Health Perspect.* 2006; **114**(4): 567–72.
4 Godfrey KM, Barker DJ. Fetal nutrition and adult disease. *Am J Clin Nutr.* 2000; **71**(5 Suppl.): S1344–52.
5 Godfrey K, Robinson S, Barker DJP, *et al.* Maternal nutrition in early and late pregnancy in relation to placental and fetal growth. *BMJ.* 1996; **312**: 410–14.
6 Mathews F, Yudkin P, Neil A. Influence of maternal nutrition on outcome of pregnancy: prospective cohort study. *BMJ.* 1999; **319**: 339–43.

7 Jackson AA. Nutrients, growth, and the development of programmed metabolic function. *Adv Exp Med Biol.* 2000; **478**: 41–55.

8 Duggleby SL, Jackson AA. Relationship of maternal protein turnover and lean body mass during pregnancy and birth length. *Clin Sci (Lond).* 2001; **101**(1): 65–72.

9 Kramer MS. Balanced protein/energy supplementation in pregnancy. *Cochrane Database Syst Rev.* 2003; **4**: CD000032.

10 Rayco-Solon P, Fulford AJ, Prentice AM. Maternal preconceptional weight and gestational length. *Am J Obstet Gynecol.* 2005; **192**(4): 1133–6.

11 Kind KL, Moore VM, Davies MJ. Diet around conception and during pregnancy – effects on fetal and neonatal outcomes. *Reprod Biomed Online.* 2006; **12**(5): 532–41.

12 Stein AD, Ravelli AC, Lumey LH. Famine, third-trimester pregnancy weight gain, and intrauterine growth: the Dutch Famine Birth Cohort Study. *Hum Biol.* 1995; **67**(1): 135–50.

13 Lumey LH. Decreased birthweights in infants after maternal in utero exposure to the Dutch famine of 1944–1945. *Paediatr Perinat Epidemiol.* 1992; **6**(2): 240–53.

14 Stein AD, Lumey LH. The relationship between maternal and offspring birth weights after maternal prenatal famine exposure: the Dutch Famine Birth Cohort Study. *Hum Biol.* 2000; **72**(4): 641–54.

15 Ross MH, Romrell LJ, Kaye GI. *Histology – A Text and Atlas.* 3rd ed. (International ed.). Baltimore: Williams and Wilkins; 1995. pp. 702–6.

16 Baschat AA, Cosmi E, Bilardo CM, *et al.* Predictors of neonatal outcome in early-onset placental dysfunction. *Obstet Gynecol.* 2007; **109**(2 Pt. 1): 253–61.

17 Rennie JM, Roberton NRC. *A Manual of Neonatal Intensive Care.* 4th ed. London: Hodder Arnold; 2002.

18 ESPGHAN. Guidelines on Paediatric Parenteral Nutrition of the European Society of Paediatric Gastroenterology, Hepatology and Nutrition (ESPGHAN) – Energy. *J Pediatr Gastroenterol Nutr.* 2005; **41**(2): S5–11.

19 Ambalavanan N. *Fluid, electrolyte and nutrition management of the newborn.* Available at: www.emedicine.com (accessed 14 April 2009).

20 Pierro A. Metabolism and nutritional support in the surgical neonate. *J Pediatr Surg.* 2002; **37**(6): 811–22.

21 ESPGHAN. Guidelines on Paediatric Parenteral Nutrition of the European Society of Paediatric Gastroenterology, Hepatology and Nutrition (ESPGHAN) – Amino Acids. *J Pediatr Gastroenterol Nutr.* 2005; **41**(2): S12–18.

22 ESPGHAN. Guidelines on Paediatric Parenteral Nutrition of the European Society of Paediatric Gastroenterology, Hepatology and Nutrition (ESPGHAN) – Carbohydrates. *J Pediatr Gastroenterol Nutr.* 2005; **41**(2): S28–32.

23 ESPGHAN. Guidelines on Paediatric Parenteral Nutrition of the European Society of Paediatric Gastroenterology, Hepatology and Nutrition (ESPGHAN) – Lipids. *J Pediatr Gastroenterol Nutr.* 2005; **41**(2): S19–27.

24 Kalhan SC, Kilic I. Carbohydrate as nutrient in the infant and child: range of acceptable intake. *Eur J Clin Nutr.* 1999; **53**(Suppl. 1): S94–100.

25 Lafeber HN, Sulkers EJ, Chapman TE, *et al.* Glucose production and oxidation in preterm infants during total parenteral nutrition. *Pediatr Res.* 1990; **28**(2): 153–7.

26 Sauer PJ, Van Aerde JE, Pencharz PB, *et al.* Glucose oxidation rates in newborn infants measured with indirect calorimetry and [U-13C] glucose. *Clin Sci (Lond).* 1986; **70**: 587–96.

27 Donnell SC, Lloyd DA, Eaton S, *et al.* The metabolic response to intravenous medium-chain triglycerides in infants after surgery. *J Pediatr.* 2002; **141**: 689–94.

28 Radermacher P, Santak B, Strobach H, *et al.* Fat emulsions containing medium-chain trig-lycerides in patients with sepsis syndrome: effects on pulmonary hemodynamics and gas exchange. *Intensive Care Med.* 1992; **18**: 231–4.

29 Roth B, Ekelund M, Fan BG, *et al.* Biochemical and ultra-structural reactions to parenteral nutrition with two different fat emulsions in rats. *Intensive Care Med.* 1998; **24**: 716–24.

30 Yeh SL, Lin MT, Chen WJ. MCT/LCT emulsion ameliorate liver fat deposition in insulin-treated diabetic rats receiving total parenteral nutrition. *Clin Nutr.* 1998; **17**: 273–7.

31 Pierro A, Carnielli V, Filler RM, *et al.* Metabolism of intravenous fat emulsion in the surgical newborn. *J Pediatr Surg.* 1989; **24**: 95–101.

32 ESPGHAN. Guidelines on Paediatric Parenteral Nutrition of the European Society of Paediatric Gastroenterology, Hepatology and Nutrition (ESPGHAN) – Iron, Minerals and Trace Elements. *J Pediatr Gastroenterol Nutr.* 2005; **41**(2): S39–46.

33 Patruta SI, Hörl WH. Iron and infection. *Kidney Int Suppl.* 1999; **69**: S125–30.

34 Ono J, Harad K, Kodaka R, *et al.* Mananganese deposition in the brain during long-term parenteral nutrition. *J Parenter Enteral Nutr.* 1995; **19**: 310–12.

35 Kafritsa Y, Fell J, Long S, *et al.* Long-term outcome of brain manganese deposition in patients on home parenteral nutrition. *Arch Dis Child.* 1998; **79**: 263–5.

36 ESPGHAN. Guidelines on Paediatric Parenteral Nutrition of the European Society of Paediatric Gastroenterology, Hepatology and Nutrition (ESPGHAN) – Vitamins. *J Pediatr Gastroenterol Nutr.* 2005; **41**(2): S47–53.

37 Buckler JM, Green MA. Comparison of the early growth of twins and singletons. *Ann Hum Biol.* 2004; **31**: 311–12.

38 Alexander GR, Kogan M, Martin J, *et al.* What are the fetal growth patterns of singletons, twins and triplets in the United States? *Clin Obstet Gynecol.* 1998; **41**: 115–25.

39 Butte NF, Wong WW, Hopkinson JM, *et al.* Infant feeding mode affects early growth and body composition. *Pediatrics.* 2000; **106**(6): 1355–66.

40 Dewey KG. Growth patterns of breastfed infants and the current status of growth charts for infants. *J Hum Lact.* 1998; **14**(2): 89–92.

41 Wright CM, Parkinson KN. Postnatal weight loss in term infants: what is normal and do growth charts allow for it? *Arch Dis Child Fetal Neonatal Ed.* 2004; **89**(3): F254–7.

42 Sauer PJ. Can extrauterine growth approximate intrauterine growth? Should it? *Am J Clin Nutr.* 2007; **85**(2): S608–13.

43 Hemachandran AH, Klebanoff MA. Use of serial ultrasound to identify periods of fetal growth restriction in relation to neonatal anthropometry. *Am J Hum Biol.* 2006; **18**(6): 791–7.

44 Kan E, Roberts G, Anderson PJ, *et al.* Victorian Infant Collaborative Study Group. The association of growth impairment with neurodevelopmental outcome at eight years of age in very preterm children. *Early Hum Dev.* 2008; **84**(6): 409–16.

45 Mahajan SD, Aalinkeel R, Singh S, *et al.* Endocrine regulation in asymmetric intrauterine fetal growth retardation. *J Matern Fetal Neonatal Med.* 2006; **19**(10): 615–23.

46 Akinyinka OO, Sanni KA, Falade AG, *et al.* Arm area measurements as indices of nutritional reserves and body water in African newborns. *Afr J Med Sci.* 1999; **28**(1–2): 5–8.

47 Hediger ML, Overpeck MD, Kucxmarski RJ, *et al.* Muscularity and fatness of infants and young children born small- or large-for-gestational-age. *Pediatrics.* 1998; **102**(5): E60.

48 Sann L, Durand M, Picard J, *et al.* Arm fat and muscle areas in infancy. *Arch Dis Child.* 1988; **63**(3): 256–60.

49 Olhager E, Forsum E. Assessment of total body fat using the skinfold technique in full-term and preterm infants. *Acta Paediatr.* 2006; **95**(1): 21–8.

50 Excler JL, Sann L, Lasne Y. Anthropometric assessment of nutritional status in newborn infants. Discriminative value of mid arm circumference and of skinfold thickness. *Early Hum Dev.* 1985; **11**(2): 169–78.

51 Yau KI, Chang MH. Growth and body composition of preterm, small-for-gestational-age infants at a postmenstrual age of 37–40 weeks. *Early Hum Dev.* 1993; **33**(2): 117–31.

52 Behrman RE, Kliegman RM, Jenson HB. *Nelson Textbook of Pediatrics.* 16th ed. Saunders; 2000.

53 Austgen L. *Brown adipose tissue.* Available at: www.vivo.colostate.edu/hbooks/pathphys/misc_topics/brownfat.html (accessed 14 April 2009).

54 Klaus S. Functional differentiation of white and brown adipocytes. *Bioessays.* 1997; **19**(3): 215–23.

55 Cannon B, Nedergaard J. Brown adipose tissue: function and physiological significance. *Physiol Rev.* 2004; **84**(1): 277–359.

56 Zancanaro C, Carnielli VP, Moretti C. An ultrastructural study of brown adipose tissue in pre-term human newborns. *Tissue Cell.* 1995; **27**(3): 339–48.

57 Budge H, Dandrea J, Mostyn A, *et al.* Differential effects of fetal number and maternal nutrition in late gestation on prolactin receptor abundance and adipose tissue development in the neonatal lamb. *Pediatr Res.* 2003; **53**(2): 302–8.

58 Budge H, Edwards LJ, McMillen IC, *et al.* Nutritional manipulation of fetal adipose tissue deposition and uncoupling protein 1 messenger RNA abundance in the sheep: differential effects of timing and duration. *Biol Reprod.* 2004; **71**(1): 359–65.

59 Georgieff MK. Nutrition and the developing brain: nutrient priorities and measurement. *Am J Clin Nutr.* 2007; **85**(2): S614–20.

60 Georgieff MK, Hoffman JS, Pereira GR, *et al.* Effect of neonatal caloric deprivation on head growth and 1-year developmental status in preterm infants. *J Pediatr.* 1985; **107**: 581–7.

61 Latal-Hajnal B, von Siebenthal K, Kovari H, *et al.* Postnatal growth in VLBW infants: significant association with neurodevelopmental outcome. *J Pediatr.* 2003; **143**(2): 163–70.

CHAPTER 11

An overview of haemostasis

Bashir A Lwaleed and Rashid Kazmi

CONTENTS

INTRODUCTION

The function of normal haemostasis is to prevent blood loss from injured vessels. The process ensures that blood remains fluid in the vessels and clots at the site of injury. It is quick, localised and finely regulated. Once a clot has served its purpose, it is removed, the circulation is re-established and tissues remodelled. It is not difficult to envisage that any disruption in this process may tip the balance and lead to either a haemorrhagic or thrombotic tendency.

A complex interplay of three components achieves haemostasis. These include the vessel wall, intravascular components (platelets and coagulation factors) and fibrinolysis (the process of breaking the clot). Together, they regulate the haemostatic process by clot formation to prevent bleeding, and later on, clot dissolution through the fibrinolytic system. The system is also closely linked to other defence mechanisms in the body, including the immune system and inflammatory response.

NORMAL HAEMOSTASIS

Injury results in a transient constriction of the vessel. This is caused by a local contractile response of the vascular wall to trauma and is followed by a highly complex process of haemostasis, which for the ease of description, can be divided into the steps described below.

Formation of the platelet plug

Platelets are anucleate fragments of megakaryocytes and circulate in blood as disc-shaped cells. They have a number of membrane glycoproteins, which are involved in adhesion and aggregation. The most important of these are GPIIb-IIIa and GPIb-V–IX. Within platelets a number of granules are found. Of these, *alpha granules* contain a large number of proteins. The second type of granules, *dense granules*, contain a number of substances capable of stimulating other platelets on release. Under normal circumstances, platelets have no contact with sub-endothelial tissue and remain quiescent. A breach in the endothelium exposes collagen and causes platelets to adhere to it. This is mediated through von Willebrand factor (vWF), which is a large glycoprotein and bridges platelets to collagen only at the site of injury. Circulating vWF is unable to bind platelets. However, when sub-endothelial collagen is exposed, vWF binds to this and in doing so undergoes a conformational change. Platelets can now bind to this through their GPIb-V–IX glycoprotein.

The initial step in haemostasis is, therefore, the binding of inactive platelets to vWF attached to sub-endothelial collagen. This contact induces a change in their shape. From a disc they become a sphere with multiple pseudopods making them adhesive and facilitating contact with other platelets. Subsequent to this they synthesise thromboxane A2 and release this together with adenosine diphosphate (ADP) contained in dense granules. These act as strong stimulants for neighbouring platelets causing a similar sequence of events in them. As a result, a platelet plug is formed at the site of injury and serves to seal this. This, however, is fragile and needs to be strengthened. The consolidation occurs through coagulation system.

Consolidation of the platelet plug: the blood coagulation system

The platelet plug prevents bleeding from small wounds but needs to be stabilised. A complex series of reactions produces fibrin, which is the final product of the blood coagulation system. This not only consolidates the platelet plug but is also needed for securing haemostasis from larger wounds. The production of fibrin depends on the generation of thrombin, which is achieved through a cascade of reactions where there is sequential activation of inactive clotting factors (*see* Table 11.1) in a stepwise fashion.

Classically this was described as two distinct pathways, extrinsic and intrinsic, joining together at a common pathway (*see* Figure 11.1). While this concept is still useful, especially for understanding routine clotting tests, it is inadequate in answering a number of questions. The cell-based model of haemostasis is the accepted mechanism now (*see* Figure 11.2). According to this model, coagulation proceeds in relation to two cell surfaces – exposed sub-endothelial tissue and activated platelets.

TABLE 11.1 Coagulation factors, common names and sources. Although the Roman numerical system is used for blood coagulation factors now, a number of synonyms were in use previously. The table shows current numerical system and previous terminology together with main source of synthesis in the body.

Factor number	Descriptive name(s)/former terminology	Source
Factor I	Fibrinogen	Liver
Factor II	Prothrombin	Liver
Factor III	Tissue factor (thromboplastin)	Damaged tissues or cells, activated platelets
Factor IV	Ionised calcium (Ca^{++})	Diet, bones and platelets
Factor V	Proaccelerin or labile factor	Liver
Factor VI	Initially used to describe what is now recognised as activated factor V (FVa). This numerical is not used now.	
Factor VII	Proconvertin or stable factor	Liver
Factor VIII	Antihaemophilic factor	Liver. Significant extra-hepatic synthesis
Factor IX	Plasma thromboplastin component, Christmas factor	Liver
Factor X	Stuart-Prower factor	Liver
Factor XI	Plasma thromboplastin antecedent	Liver
Factor XII	Hageman factor	Liver
Factor XIII	Fibrin-stabilising factor	Liver and platelets

The first step is the exposure of tissue factor (TF) on the sub-endothelial cells: TF is a transmembrane protein and is constitutively expressed on the surface of fibroblasts in the sub-endothelium. Normally it does not come in contact with circulating blood but gets exposed with vascular injury or damage. It then makes a complex with circulating factor VII (FVII), which is subsequently auto-cleaved within the complex to its active form, FVIIa. The TF-FVIIa complex binds a small amount of FX and activates it to become FXa. This new complex (TF-FVIIa-FXa) is capable of activating a small amount of prothrombin to its active form thrombin. Although the conversion of fibrinogen to fibrin is carried out by thrombin, the amount of thrombin at this stage is insufficient for the large-scale production of fibrin. Instead, thrombin at this point activates platelets and a number of other clotting factors including FV and FVIII. This is the 'initiation' of coagulation and is a prelude to the 'thrombin burst' that occurs on the surface of activated platelets and is necessary for the production of fibrin.

In addition to activating FX, TF-FVIIa complex also activates FIX: activated FIX (FIXa) complexes with FVIIIa (activated by thrombin in the 'initiation' stage) on the surface of activated platelets. Like TF-FVIIa complex, this activates FX, occurring this time on the surface of activated platelets. Alpha granules in platelets contain a number of clotting factors that are acquired by pinocytosis. On activation, platelets

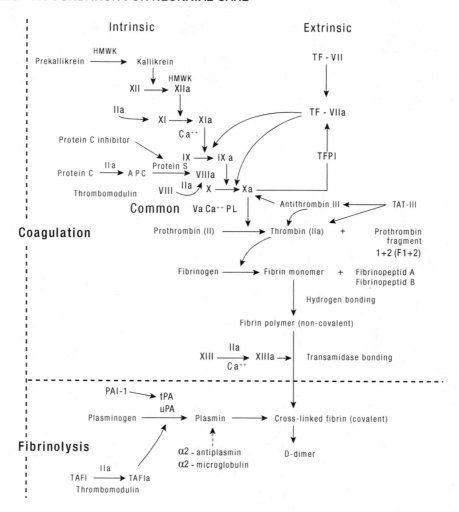

FIGURE 11.1 Schematic representation of the haemostatic system.

The coagulation system

Intrinsic pathway (contact system) is initiated when contact is made between blood and exposed negatively charged surfaces. High-molecular-weight kininogen (HMWK) converts prekallikrein to kallikrein and factor XII (FXII) to FXIIa. The latter converts FXI to FXIa that activates FIX. Activated FIX converts FX to FXa, which with its co-factors FVa, FVIIIa, phospholipids (PL) and Ca++ form 'the prothrombinase' complex. This activates prothrombin (II) to thrombin (IIa).

Extrinsic pathway (cellular injury) is triggered upon vascular injury, which leads to tissue factor (TF) exposure. FVII binds endothelium-TF and is activated to FVIIa. The TF-FVIIa complex activates FX and FIX.

Common pathway is the final step of the coagulation process where, thrombin is formed from FII (prothrombin) through the action of FXa, FVa, Ca++ and phospholipids (PL). Tissue factor pathway inhibitor (TFPI) inactivates TF-FVIIa complex in concert with FXa. Thrombin activates FXI, which in turns converts FIX to FIXa. The generation of FXa is then amplified through the action of FIXa and co-factor FVIIIa. Ultimately, FIIa converts fibrinogen to fibrin and activates FXIII, which cross-links fibrin polymers to solidify the clot.

Fibrinolytic system

Fibrinolysis is initiated when plasminogen is converted to plasmin by tissue-type plasminogen activator (t-PA). Subsequently, plasmin degrades the fibrin clot into soluble fibrin degradation

(continued)

products. The formation of plasmin is enhanced by a positive feedback loop. Thrombin-activatable fibrinolysis inhibitor (TAFI) is activated by an array of haemostatic factors including thrombin, thrombin/thrombomodulin complex or plasmin to its active form (TAFIa), which inhibits fibrinolysis. TAFIa down-regulates fibrinolysis in vivo via the removal of carboxy-terminal lysine and arginine residues from partially-degraded fibrin which acts as a key proponent of the positive feedback in the fibrinolytic cascade. In doing so TAFIa therefore inhibits further plasminogen activation by abrogating the required fibrin co-factor function for t-PA-mediated plasminogen activation, thus resulting in a decreased rate of plasmin formation. This in turn results in decreased fibrinolytic activity. (Adapted from: Lwaleed BA, *et al.* Seminal hemostatic factors: then and now. *Semin Thromb Hemost.* 2007; **33**(1): 3–12.)

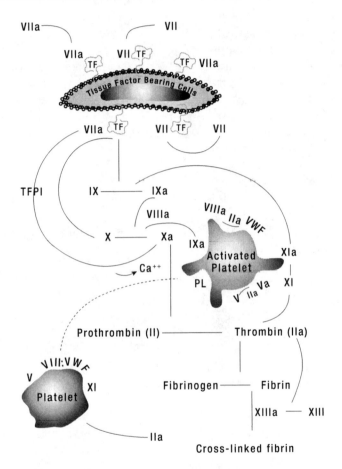

FIGURE 11.2 Cellular tissue factor initiated coagulation

Factor VII (FVII) binds tissue factor (TF) on TF-bearing cells and is auto-activated to FVIIa. A trace amount of FVIIa is also found in the circulation. The resulting complex (TF-FVIIa) activates FX and FIX. The activated FX generates a small amount of thrombin (IIa). In a FXa-dependent feedback system, tissue factor pathway inhibitor (TFPI) almost immediately binds and inhibits the TF-FVIIa complex. However, initial production of thrombin activates platelets and FV and releases and activates FVIII from being bound to von Willebrand (vWF). Additionally it activates FXI. Activated FIX (FIXa) binds to the activated platelets and activates FX. Platelets-generated-FXa then generates large amounts of thrombin, which is needed to form the fibrin clot.

Source: Lwaleed BA, *et al.*, op. cit.

release their FV that, together with circulating FV, is activated by thrombin (generated in the 'initiation step'). Activated factor V (FVa) binds FXa to make prothrombinase complex which catalyses the conversion of prothrombin to thrombin. This 'thrombin burst' is sufficient for converting fibrinogen into fibrin monomers. These are cross-linked by FXIII to make a stable clot. The whole process proceeds at the site of endothelial injury on the surface of activated platelets. Platelet activation, therefore, is crucial to maintenance of normal haemostasis. There is evidence that production of thrombin occurs much more rapidly on the platelet surface than in the fluid phase or on artificial lipid micelles. In addition to the generation of fibrin, thrombin also activates several other clotting factors including FXI and FXIII.

Thrombin generation depends on the assembly of prothrombinase complex on the surface of platelets and requires ongoing activation of FIX: under basal conditions this is achieved by TF-VIIa complex. However, this may be compromised in situations of high haemostatic demands. In these circumstances FXI, which is activated by thrombin, catalyses the activation of FIX. This route thus serves as an adjunctive pathway for generating prothrombinase and assumes significance in securing haemostasis in the setting of increased load on the haemostatic system, e.g. in the post-operative period.

Regulation of haemostasis

By virtue of its potentially explosive nature, coagulation – if unrestricted – could encroach on intact endothelium and lead to widespread thrombosis. There are three main pathways to ensure that the procoagulant activity does not spread beyond the confines of endothelial injury.

Tissue factor pathway inhibitor (TFPI)

As has been seen, the initiation of thrombin production is via activation of FX by TF-FVIIa. TFPI, a plasma protein, is a specific inhibitor of this pathway. It inhibits FXa in two ways. Firstly, any FXa that diffuses away from the site of injury is directly inhibited by TFPI. In addition, TFPI targets TF-FVIIa complex thus switching off further activation of FX. While TFPI reacts directly with TF-FVIIa complex, the efficiency of this reaction is significantly increased after TFPI binds FXa.

Antithrombin pathway

Antithrombin is a glycoprotein synthesised in the liver. As the name suggests, it binds and neutralises thrombin. It also inhibits several other activated clotting factors including FIXa and FXa. The rate of these reactions is slow but is immensely augmented by heparin. This forms the basis of therapeutic use of heparins as an anticoagulant.

Protein C/protein S pathway

Protein C is a vitamin-K-dependent serine protease. It is synthesised in the liver and circulates in an inactive form. The activation of protein C is brought about by thrombin. Whereas other activities of thrombin are procoagulant, the activation of protein C elicits anticoagulant function. This paradoxical role of thrombin is dependent on binding an integral membrane protein – thrombomodulin – that is expressed abundantly on normal endothelial cells of the microcirculation but is lost from damaged endothelium. As thrombin diffuses away from the site of injury, it encounters thrombomodulin on intact endothelium and binds it with a high degree of affinity. This leads to a conformational change in thrombin, changing its substrate specificity from fibrinogen to protein C. The resultant complex activates protein C which, together with its co-factor, protein S, inactivates FVa and FVIIIa.

Fibrinolysis

Not only is there a need for the fibrin clot to be limited to the site of injury, it is also essential that the clot is removed and circulation to the tissues re-established. The process of dissolution of fibrin deposit and clot is called fibrinolysis. It is essential for tissue repair and wound healing. Like coagulation, fibrinolysis is a complex system which is modified by many activators and inhibitors (*see* Figure 11.1). Just as thrombin is at the heart of the process of coagulation, fibrinolysis mainly centres on fibrin cleaving serine protease, plasmin. This enzyme is produced from its inactive precursor, plasminogen – a β-globulin proenzyme – by the action of two activating enzymes. Tissue plasminogen activator (t-PA) is the primary plasminogen activator within the vascular circulation. It is released from perturbed endothelial cells near the site of vascular injury and converts plasminogen in blood and tissue fluid to plasmin.

The second plasmin activator is urokinase that is secreted by epithelial cells and keeps hollow organs such as ureters free of clots. Plasmin acts by hydrolysing arginine and lysine bonds in a number of substrates. Its major effect is degradation of fibrin and fibrinogen. The plasmin-generating potential of plasma is enormous and capable of degrading the total amount of circulating fibrinogen in a short period of time. This is circumvented by inhibition of plasmin and is brought about by two mechanisms. Firstly, α-2-antiplasmin – a single-chain glycoprotein synthesised by the liver – specifically inhibits plasmin directly by forming a 1:1 complex with plasmin. Secondly, the generation of plasmin is inhibited indirectly by inactivation of plasminogen activators (*see* Figure 11.1).

There are three types of plasminogen activator inhibitor (PAI), of which plasminogen activator inhibitor-1 (PAI-1) seems to be most important. Thus the inhibition of fibrinolysis may occur either by direct inhibition of plasmin by α-2 antiplasmin, or by inactivation of plasminogen activators (t-PA and urokinase) by PAI-1. Inappropriate activation or inadequate inhibition of plasmin leads to ongoing fibrinolytic activity. Rare genetic conditions of deficiency PAI and α-2-antiplasmin which confer a bleeding tendency are examples of the latter.

There is yet another enzyme, thrombin-activatable fibrinolysis inhibitor (TAFI) which down-regulates fibrinolysis. As fibrin becomes degraded by plasmin, new C-terminal lysine and lysine residues are exposed in the partially digested clot. These further enhance activation of plasminogen to plasmin. TAFI is a metallocarboxypeptidase that strengthens fibrin clot by removing these residues and thus helps limit fibrinolysis. TAFI is activated by an array of haemostatic factors including thrombin, thrombin/thrombomodulin complex and plasmin. Inhibition of TAFI, therefore, increases the rate of fibrinolysis (*see* Figure 11.1).

ASSESSMENT OF HAEMOSTASIS

Problems in the haemostatic mechanism can be due to either a failure of haemo-static plug formation and stabilisation, inappropriate activation and propagation of coagulation, or deranged fibrinolysis. A bleeding tendency can result from a defect in the blood vessels, low platelet number, defective platelet function, deficiency of blood coagulation factors and excessive fibrinolysis. On the other hand, a thrombotic tendency ensues when there is a loss of inhibitory controls on coagulation.

The approach to a bleeding patient requires a careful history and thorough physical examination. These help to distinguish between defects affecting different components of haemostasis. For instance, mucocutaneous bleeding is characteristic of thrombocytopaenia or defective platelet function. On the other hand, bleeding into synovial joints and soft tissues is the hallmark of coagulation factor deficiencies, such as haemophilia. While the commonly used coagulation tests do not reflect the complexity of haemostasis in the body, it is important to have an understanding of *in vitro* coagulation. Only then is the correct interpretation of laboratory coagula-tion tests possible.

Although initially the 'waterfall' model of coagulation was proposed to explain physiological haemostasis its relevance now is limited to the understanding of labora-tory results. According to this, coagulation occurs as a series of amplifying proteolytic reactions culminating in the formation of a fibrin clot. The process starts as two distinct pathways, intrinsic and extrinsic, joining to form the common pathway. The intrinsic pathway is activated when blood comes in contact with a foreign sur-face such as glass. Contact with a non-endothelialised surface causes activation of a number of 'contact factors'. These include high-molecular-weight kininogen, prekal-likrein and FXII. Activated FXII (FXIIa) in turn leads to activation of FIX to FIXa. This subsequently, in the presence of FVIII, activates FX to FXa. At this juncture the extrinsic pathway joins the intrinsic pathway to form the common pathway.

The addition of certain tissue extracts to blood activates the extrinsic pathway. Thromboplastin in the tissue extract binds to FVII and the resulting complex acti-vates FX to FXa. This is the joining point of the two pathways to form the common pathway. FXa in the presence of FV activates prothrombin to thrombin, which con-verts fibrinogen to fibrin. As discussed below, the concept of a coagulation 'cascade' with two different pathways is utilised in interpretation of routinely used coagulation tests.

Laboratory tests

Assessment of haemostatic function falls into three categories, as discussed below.

Platelet function tests

Platelets have a key role in haemostasis and assessment of their function is vital for evaluation of haemostasis. Measurement of platelet function is, however, fraught with problems. This is because, firstly, physiological conditions are not simulated *in vitro* and, secondly, platelets are easily activated on manipulation.

While a number of sophisticated tests have come up in recent years, the first and most important evaluation of platelet function is the platelet count. Automated cell counters give a rapid and reliable platelet count but tend to overestimate the platelet count in situations where there is cell debris, e.g. in thalassaemias and thrombotic thrombocytopenic purpura. On the other hand, the count is underestimated in conditions with large platelets, e.g. in immune thrombocytopaenia. Optical counting methods work on the principle of the light-scattering property of platelets and generate more accurate results. Examination of a peripheral blood film is an invaluable part of assessment of platelet function as this gives information not only about platelet count but also about platelet morphology.

Platelets can aggregate *in vitro* when challenged with agonists. The response is an increase in light transmission of platelet-rich plasma and can be recorded by a photocell as a function of time after addition of the agonist. Platelet aggregation studies are used to diagnose inherited and acquired disorders of platelet function. The test can be affected by a number of drugs of which the most notable are aspirin and other non-steroidal anti-inflammatory agents.

The bleeding time has been used to assess *in vivo* haemostasis for almost a century. Caution is required in undertaking this as it can be difficult to interpret and is poorly reproducible. The platelet function analyser (PFA-100®) is a simple, *in vitro* test for assessing haemostasis and could eventually replace the bleeding time. Its specificity, however, does not seem to be any better than the bleeding time.

Coagulation tests

Despite major advancements in the understanding of haemostasis it remains a dauntingly complex process. Not surprisingly there is still no truly satisfactory laboratory test for its global assessment. While the available tests measure coagulation in fragmented parts and do not reflect physiological haemostasis, they remain valuable from a diagnostic point of view. The concept of a 'waterfall model' is essential to an understanding and interpretation of these tests. Coagulation is initiated *in vitro* by the addition of calcium plus an activating agent to plasma, and the time required for the formation of a clot is measured.

PROTHROMBIN TIME (PT)

This is a measure of the integrity of the extrinsic and common pathways of coagulation, and therefore measures the activities of FII, FV, FVII, FX and fibrinogen. TF in the form of 'thromboplastin', together with calcium, is added to citrated plasma. This initiates clotting by activating FVII and therefore completely bypasses the intrinsic pathway. Variations in PT occur due to different preparations of thromboplastin and instrumentation. As PT is used to monitor oral anticoagulation therapy this posed a major problem in the management of these patients. To overcome this, the International Normalised Ratio (INR) was developed. This is a mathematical derivative of PT and takes into account the sensitivity of the thromboplastins used. INR has therefore replaced PT for the monitoring of oral anticoagulants.

ACTIVATED PARTIAL THROMBOPLASTIN TIME (APTT)

This is a measure of the intrinsic and common pathways. Phospholipids, which lack TF (hence the name 'partial thromboplastin') together with an activator of contact factors and calcium, are added to plasma. The APTT is prolonged in deficiencies of all clotting factors except FVII and FXIII. There are special tests for the latter, as described below.

THROMBIN TIME (TT)

This is the simplest coagulation test. It is performed by adding thrombin to plasma and is a measure of rate of conversion of fibrinogen to fibrin. It is prolonged when there is a deficiency of fibrinogen or in the presence of inhibitors of the conversion reaction, e.g. heparin or fibrin degradation products.

CLOT SOLUBILITY TEST

The three tests described so far measure the amount of time for the formation of fibrin. Because FXIII acts when fibrin monomers have already formed it is not detected by these tests. In this test, the clot is resuspended in diluted urea or monochloroacetic acid. A normal clot takes a prolonged period of time to dissolve whereas subjects with FXIII deficiency make a fragile clot that dissolves quickly.

It is recognised that a deficiency of a coagulation factor invariably results in a prolonged clotting time (PT, APTT or TT). Whereas in most cases a bleeding tendency ensues, it is well established that deficiencies or complete absence of 'contact factors' – that is, FXII, prekallikrein and high-molecular-weight kininogen – despite causing a prolongation of APTT, do not cause any clinical haemostatic problem. Current evidence suggests that these factors may have a role in inflammation and the immune response.

Fibrinolytic tests

Fibrinolysis is difficult to detect in normal individuals. However, it is greatly accelerated in certain disease conditions and the 'euglobulin clot lysis time' is shortened in hyperfibrinolysis. Active fibrinolysis can also be determined by measuring fibrin degradation products (e.g. plasma D-dimer). D-dimer is only produced from a clot, thus an elevated level of D-dimer is strong evidence that a previously formed clot is undergoing dissolution.

Coagulation factor inhibitor tests

Haemostatic abnormalities may arise from the formation of autoantibodies directed against specific coagulation factors. These can arise in association with other autoimmune conditions, such as rheumatoid arthritis or systemic lupus erythematosus; certain malignant conditions, or they may occur spontaneously. The screening test (PT or APTT) is prolonged and fails to correct with addition of normal plasma in a 1:1 mix. Specific factor assays are needed for a definitive diagnosis.

Thromboelastography (TEG)

More than 90% of the coagulation process takes place after the initiation of clot formation and evaluation of whole blood provides a valuable tool in assessing continuous changes of the overall properties of the developing clot. TEG measures the viscoelastic properties of whole blood and provides information on the entire process of coagulation including initiation and speed of clot formation, clot strength, platelets and fibrinolysis. The test is performed on a small amount of blood placed in a cylindrical cup. As the clot forms, a characteristic tracing is generated by a pin suspended in the blood. Different components of the tracing reflect various activities of the haemostatic process and can indicate different abnormalities of the process. Although used widely as point-of-care test in cardiac and other surgical fields, its utility in general haematologic practice is still undefined.

Specific factor assays (functional and immunological)

There are assays commercially available for the quantification of individual haemo-static factors in plasma or serum. These are often performed to pinpoint the defect responsible for a specific haemostatic disorder. Functional results usually agree with the immunological ones but occasionally there is a discrepancy with the immuno-logical values exceeding the functional concentrations. This suggests the presence of an abnormal clotting factor that is immunologically close to normal but functionally defective. The interpretations of the results using these types of system may vary with the type of assay used.

DISORDERS OF THE HAEMOSTATIC SYSTEM

Platelet disorders

Not only do platelets play a key role in primary haemostasis by making a platelet plug but, it must be emphasised, the conversion of fibrinogen to fibrin by 'thrombin burst' occurs on the surface of activated platelets. An inadequate number or defec-tive function of platelets can, therefore, have serious haemostatic effects. Conversely, perturbations of platelet activity can lead to pathological thrombus formation and vascular occlusion resulting in thrombotic events such as stroke or acute coronary syndromes. Platelet disorders can be due to either abnormal number or function. Both kinds of disorder can be inherited or acquired. While congenital disorders are uncommon, acquired disorders are encountered frequently in clinical practice.

Inherited disorders

Inherited platelet disorders can be grouped as follows.

FAMILIAL THROMBOCYTOPAENIAS

These constitute a heterogeneous group of conditions with the common theme of a low platelet count causing bleeding. The pathogenetic mechanisms are varied and include defects of transcription factors, megakaryocyte production and cytoskeleton.

DISORDERS OF ADHESION

Platelets adhere to the sub-endothelial collagen of the damaged vessel wall through GPIb-V–IX. The interaction is mediated by vWF that acts as a bridge between GPIb-V–IX and sub-endothelium. If either the GPIb-V–IX or vWF is deficient or defective, adhesion will not proceed properly.

Bernard-Soulier syndrome

A rare autosomal recessive disorder due to an abnormality in GPIb-V–IX complex. The distinctive feature is thrombocytopaenia with giant platelets. Clinical features are characteristic of platelet dysfunction with mucocutaneous bleeding such as epistaxis, gingival bleeding and menorrhagia. Fortunately major bleeding in the absence of trauma is uncommon.

von Willebrand disease (vWD)
In addition to mediating platelet adhesion, another major function of vWF is to carry FVIII. Therefore, disorders affecting vWF not only cause defective platelet adhesion but also lead to defective coagulation. vWD is usually inherited as autosomal domi-nant although a number of subtypes display autosomal recessive inheritance – *see* 'Coagulation disorders' below.

DISORDERS OF AGGREGATION

Platelet–platelet interaction is mediated through fibrinogen and its platelet receptor glycoprotein GPIIb-IIIa. Two congenital disorders affect this interaction and cause defective platelet aggregation.

Glanzmann thromasthenia
Platelet activation changes the conformation of glycoprotein GPIIb-IIIa and trans-forms it into a competent fibrinogen receptor. Glanzmann thromasthenia is a rare autosomal recessive disorder characterised by a qualitative or quantitative defect in GPIIb-IIIa. Clinical features include significant mucocutaneous bleeding despite normal platelet count and morphology. Presentation is early in life and severity of haemostatic problems tends to improve with age.

Congenital afibrinogenaemia
It is a rare condition and is usually inherited in an autosomal recessive fashion. Platelet function and coagulation are both impaired and the resultant bleeding tendency can be catastrophic. Clinical features include prolonged umbilical cord, mucosal, musculoskeletal and intracranial bleeding. In females recurrent miscar-riages can occur. PT, APTT and TT are all prolonged. Diagnosis is confirmed by showing absence of immunoreactive fibrinogen in plasma.

DISORDERS OF SECRETION

This is a heterogeneous group where the defect lies in the contents or secretion of intracellular granules which causes impairment of platelet aggregation. The problem may extend to other cell types in some disorders.

Granules disorders
Two disorders are worth mentioning in this group. In *Gray platelet syndrome*, α granules are absent. This is inherited as an autosomal recessive disorder although autosomal dominant inheritance has also been described. The bleeding manifesta-tions are mucocutaneous and generally mild. *Quebec disorder*, a rare autosomal dominant disorder, is characterised by the absence of FV in α granules.

Dense granule disorders
Dense granules contain serotonin, adenosine triphosphate (ATP), ADP and lysosomal membrane proteins. On platelet activation, these fuse with the plasma membrane and are secreted to activate further platelets. Congenital deficiency of these causes a bleeding tendency of variable severity. Sometimes the deficiency extends to other lysosome-related organelles and produces a characteristic clinical picture. In *Hermansky-Pudlak syndrome*, in addition to a mild bleeding tendency, patients dem-onstrate oculocutaneous albinism. In *Chediak-Higashi syndrome*, a bleeding tendency

occurs together with oculocutaneous albinism, marked immune dysfunction and progressive neurologic dysfunction. Giant inclusion bodies are seen in neutrophils and other granule-containing cells.

DISORDERS OF SIGNALLING PATHWAY

This is a heterogeneous group in which a defect in any component of signal transduction – from abnormal cell surface receptor through to the activation of G-proteins and the release of intracellular messengers, causes impaired platelet aggregation. This usually results in a mild bleeding tendency.

SCOTT SYNDROME

There is a failure of thrombin generation on the surface of activated platelets in this rare condition.

Acquired disorders

These can be grouped as follows.

DRUGS

Acquired platelet dysfunction is most frequently a result of drug usage. Aspirin and other non-steroidal anti-inflammatory drugs are the most common agents. Aspirin interferes with platelet aggregation by inhibiting platelet cyclo-oxygenase irreversibly. In contrast, the inhibition by other conventional non-steroidal anti-inflammatory drugs is reversible and usually short lived. Clopidogrel and ticlopidine are non-competitive inhibitors of ADP receptor on platelets. Like aspirin, they are used extensively in clinical practice for the treatment of arterial thrombotic disease. Regardless of the stimulus, GPIIb-IIIa acts as the final common pathway for platelet aggregation. Antagonists of GPIIb-IIIa such as abciximab, tirofiban and eptifibatide are used widely in interventional coronary artery procedures.

SYSTEMIC DISORDERS

Platelet dysfunction can occur in a number of medical conditions including uraemia, liver disease and paraproteinaemia. In myelodysplasia and myeloproliferative disorders platelets may be intrinsically abnormal due to a defect at the level of megakaryocytes.

Coagulation disorders

These can be either inherited or acquired, as discussed below.

Inherited disorders

While deficiencies of all coagulation factors are known to occur, haemophilia A, haemophilia B and vWD make up about 95% of inherited coagulation disorders.

HAEMOPHILIA A AND B

These occur due to a congenital deficiency of FVIII and FIX, respectively. They are inherited as X-linked recessive disorders. The incidence of haemophilia A is about 1 in 5000, and of haemophilia B 1 in 25 000 live male births. The severity of the disease depends on the baseline factor level. A level of < 1% is regarded as severe, a level of 1% to 5% as moderate, and a level of > 5% to < 40% as mild haemophilia. Females with one defective copy of the gene are carriers. They can have a low factor level similar to mild haemophiliacs and experience bleeding complications.

Fortunately haemostatic problems in moderate and mild cases usually arise only in relation to trauma or surgical procedures. Bleeding occurs spontaneously in severe disease and is mainly musculoskeletal although can occur in any location. Spontaneous haemarthrosis, occurring in large joints, is the hallmark of severe disease. Repeated joint bleeding leads to permanent damage resulting in severe arthropathy. The fact that a factor level of just 1% prevents spontaneous bleeding has formed the basis of replacement therapy. Regular prophylactic treatment two or three times a week with FVIII (haemophilia A) or FIX (haemophilia B) concentrates can effectively prevent spontaneous bleeding.

Presentation in the neonate may result from a known family history, because of bleeding after invasive procedures, or from bleeding and bruising following the routine intramuscular injection of vitamin K. In babies in whom haemophilia is known or suspected to be present, vitamin K should be given orally.

VON WILLEBRAND DISEASE
vWF is a glycoprotein synthesised by endothelial cells and megakaryocytes. It is required for platelet adhesion and also acts as a carrier protein for FVIII. A deficiency or qualitative abnormality of this causes vWD. It is the most common inherited bleeding disorder. Population screening has shown the prevalence to be up to 1%, although symptomatic disease is much less common, affecting about 0.01% of the population.

Haemostatic manifestations are mainly due to defective platelet plug formation with mucocutaneous bleeding dominating the clinical picture. vWD is classified into three types based on results of laboratory investigations. Type 1 is a quantitative deficiency of vWF and makes up about 75% of cases. Type 2 is divided in four subtypes. Of these, types 2A, 2B and 2M are due to qualitatively abnormal vWF and are inherited in an autosomal dominant manner. Type 2N is due to a defect in the FVIII binding site of vWF. The resulting phenotype is of mild haemophilia A but the genetics are distinctly different, with an autosomal pattern. Type 3 results from an absence or severe reduction of vWF and is inherited in a homozygous or doubly heterozygous fashion.

Although presentation of vWD in the neonatal period has been described, it more commonly presents as frequent bruising or nosebleeds in older children or adults.

RARE COAGULATION DISORDERS
Deficiencies of other coagulation factors are rare, making up about 3–5% of all inherited deficiencies of coagulation factors. Inheritance pattern is autosomal with homozygotes or compound heterozygotes having a severe clinical course due to a marked deficiency of coagulation factor. Deficiencies of all coagulation factors are known including fibrinogen, FII, FV, FVII, FXI and FXIII. Deficiencies of FXII and other contact factors (prekallikrein and high-molecular-weight kininogens) are well

known but despite causing prolongation of activated partial thromboplastin time, do not cause haemostatic problems and are therefore of no clinical significance.

Acquired disorders

These are far more common than inherited disorders. Whereas inherited disorders are characterised by deficiency of a single coagulation factor, acquired disorders are associated with deficiencies of multiple clotting factors.

LIVER DISEASE

The liver is the site of synthesis of all coagulation factors, although FVIII displays significant extra-hepatic synthesis. It is, therefore, not surprising that severe disturbances of haemostasis can occur in hepatocellular failure. Not only is there impaired synthesis of coagulation factors, but degradation of activated coagulation factors is compromised as well. This can cause disseminated intravascular coagulation (DIC) that further augments the coagulopathy. Moreover, there is accelerated fibrinolysis which, together with thrombocytopaenia (resulting from portal hypertension and congestive splenomegaly), provides all the ingredients for a profound haemostatic compromise.

DISSEMINATED INTRAVASCULAR COAGULATION

This is not a disease in itself and is always secondary to another underlying disorder capable of initiating coagulation. A multitude of disorders promoting the expression of TF on endothelium or mononuclear cells can cause DIC. These include sepsis, trauma, malignant disorders, snakebites, transfusion reactions and obstetrical complications, such as amniotic fluid embolism and placental abruption. Irrespective of the underlying disorder, there is a sustained and uncontrollable generation of thrombin causing widespread intravascular deposition of fibrin, producing tissue ischaemia. This, in turn, activates plasminogen to plasmin and secondary fibrinolysis ensues. Ongoing coagulation leads to depletion of platelets and coagulation factors that, together with continual fibrinolytic activity, produce a haemorrhagic state in the face of thrombosis in the microcirculation. The result is a paradoxical picture of end-organ damage due to thrombosis in a bleeding patient.

The clinical and laboratory picture depends on the severity and on whether DIC is acute or chronic. In acute DIC, the platelet count and the levels of coagulation factors V, VIII and fibrinogen are reduced. Coagulation studies show the clotting times (PT, APTT and TT) to be prolonged, due to consumptive coagulopathy of the coagulation factors. In certain situations DIC can be chronic and may not lead to any derangement in these parameters. As the ongoing production of fibrin with its subsequent degradation to D-dimers underlies the pathophysiology – whether it is acute or chronic – D-dimer levels are always elevated in DIC. The level of fibrinogen would be expected to fall and it does so in acute DIC where the rate of destruction exceeds production. However, in chronic DIC it may remain normal or can even be elevated. This is explained by the fact that fibrinogen is an acute phase reactant and its synthesis goes up in inflammatory conditions. Thus its level depends on the balance of production and degradation, which in chronic cases can be tilted towards a relatively increased production in comparison with degradation.

ACQUIRED CIRCULATING COAGULATION INHIBITORS

A serious bleeding tendency can ensue due to the development of inhibitory antibodies against coagulation factors. Most commonly this occurs against FVIII although auto antibodies against all clotting factors have been described. Acquired haemophilia is a rare disorder, occurs in adult life and affects both sexes. It has a distinct clinical picture and, in contrast to the musculoskeletal bleeding that is the hallmark of congenital haemophilia, severe mucocutaneous and soft-tissue bleeding dominates the clinical picture. While 50% of cases are idiopathic, an association is well recognised with other auto immune conditions, malignant disease and pregnancy.

Inhibitory antibodies against coagulation factors can also arise in patients with congenital bleeding disorders on treatment with factor concentrates or blood products. In haemophilia A, for example, the immune system perceives exogenous FVIII as 'non-self' and launches an immune response against it. The development of inhibitory antibodies in both settings poses immense therapeutic challenges as any exogenous clotting factor is neutralised immediately. Definitive treatment is eradication of these antibodies through immune suppression. Management of bleeding complications requires treatment with activated prothrombin complex concentrates or recombinant activated FVII.

VITAMIN K DEFICIENCY

Haemostasis proceeds by binding of coagulation factors to platelet surface. For FII, FVII, FIX and FX – the vitamin-K-dependent coagulation factors – this occurs through their gamma-carboxylglutamic acid residues that recognise platelet phospholipids and bind to them. The residues, essential for biological activity of these factors, are a result of post-translational modification of the glutamic acid residues. The reaction, in which glutamic acid residues are converted to gamma-carboxyglutamyl acid residues, depends on a hepatic enzyme – gamma-glutamyl carboxylase – that requires biologically active vitamin K as an obligatory co-factor. Vitamin K deficiency or unavailability of biologically active vitamin K (as a result of oral anticoagulant therapy), produce a bleeding tendency by inhibiting the activity of gamma-glutamyl carboxylase.

Vitamin K is widely distributed in plants and its deficiency in an otherwise healthy adult is rare. As it is fat-soluble, conditions affecting absorption of fat such as chronic pancreatitis or biliary cirrhosis result in its deficiency. Patients tend to bruise easily and have mucosal bleeding.

HAEMOSTASIS IN THE NEONATE

It is recognised that the haemostatic system in the newborn is significantly different from that of the adult. While several unique features confer certain advantages (for example, venous and arterial thromboembolism are distinctly uncommon), the immaturity of the system at birth makes the neonate susceptible to haemostatic disorders such as haemorrhagic disease of the newborn secondary to vitamin K deficiency.

As there is essentially no transplacental passage of coagulation proteins from the mother, the levels of all components of haemostasis reflect fetal synthesis. Age-specific ranges of coagulation parameters and haemostatic factors have been published for premature and full-term babies. The main maturation of the haemostatic system in the fetus occurs before the thirtieth week of gestation. Therefore, only minor differences are found at birth between the haemostatic parameters of premature and full-term babies. Moreover, a rapid rate of maturation is observed in the premature compared with full-term infants.

In the healthy premature infant, while a wider range of PT is found, mean values are similar to those of adults. Likewise, in the healthy full-term infant, the PT remains comparable to adult values throughout, although shows significant shortening in the first month, which is mainly a result of rise in FVII level.

The APTT, on the other hand, is prolonged at birth regardless of maturity and in full-term infants reaches adult values at 3 months of age. Fibrinogen is normal at birth and shows a significant rise on the fifth day of life. The levels of the vitamin-K-dependent factors are only 50% of the adult values and rise to normal adult values by the sixth month of life. Whereas the rise in FII, FIX and FX is gradual, the FVII level goes up more quickly. FV level is normal at birth. The levels of FVIII and vWF are similar or increased compared with adult values, with the latter showing a continuous rise for a few months after birth. FXI and FXII are low at birth and gradually rise into the adult range by 6 months. The reduced levels of procoagulants impair thrombin generation during childhood. This, however, does not seem to lead to a bleeding tendency but may serve to prevent thromboembolism in this population.

The concentrations of antithrombin, protein C and protein S are significantly reduced during infancy and childhood. Antithrombin levels reach adult values by 3 months. Protein C and protein S, on the other hand, remain depressed during childhood. In adults, about 50–60% of protein S circulates in its inactive form, bound to complement component C_4B protein. However, since neonates do not have C_4B protein, virtually all protein S circulates in the free active form. Thus, a prothrombotic state that would otherwise follow from a deficiency of protein S is counterbalanced. The prothombotic state caused by the deficiency of antithrombin is offset by a different mechanism. The activity of thrombin is also inhibited by another plasma protein, α_2-macroglobulin (α_2-M). The levels of this are elevated in the newborn and continue to rise until 6 months of age. Whereas plasma antithrombin levels normalise by the third month, α_2-M continues to remain high throughout childhood and serves to guard against thromboembolism.

While the ultrastructure of neonatal platelets shows no difference from that of platelets in adults, they display *in vitro* hyporesponsiveness to a number of agonists that results from a relative defect in signal transduction. At the same time platelet adhesion, by virtue of abundance of large vWF multimers, is significantly increased and may compensate for diminished activation.

IMPLICATIONS FOR DIAGNOSIS

Differences in the levels of haemostatic proteins in the neonate compared with those in adults have significant diagnostic implications. The plasma levels of fibrinogen, FV, FVIII and vWF are either normal or raised at birth. It is well recognised that the level of fibrinogen goes up in response to inflammatory conditions such as sepsis. However, in a normal neonate, plasma fibrinogen level rises on the fifth day of life, and a raised level at this stage does not necessarily indicate sepsis.

The laboratory diagnosis of haemophilia A depends on demonstrating a low plasma level of FVIII. As FVIII level is generally normal, and never < 30% in the neonate, the diagnosis of severe (< 1%) and moderate (1% to 5%) haemophilia A can be established confidently if the FVIII level is correspondingly low. It is well recognised that FVIII level rises in response to a number of physiological and pathological stimuli. Therefore milder forms of haemophilia A may not be excluded due to the possibility that the FVIII level may have gone up into the normal neonatal range transiently because of neonatal stress.

The levels of FXII and vitamin-K-dependent factors are about half the adult values. Whereas this precludes reliable diagnosis of moderate and mild forms of haemophilia B, a credible diagnosis of severe haemophilia B can be established if the FIX level is <1%.

As the concentrations of antithrombin, protein C and protein S are markedly reduced in the newborn, it is imprudent to diagnose their deficiency state at this stage.

HAEMORRHAGIC DISEASE OF THE NEWBORN

A bleeding tendency in the newborn (unrelated to trauma or haemophilias) has been known for more than a century. The most significant cause of this is inadequate activity of vitamin-K-dependent coagulation factors, consequent upon a deficiency, or unavailability of the biologically active form of vitamin K. Most frequently this occurs in the first week of life, after 24 hours after birth, and is known as the 'classical type'. However, early-onset (occurring within 24 hours of birth), and late-onset (occurring at any time after the first week but within six months) presentations are well known to occur.

There is poor transfer of vitamin K across the placenta and consequently in case of inadequate intake it gets depleted quickly in the newborn. Due to the low content of vitamin K in breast milk the incidence of classic haemorrhagic disease of newborn is much higher in those who are breastfed solely. Early-onset disease is almost exclusively a result of transplacental passage of drugs affecting vitamin K activity. These include anticonvulsants (carbamazepine, phenytoin and barbiturates), oral anticoagulants and some antimicrobials (cephalosporins, rifampicin and isoniazid).

Late-onset disease occurs most commonly in those infants who have prolonged breastfeeding without supplemental vitamin K. Bleeding, either spontaneous or iatrogenic, can occur at any site commonly affecting skin, mucus membranes, gastrointestinal and urinary tracts and retroperitoneal cavity. The most serious complication is intracranial haemorrhage, which can affect a significant number of cases.

The diagnosis is strongly suspected upon finding a clearly prolonged PT together with a normal fibrinogen level and platelet count, and is confirmed by normalisation of PT within an hour of administering vitamin K. Haemorrhagic disease of the newborn can be successfully prevented by prophylactic administration of vitamin K at birth and supplementation of infant formulas with vitamin K. Prevention of early-onset disease may necessitate stopping or replacing the offending drug in the mother, or maternal vitamin K prophylaxis during pregnancy.

KEY POINTS FOR PRACTICE

1 PT mean values in both preterm and full-term babies are similar to those of adults but have a wider range.

2 APTT values are prolonged in both preterm and full-term babies for up to three months.

3 The plasma concentrations of the vitamin-K-dependent factors (FII, FVII, FIX and FX) at birth are only about 50% of those of adults and may not reach adult values until the infant is about six months old. The low FIX levels may interfere with the diagnosis of haemophilia B.

4 The plasma concentrations of fibrinogen, FV, FVIII and vWF are normal or raised at birth. An increase in fibrinogen concentrations occurs on day five.

5 Plasma concentrations of Factor VIII increase in response to stress and other physiological stimuli. This may mask the diagnosis of milder forms of haemophilia A.

6 Plasma concentrations of antithrombin, protein C and protein S are low in infancy and childhood but, in the case of protein S, this is counterbalanced by the absence of C_4B protein, which means that almost all protein S circulates in its unbound, active form.

7 Vitamin K should not be administered intramuscularly if there is a possibility of haemophilia or other coagulation disorders.

FURTHER READING

Andrew M, Paes B, Milner R, *et al.* Development of the human coagulation system in the full-term infant. *Blood.* 1987; **70**(1): 165–72.

Andrew M, Paes B, Milner R, *et al.* Development of the human coagulation system in the healthy premature infant. *Blood.* 1988; **72**(5): 1651–7.

Furie B, Furie BC. Mechanisms of thrombus formation. *N Engl J Med.* 2008; **359**(9): 938–49.

Lwaleed BA, Bass PS. Tissue factor pathway inhibitor: structure, biology and involvement in disease. *J Pathol.* 2006; **208**(3): 327–9.

Lwaleed BA, Cooper AJ, Voegeli D, *et al.* Tissue factor: a critical role in inflammation and cancer. *Biol Res Nurs.* 2007; **9**(2): 97–107.

Lwaleed BA, Goyal A, Delves GH, *et al.* Seminal hemostatic factors: then and now. *Semin Thromb Hemost.* 2007; **33**(1): 3–12.

Roberts HR, Hoffman M, Monroe DM. A cell-based model of thrombin generation. *Semin Throm Hemost.* 2006; **32**(Suppl. 1): 32–8.

Rodriguez NI, Hoots WK. Advances in hemophilia: experimental aspects and therapy. *Pediatr Clin North Am.* 2008; **55**(2): 357–76.

CHAPTER 12

Clinical decision making

Magi Sque, Max Chipulu and Debra McGonigle

CONTENTS

INTRODUCTION

Decision making is at the heart of clinical encounters or operational decisions (decisions that generate action). It therefore follows that the better our decisions, the more successful and effective our clinical practice will be. Sound decision making and operational decisions depend upon fully informed assessments and astute, analytic judgements. Clinicians should be concerned about their decision making as a means of improving accuracy and agreement among health professionals, and of ensuring professional accountability. There is also the need to be aware of and recognise the types of heuristics and biases[1-4] that can influence judgement choices and decision making.[2,4,5]

Clinical decisions span at least three areas of practice as clinicians make decisions about diagnosis, monitoring and interventions. Diagnoses are determined for the purpose they are required, for example identification of a state or condition, its trajectory, the pattern of distress and severity, its treatment or prognosis. Monitoring is largely concerned with detecting changes in the practice situation and tends to ask the questions: Is the patient getting better or worse? Is an intervention working? Is there cause for revision of particular therapy? Are further diagnostic investigations appropriate? Decisions about interventions underpin care, treatment and referral options.

The aim of this chapter is to encourage reflection on the underpinning theories of clinical decision making so that you will be able to acknowledge the processes that influence the ways in which decisions are made. The chapter starts with a discussion about the important elements that underpin clinical decisions, highlighting the significance of the assessment process, judgements, information processing, heuristics and intuition. It moves to a discussion covering humanistic intuitive discourses, Brunswik's Lens Model,[6,7] social judgement theory[6,8,9] and the cognitive continuum.[6,7] The final part of the chapter addresses decision analysis, rational theories of decision making, risk, uncertainty, and probability and decision trees.

Reflection on decisions made in clinical practice is important if we are to learn from the experience and look to improving the ways decisions are made. There is a need for everyone to be able to provide a clear rationale for the decisions made in terms of professional accountability and also to ensure that, whenever possible, decisions are based on the best available evidence. To demonstrate application of some of the more theoretical elements of clinical decision making, a decision from clinical practice has been used.

It is thought that decisions made in clinical practice are made 'on-the-spot' often without much time, and the case used here (*see* Box 12.1) is a good example of this. However, retrospective reflection on the decision clearly demonstrates how quickly the many elements (including personal experience, knowledge, assessment, cues) underpinning the decision are subconsciously assimilated and synthesised before a reasoned decision is made.

DEFINING CLINICAL DECISION MAKING

Clinical decision making is a cognitive process concerned with problem recognition through the identification of cues or of relevant clinical features, data gathering, assimilation, analysis, evaluation and choice, to produce an operational decision. Data gathering, assimilation and analysis are part of the **assessment** process. Evaluation and choice are part of the **judgement** process. Clinical judgement is the outcome of the assessment. Clinical judgement uses the skills of critical analysis, through which the clinician makes an evaluation of the status and quality of the presenting phenomenon or condition and forms an opinion or conclusion (inference) about what is (or will be) needed for an **operational decision**; it is an evaluation and choice between alternative courses of action.

Judgements can be:
▶ **descriptive** – attributes observed directly or from other sources
('the jaundiced baby was as orange as orange juice')
▶ **evaluative** – expresses a qualitative difference
('the baby's temperature is normal today after the pyrexia recorded yesterday')
▶ **causal** – attributes that explain a problem
('the baby's weight gain can be attributed to increased feeding')

BOX 12.1 THE CLINICAL DECISION

Edward was born in a district general hospital at 36 weeks' gestation, weighing 2.6 kilograms. He was transferred to the regional neonatal surgical centre with a diagnosis of oesophageal atresia and a tracheo-oesophageal fistula. Surgery to correct these anomalies took place the following afternoon and Edward returned from theatre ventilated via an endotracheal tube (ETT), and sedated with 20 µg/kg/h of morphine. Operation notes indicated that the anastomosis was under some tension. Edward was nursed on the neonatal unit in the intensive care room where four nurses were caring for seven other babies.

The Senior Sister in charge on the night of Edward's operation was made aware of difficulties relating to his airway management, when asked to prepare drugs for his reintubation. The unit was full, with 23 patients. Medical cover consisted of an on-site Senior House Officer who was attending a delivery one floor below, a Neonatal Registrar who had just finished a period of supervised practice because of concerns relating to her competency, and an on-call Consultant who was a 15-minute drive away. Edward's allocated nurse, although experienced in caring for neonates, had limited surgical experience.

Edward was bradycardic (heart rate of 60 beats per minute) and oxygen saturation was 75% with no chest movement despite the Registrar giving ambubag ventilation via his endotracheal tube. The Sister checked with the nurse caring for Edward that she had checked his ETT for secretions and according to the nurse the tube was patent. Rather than prepare reintubation drugs and remove the ETT, the Sister decided to instil 0.5 mL of 0.9% sodium chloride into the ETT prior to performing ETT suction again to clear any possible obstruction. She had major concerns relating to reintubation in terms of its effect on the anastomosis site and the ability of the Registrar to perform the procedure.

▶ **inference** – not based on facts gathered from the patient
('if there is an increase in preterm deliveries then admissions to the neonatal unit may be higher')
▶ **predictive** – what might happen to the patient
('if the term ventilated baby remains poorly sedated, he may develop a pneumothorax').

An **operational decision** is what you do or do not do as a consequence of your judgement. Operational decisions are made in the course of managing and delivering care. They are the reasons for assessment and could be described as the assessment goal. An **operational decision** is about **acting** on a judgement **choice**. Operational decisions are concerned with **action**.

Rules of thumb, heuristics and bias

When making judgements and, consequently, decisions, we need to access the vast amount of knowledge and information in our memories. To achieve this, heuristics or 'rules of thumb' are frequently used as short cuts to this information.[1-4] However, the inappropriate use of such selective information can be problematic. Heuristics have been intensively and extensively studied in psychology, sociology, economics and computer science.[1,10] The work in psychology of Kahneman and Tversky[11] is notable in this area. Heuristics may lead to a quick, feasible solution but may also cause system bias so that the way in which information is processed is imperfect. The most common of these heuristics, availability, representativeness and anchoring, and adjustment, are described by Cioffi.[12]

The availability heuristic tends to use information closest to hand. Evidence demonstrates that the way individuals judge events is based on the evidence available to them. For this reason, events that can be easily visualised or recalled may be judged to be more likely than they are. Individuals also appear to judge events based on how 'typical' of the class of the event they are judging the event in question appears, regardless of other evidence outside their own experience of 'typical'.

The representative heuristic involves reasoning influenced by prior experiences of similar events which may lead to over-reliance on certain evidence while other facts are ignored. As a consequence of using selective heuristics, people, including clinicians, sometimes make substantial decision errors.[13]

Anchoring and adjustment heuristics draw on anchors, usually in the form of cognitive reference points;[9,12] for example, a poorly perfused neonate like Edward could be expected to have a bluish complexion, indicative of cyanosis.

Intuition

In clinical decision making some health professionals have repeatedly stated reliance on intuitive judgement.[14] However, there appears to be endless debate about what intuition is and whether it deserves recognition and legitimacy in praxis. Harbison[15] describes a logic underlying intuitive judgement but it has been explained by others as an inability to articulate the decision-making process. Hams[14] explains that a deeply grounded knowledge base, developed through critical thought, helps experienced practitioners to practise intuitively. Therefore each clinical experience becomes a lesson, which informs the next one. Buckingham and Adams[16] discuss how cues can stimulate recall and describe the term 'pattern recognition' as the linking of cues with diagnostic categories. Intuition is seen by some as the skill of pattern recognition involving the rapid, unconscious processing of cues; giving rise to an inability to articulate the decision-making process. Gobet and Chassy[17] describe the work done by Benner[18] in the 1980s as being 'too simple' to account for the complexities of expert intuition. They explain how intuitive decision making is linked to individual perception and analytic and conscious problem solving at the expert level aided by chunks of related information[19] and complex data structures or templates[20] that are associated with long-term memory information.

McKinnon,[21] on the other hand, argues that stored emotional interpretation of clinical phenomena and its interface with reasoning, via neural pathways, creates intuitive responses by the expert practitioner. He stresses the importance of the link between cognition and emotion to explain intuitive thought and response. McKinnon[21] claims that: 'Emotion stands at the helm of memory guidance, consolidation, storage and retrieval. Cognition is emotion gated' (p. 42). Emotion is therefore suggested to be the precursor to thought and response; that is, we feel before we think.[22] It would appear, therefore, that intuition is much more than a 'gut feeling'. It appears to have a deeply grounded knowledge base but because of its often very rapid and unconscious nature, this becomes difficult to articulate. Later we will see how intuition is used in practice.

Assessment

Assessment is the first stage of the decision-making process and it is used to 'build a picture' of the patient's situation and it is fundamental and crucial to accurate clinical judgements and reliable operational decisions. Key data-gathering strategies of the assessment process are: listening, asking, observing, doing, filtering and finally synthesising and interpreting. More specifically, data gathering will include exploring the history of the clinical event, which may involve asking questions, both general and focused, of individuals who are able to give an accurate account of events. This may be the patient or, in the case of the neonate, the parent or relevant health professional. A thorough examination of the patient through observation, using look, feel and move strategies, and both visual and non-visual cues (*see* Box 12.2) and investigations to help confirm or refute suspicions will complete the data-gathering process.

Awareness of the need for assessment in Edward's case was brought about by the request from clinical staff for the Sister to prepare medication for reintubation. One of the medications, a muscle relaxant, would require the use of bag-and-mask ventilation and replacing Edward's endotracheal tube would require extension of his neck.

BOX 12.2 THE VISUAL AND NON-VISUAL CUES USED DURING THE ASSESSMENT PROCESS OF EDWARD

Visual cues

- Mechanical ventilation via an endotracheal tube
- Heart rate 60 BPM
- No chest movement
- Cyanotic
- Sedated on a continuous morphine infusion
- Surgical wound
- Night time – reduced personnel and services

Non-visual cues

- Post-operative oesophageal atresia and tracheo-oesophageal repair
- Recent anaesthetic
- Anastomotic tension
- Bag-and-mask ventilation to be avoided if at all possible
- Senior House Officer attending a delivery elsewhere
- Inexperienced Registrar – recent period of supervised practice
- On-call Consultant off site – approximately 15-minute drive away
- Relatively inexperienced nurse caring for Edward

Both of these actions were perceived by the Sister as having a detrimental effect on the anastomosis site. The first step in the Sister's decision making and a fundamental part of the assessment process was that of cue acquisition. In a very brief period of time, both visual and non-visual cues (Box 12.2) led the Sister to an assessment of Edward's situation and the need for a course of action or an operational decision.

Building a picture of the patient situation is the cognitive processing element of assessment. It involves matching past experience with the present case, which could be flawed.[9] The literature suggests that there are significant inadequacies in the assessment process caused by *inadequate data search* and *early closure* of the consultation.[2] Assessment is not only about data gathering. Knowledge is fundamental to the ability to accurately interpret and synthesise data. Table 12.1 identifies six broad types of knowledge that impact on the assessment process and consequent decision making.[23–25] The table also demonstrates how these types of knowledge were applicable to the Sister's decision making in Edward's case.

TABLE 12.1 Types of knowledge applied in Edward's case

Type of knowledge	Definition	Sources and relevance	Application to the decision made
Empirical[23]	Scientific, technical or factual knowledge that underpins clinical practice and may take the form of science, learning theories, organisation of facts, describing and explaining phenomena.	Literature, formal education, research or clinical audit. Relevance to health assessment, physical examination, diagnosis, prognosis, treatment.	Knowledge used in relation to neonates, oesophageal atresia, surgical treatment, complications, and ventilation obtained from specialist courses, study days, journals.
Ethical[23]	Moral experience gained through life, knowing what is right and wrong.	Experience, custom and passing on of values and beliefs, through observation and teaching. Moral framework that underpins clinical action.	Principles of rights and responsibilities, beneficence and non-maleficence applied; to respect Edward's right to life, to act responsibly to do positive good for Edward and to do him no harm.
Aesthetic[23]	Aesthetic knowledge appears to have no rational or logical explanation. It is individualised through experience and is regarded as 'intuitive'.	Gained through experience and the individual characteristics of the person such as their values and beliefs. Decisions are made rapidly without apparent rationale or logical reasoning. Commonly part of the repertoire of the expert practitioner.	Neonatal surgical experience over many years leading to 'intuitive' reasoning.

(continued)

Type of knowledge	Definition	Sources and relevance	Application to the decision made
Personal[23]	Self-knowledge, knowing oneself, individual perceptions, feelings, prejudices or biases.	Experience, learning from self and others. Awareness of one's own perceptions, feelings, prejudices or biases.	Aware of own personal limitations (strengths and weaknesses). Acknowledges bias towards Registrar because of recent concerns about capability.
Socio-political[24]	Social, economic, political considerations relevant for a particular society. It is about the bigger context than an individual patient.	Awareness, experience. How the individual patient fits within the bigger picture.	Clinical governance issues: risk and quality. Economic: issue of increased financial and personal cost related to any post-operative complications.
Woman's[25]	Feminist perspective over science as male dominated. Argues that science and technology undermine feminist knowledge, which involves women's life instincts and the humanness of relationships.	Women's life experiences. Women's socialisation into the role of health professional.	Not knowingly aware of its application in this decision.

Of particular importance to the Sister's decision were empirical, ethical, personal and aesthetic knowledge. The confidence that comes with knowledge, experience and knowing one's personal limitations led the Sister directly and quickly to the decision. Equally important was personal knowledge of the Registrar in relation to clinical capability, the absence of the Senior House Officer and the time factor in summoning the on-call Consultant. However, it appears the most important type of knowledge used was aesthetic, in the form of 'intuition'. The need for immediate action to re-establish ventilation and consequently improve Edward's heart rate and colour meant the decision-making process advanced rapidly over a period of 10–15 seconds. The large numbers of simultaneous cues were used intuitively to make the decision **not to remove the ETT but to ensure patency by instilling 0.5 mL of 0.9% sodium chloride and applying suction.**

Underpinning all clinical decision making, as in the Sister's operational decision, is ethical knowledge. Making ethical clinical decisions is facilitated through cognition and objectivity, which is more than merely following rules or acting intuitively. Applying ethical knowledge is about positively deciding the correct action to take in a given situation that will be in the best interest of the patient. This requires the ability to facilitate dialogue based on options and optimal solutions, the ability to anticipate circumstances and recognise the subtleties of moral issues. Clearly underpinning the Sister's decision was Edward's right to life and her professional responsibility to exert beneficence; to take action that would potentially have the safest positive outcome for Edward, i.e. ensuring patency of the endotracheal tube, whilst upholding the principle of non-maleficence 'to do no harm' through not causing a potential rupture of the anastomosis and further post-operative complications through the act of reintubation.

Two other important domains that impact on the assessment and decision-making process are domain-specific knowledge and prior knowledge of the patient and their circumstances.[26] Clearly a neonatal practitioner will have specific domain knowledge that will assist them in making appropriate decisions about their tiny clients. Clinical staff will also develop a familiarity with the particular baby and their individual responses so they are better able to make judgements about clinical signs and the illness trajectory. Specific knowledge and expectations about a neonate's family situation that might affect decisions about support issues such as discharge planning, are also very important.

To access this knowledge from memory, we must apply heuristics, pattern recognition or rules. A combination of cues may bring hypotheses to mind and they can be easily retrieved from memory. Therefore, to make sense of cue gathering to inform the reasoning process, hypotheses generation and consequent judgements, cues need to be sorted and 'chunked' or coalesced.[19] Box 12.3 shows the sorting and coalescing of Edward's assessment cues.

Judgements

It could be argued that, in making the decision not to remove Edward's ETT, the Sister used both anchoring and representative heuristics. The cognitive reference points of low heart rate, cyanosis and no chest movement immediately led the Sister to the judgement that the endotracheal tube was blocked, whilst there was recognition of a similarity between Edward's situation and previous experience of caring for babies with oesophageal atresia. Whilst heuristics are perceived as an aid to reducing uncertainty, they can also be the cause of poor decision making and bias.[1-4,9] Biases such as ignoring base rates (prevalence), hindsight or stereotyping may occur for numerous reasons including over-confidence, time pressures or one's own values and beliefs.[2] On reflection, the Sister's bias in relation to the ability of the Registrar to reintubate Edward carried some weight in the decision.

The information processing theory is perhaps the most influential theory which describes how decisions are made. Bohinc and Gradisar[27] state that its basis is in studies on human problem solving, but in healthcare it is defined as a process of hypothetical-deductive reasoning. Thompson and Dowding[9] cite Elstein et al.'s[28] hypothetico-deductive model, listing the four-stage process as: cue acquisition, hypothesis generation, cue interpretation and hypothesis evaluation. Thompson and Dowding[9] discuss the generation of between four and six initial and tentative hypotheses as a norm. They argue, however, that these may be flawed, as human reasoning is 'bounded' by the capacity of the human memory. There is also the danger of being too focused and missing potential outcomes. Table 12.2 shows the tentative hypotheses generated by the Sister from the coalescence of cues.

BOX 12.3 CHUNKING AND COALESCING OF EDWARD'S ASSESSMENT CUES

Clinical history

- Repair of oesophageal atresia and tracheo-oesophageal fistula 12 hours previously
- Anastomotic tension
- Bag-and-mask ventilation to be avoided if at all possible

Current status

- Preterm baby 36/40
- Recent anaesthetic
- Continuous morphine infusion
- Mechanically ventilated

Clinical observations

- Heart rate 60 BPM
- No chest movement
- Cyanotic

Staffing context

- Inexperienced Registrar present
- Senior House Officer elsewhere
- On-call Consultant off site
- Inexperienced attending nurse
- Night-time – less urgent care support

TABLE 12.2 The hypotheses generated from coalescence of cues

Coalescence of cues	Tentative hypotheses
• Repair of oesophageal atresia and tracheo-oesophageal fistula 12 hours previously • Anastomotic tension • Bag-and-mask ventilation to be avoided if at all possible	Risk of anastomotic breakdown
• Preterm baby 36/40 • Recent anaesthetic • Continuous morphine infusion • Mechanically ventilated	Edward is unlikely to breathe if endotracheal tube removed
• Heart rate 60 BPM • No chest movement • Cyanotic	Blocked ETT

(continued)

Coalescence of cues	Tentative hypotheses
<ul><li>Inexperienced Registrar</li><li>Senior House Officer elsewhere</li><li>On-call Consultant off site</li><li>Inexperienced attending nurse</li><li>Night-time – less urgent care support</li></ul>	Risk of failure to reintubate

These tentative hypotheses form first-order judgements, which become second-order cues. Interpretation of the second-order cues and whether to accept the opinion and the probability that the opinion is correct leads to second-order judgements and the choice of an operational decision. The Sister's decision-making process using the hypothetico-deductive process is illustrated in Figure 12.1.

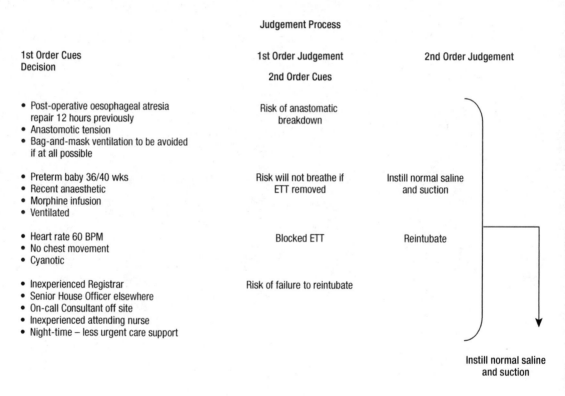

FIGURE 12.1 Demonstrates the decision-making process using the hypothetico-deductive process

However, it is possible for clinicians to come to different decisions even though they are presented with the same set of cues. One way of explaining this is through social judgement theory.[6]

Social judgement theory

Using social judgement theory we can answer the question: Did the clinician get it right? This theory helps us to evaluate and learn from our decisions to improve our decision making. Social judgement theory considers the relationship between judgement and the selection of information. Judgements are analysed, after they have been made, for their accuracy and the relative importance given to each cue. Both the patient and the clinical context need to be considered equally.

The theoretical foundation for this judgement analysis is the Brunswik's Lens Model.[6,8] In 1943[6] Brunswik, an Austrian psychologist, proposed the Len's Model that functions like a convex lens. The model applied to the clinical situation assumes the actual state of the patient offers a clinician tangible surface cues, i.e. signs and symptoms of their intangible states. The outcome of the assessment, judgement and decision, in this example, not to remove the ETT but to instil 0.5 mL 0.9% sodium chloride and apply suction, depended on the qualities of the judge, in this case the Sister; the qualities of the patient, Edward; and the quality of the interaction. Because tangible cues do not indicate the depth of conditions with certainty (inferred states such as severity or a blocked endotracheal tube), they are fallible.

Thompson and Dowding[9] explain that the outcome of a judgement is a function of how the cues are used and interpreted. During shared decision making, the Brunswik's Lens Model may be useful in that it enables clinicians to explain their rationale in terms of making a judgement by assigning different 'weights' to the presenting cues. In this context it is possible that two clinicians faced with the same patient, the same history and the same cues could make quite different judgements depending on their assessment of the patient, which might have been influenced by a number of factors including their level of knowledge, previous experience, personal biases and values.

Cognitive continuum theory

Developed by Hammond,[6] the cognitive continuum theory is a unifying theory of human judgement and decision making that acknowledges the analytical and humanistic-intuitive approaches. It focuses on the tension and distinction between intuitive and analytical thinking, recognising the diversity of individual cognitive strategies. The theory suggests that reasoning is neither purely intuitive nor purely analytical but is rather a continuum between the two poles, with judgements located at points somewhere in between,[6,9] allowing judges to alternate back and forth between analysis and intuition. The theory offers a set of interrelated predictions about task properties and cognition, suggesting that the cognitive approach of a judge relies upon three principles, namely:
- the complexity of the task to be undertaken
- the clarity of the task, and
- the way in which the task is presented.

Tasks that tend to induce intuitive judgements, as in the Sister's case, tend to be complex; lack clarity; are unstructured; present many simultaneous cues; have a variety of solutions; and require a rapid response. On the other hand, tasks to which analytical judgements best respond are clear, highly structured, have few cues that present sequentially, have definitive or few solutions and allow for time to plan a considered response.[6]

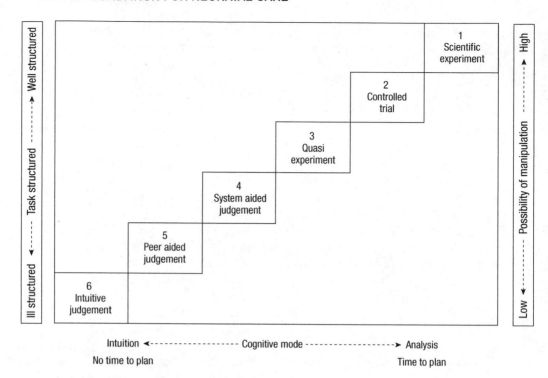

FIGURE 12.2 The cognitive continuum

The cognitive continuum theory provides a framework for clinicians to aim for accuracy in their decision making. Not adhering to its basic premise is likely to lead to judgement inaccuracies.[29] Using cognitive continuum theory we can answer the question: How did the healthcare professional get it (i.e. the judgement) right? The cognition mode to use should depend on the task structure, number of cues and time available to complete the task.[9] In the neonatal environment, mode 6 represents the position at which the articulation of evidence and Sister's cognition occurred.[15,29] Because of the large number of cues, very limited time and poorly structured task, the Sister's decision sits at mode 6 on the continuum (*see* Figure 12.2).

Kahneman *et al.*[10] cautioned that over-reliance on intuition to the exclusion of analysis can severely limit the use of knowledge and evidence. This can have detrimental effects for clinicians not producing an informed rationale to justify their decisions. The cognitive continuum highlights this need to underpin practice decisions with a sound evidence base. So we turn now to the options that allow us to calculate and provide a rational basis for clinical decisions.

THE NATURE OF DECISION ANALYSIS

As a discipline, 'Decision Analysis' is relatively new, dating back to the 1960s. In 1968 Howard Raiffa[30] published the first significant text on the subject. Usually, decision analysis involves the application of a mathematical or statistical model and is thus generally perceived as being objective and quantitative. However, this is a misconception, since decision analysis should use all types of information, some of which may be subjective. The nature of decision analysis can be summarised as:

❱ being systematic and structured
❱ integrating intuitive and subjective judgements
❱ involving qualitative and quantitative components
❱ requiring rational analysis.

Stages in decision analysis

Decision analysis uses a structured framework which enables decision making to be shared with colleagues and patients. It can provide the opportunity for numerical, quantitative evaluation of the risks and benefits associated with some decisions.

Defining the problem

At the heart of the decision is the problem to be solved. It appears an overstatement but to solve the problem effectively it is necessary to solve the right problem. To understand fully what the problem is, the scope of the problem must be known. This allows the identification of who must take part in the decision-making process. In Edward's case: Should the Sister sit in conclave with the medical staff? Should Edward's allocated nurse be involved? The Sister decided to define the problem by herself. This is how she appeared to perceive it: 'To remove or not to remove the endotracheal tube?' Would the problem definition have been different if others had been involved in defining it? Probably not, for this is an obvious problem. But bigger, less obvious strategic problems are almost entirely shaped by the worldviews of those who take part in the decision.

TABLE 12.3 Elements of the rational decision-making process applied to Edward's case

Element of the decision	Definition	Example in Edward's case
Objective(s)	The aims or goals to be achieved as a result of the solution found	Ensure patency of blocked endotracheal tube
Strategies	The alternative approaches that can be used to achieve the objective(s)	• Remove the tube immediately and reintubate • Instil 0.5 mL 0.9% sodium chloride, apply suction and reintubate later
States of the world	Environmental factors that are beyond the control of the decision maker but can influence how successfully the objectives are achieved	Success or failure could lead to: • anastomotic breakdown • tube patent but Edward's condition fails to improve • failure to reintubate
Payoffs	The value (e.g. monetary, utility or other score according to the decision maker(s)' view) of each strategy under each state of the world	E.g. a minimum score of zero if Edward's condition fails to improve, reintubation fails and help does not arrive immediately; alternatively, a maximum score of 100 if Edward's condition improves and there are no other side effects.

At the end of the problem-definition stage, the objective(s), strategies and context of the problem should be clear. This will allow the decision maker(s) to choose the most appropriate model to analyse the value of each strategy.[31]

Rational models

Rational decision models are normative but they can also be prescriptive. A very good exposition of the normative-prescriptive distinction can be found in Koehler and Harvey.[32] The aim of rational models is to maximise the 'payoff'; i.e. to choose the best strategy. To do this the decision maker must be perfectly rational and be able to perfectly calculate the 'payoff' of each strategy given. 'Perfectly rational' and 'perfect information' are two very big phrases and they point to the difficulties in applying rational models, which we will revisit below.

Certainty, uncertainty and probability

The environments in which decisions are made can be categorised as certain, risky or uncertain. Of these environments, decisions made under certainty are the easiest. The greater the lack of certainty or the greater the degree of uncertainty, the more complex the decision becomes. The idea, therefore, is that when faced with an uncertain environment, the decision maker must employ a technique that reassigns the uncertainty so that the end result is something akin to certainty. For this to happen it is necessary to gather sufficient information to allow the decision maker to quantify the degree of uncertainty or probability.

Statisticians use the word 'probability' to express numerically the degree of likelihood that a given event will happen in the future.[33] Thus, if an event is impossible, it has a probability of 0 or 0%. If an event is certain to happen, it has a probability of 1 or 100%. The degree of other uncertain events can then be measured using numbers between 0 and 1 or between 0% and 100%.

There are three generally accepted classes of probability:
- logical or classical probability
- frequentist or observed probability
- subjective probability.

Logical or classical probability

If it is possible to work out all the possible outcomes of a process and to count them, then we can logically work out with exactitude the probability of an event. This is then an exact, objective quantity.

Frequentist or observed probability

However, most events that clinicians encounter may not be easily countable or logically decomposable. What, for example, is the probability that a baby born in England may be preterm? In this situation, we may use survey or census data to estimate the probability. According to the Audit Commission,[34] 635 748 babies were born in England in 2006. Of these, 62 471 were admitted to neonatal units. Thus we can estimate:

Probability that a baby will need neonatal care = Number of babies admitted to neonatal units/Total number of babies born in England = 62 471/63 5748 = 0.1 or 10%

Again, this is an objective quantity. It is, however, not exact; it is only an estimate because it is based on survey data.

Subjective probability

However, it may not be possible to collect survey data. For example, we know in Edward's case that the Sister decided not to remove the ETT because the risk of failure to reintubate was 'high'. But what exactly was the probability of risk of failure? Box 12.4 below shows the number of factors that could have contributed to risk of failure to reintubate.

BOX 12.4 POTENTIAL INFLUENCING FACTORS ON RISK OF FAILURE TO REINTUBATE EDWARD

- Inexperienced Registrar
- Senior House Officer elsewhere
- On-call Consultant off site
- Night-time – fewer staff to manage an emergency
- Success rate of reintubation in previous cases

Whilst it is unrealistic in this case (the Sister reports that the decision was made 'in a matter of seconds'), perhaps in another context it would have been possible to go back to previous records involving cases of reintubation of babies and calculate the proportion of cases in which reintubation failed. But is this the best estimate of the chance of failure for Edward? The answer is 'No', because it is almost impossible that all the babies in previous cases were in exactly the same situation and reacted to the treatment in exactly the same way as Edward did. So what to do?

In this situation, there were a number of factors all of which could have been significantly influential. It was necessary for the Sister to use her judgement and expertise to estimate as accurately as possible the probability of failure to reintubate based on Edward's unique circumstances and taking into account all the factors. She judged the probability to be 'substantial'. Given more time, it would have been worthwhile assigning a specific number to this 'high' judgement (e.g. 10% probability), since precisely stated quantities, even when based on subjective judgement, allow for much more effective rational analysis. Now, unlike the probabilities calculated above, this quantity is neither objective nor exact. It is a subjective estimate.

The decision tree

For complex, multi-stage decision problems (unlike the case of Edward), it is often helpful to represent the options, uncertainties and outcomes in the form of a decision tree.[35] A decision tree is a mathematical, graphical illustration of all the potential possible decision options for a given choice. For each of the possible decision options, the consequences of taking that decision are quantified and expressed in terms of likelihoods and utilities. In specific clinical contexts where difficult shared decision making is important, a decision tree could offer the potential for all those involved to choose the option that best maximises benefit for the patient whilst minimising risk.

Clinical decision support systems

Clinical decision support systems (CDSS) are computer systems that integrate cues from medical and patient information sources with the aim of helping clinicians make decisions. Within the neonatal context their use is limited, a Cochrane Review reported there was insufficient evidence to enable evaluation of any potential benefit.[36] More recently, the sensitivity and speed of 'Isabel' (Isabel Healthcare Inc., USA), a new web-based clinical decision support system has been evaluated in both paediatrics[37] and in adult medicine.[38] In both studies it was reported that CDSS may have a future role as a diagnostic aid in the decision-making process.

SUMMARY

This chapter used a clinical example, Edward's case, to illustrate some of the key considerations in making judgements and decisions in the practice environment and some of the many ways in which decision making can be approached. This retrospective review of acute decisions may help either to validate such actions for the future or to influence changes in practice.

Many of the issues crucial to effective decision making have been discussed, including the importance of a sound assessment process and the ability to keep it as wide as possible and not to narrow the judgement focus too soon; the potential impact that heuristics and biases can have on creating decision errors; and the use of social judgement and the cognitive continuum as tools to both understand and analyse decisions, as a means of improving decision making. There remains much work to be done in the field, accruing evidence in the science of decision making in healthcare generally and in neonatal practice particularly. It is hoped this chapter might act as a springboard not only to improving your decision making but to deliberations with regard to contributing to further research and evidence gathering in this most important of skills.

KEY POINTS FOR PRACTICE

1   Sound assessment is based on the quality of information gathered.
2   The process of information gathering relies on cognitive searches, utilising reliable and accurate sources of information and knowledge, and the interpretation of visual and non-visual cues.
3   Judgement is a product of the assessment process and personal cognitive ability.
4   Clinicians need to reflect on the decision-making process in order that they acknowledge their personal biases, values and the role that heuristics may play.
5   Effective clinical decisions depend on sound judgements which take account of the patient's clinical needs, priorities, and values.

REFERENCES

1 Gilovich T, Griffin D, Kahneman D, editors. *Heuristics and Biases: the psychology of intuitive judgement.* Cambridge: Cambridge University Press; 2002.

2 Graber ML, Berner ES. Diagnostic error: is overconfidence the problem? *Am J Med.* 2008; **121**(5A): S2–46.

3 Elstein AS, Schwartz A. Evidence base of clinical diagnosis: clinical problem solving and diagnostic decision making: selective review of the cognitive literature. *BMJ.* 2002; **324**: 729–32.

4 Klein JG. Five pitfalls in decisions about diagnosis and prescribing. *BMJ.* 2005; **330**: 781–3.

5 Goldstein WM, Hogarth RM, editors. *Research on Judgment and Decision Making: currents, connections, and controversies.* Cambridge: Cambridge University Press; 1997.

6 Cooksey RW. *Judgement Analysis: theory, methods and applications.* London: Academic Press; 1996.

7 Standing M. Clinical judgement and decision-making in nursing – nine modes of practice in a revised cognitive continuum. *J Adv Nurs.* 2008; **62**(1): 124–34.

8 Hammond KR. How convergence of research paradigms can improve research on diagnostic judgement. *Med Decis Making.* 1996; **16**(3): 281–7.

9 Thompson C, Dowding D. *Clinical Decision Making and Judgement in Nursing.* London: Churchill Livingstone; 2002.

10 Kahneman D, Slovic P, Tversky A. *Judgement Under Uncertainty: heuristics and biases.* Cambridge: Cambridge University Press; 1982.

11 Kahneman D, Tversky A. Subjective probability: a judgment of representativeness. *Cognitive Psychology.* 1972; **3**: 430–54.

12 Cioffi J. A study of the use of past experiences in clinical decision making in emergency situations. *Int J Nurs Stud.* 2001; **38**(5): 591–9.

13 Payne JW, Bettman JR, Johnson EJ. *The Adaptive Decision Maker.* Cambridge: Cambridge University Press; 1993.

14 Hams SP. A gut feeling? Intuition and critical care nursing. *Intensive Crit Care Nurs.* 2000; **16**(5): 310–18.

15 Harbison J. Clinical decision making in nursing: theoretical perspectives and their relevance to practice. *J Adv Nurs.* 2001; **35**(1): 126–33.

16 Buckingham CD, Adams A. Classifying clinical decision making: interpreting nursing intuition, heuristics and medical diagnosis. *J Adv Nurs.* 2000; **32**(4): 990–8.

17 Gobet F, Chassy P. Towards an alternative to Benner's theory of expert intuition in nursing: a discussion paper. *Int J Nurs Stud.* 2008; **45**(1): 129–39.

18 Benner P. *From Novice to Expert.* London: Addison Wesley; 1984.

19 Gobet F, Clarkson G. Chunks in expert memory: evidence for the magical number four . . . or is it two? *Memory.* 2004; **12**(6): 732–47.

20 Gobet F, Simon HA. Five seconds or sixty? Presentations in time in expert memory. *Cognitive Science.* 2000; **24**: 651–82.

21 McKinnon J. Feeling and knowing: neural scientific perspectives on intuitive practice. *Nurs Stand.* 2005; **20**(1): 41–6.

22 Panksepp J. *Affective Neuroscience: the foundations of human and animal emotions.* Oxford: Oxford University Press; 1998.

23 Carper BA. Fundamental patterns of knowing in nursing. *Adv Nurs Sci.* 1978; **1**(1): 13–23.

24 Heath H. Reflection and patterns of knowing in nursing. *J Adv Nurs.* 1998; **27**: 1054–9.

25 Hagnell E. Nursing knowledge: women's knowledge: A sociological perspective. *J Adv Nurs.* 1988; **14**: 226–33.

26 Benner P, Tanner CA, Chesla CA. *Expertise in Nursing Practice: caring, clinical judgement, and ethics.* New York: Springer; 1996.

27 Bohinc M, Gradisar M. Decision-making model for nursing. *J Nurs Admin.* 2003; **33**(12): 627–9.

28 Elstein AS, Shulman LS, Sprafka SA. *Medical Problem Solving: an analysis of clinical reasoning.* Cambridge: Harvard University Press; 1978.

29 Cader R, Campbell S, Watson D. Cognitive Continuum Theory in nursing decision-making. *J Adv Nurs.* 2005; **49**(4): 331–447.

30 Raiffa H. *Decision Analysis: introductory lectures on choices under uncertainty.* London: Random House; 1968.

31 Goodwin P, Wright G. *Decision Analysis for Management Judgement.* 3rd ed. New York: John Wiley; 2004.

32 Koehler DJ, Harvey N, editors. *Blackwell Handbook of Judgment and Decision Making.* New York: Blackwell; 2004.

33 Rowntree D. *Probability Without Tears: a primer for non-mathematicians.* New York: Barnes & Noble; 1994.

34 Report by the Comptroller and Auditor General. *Caring for Vulnerable Babies: the reorganisation of neonatal services in England.* HC 0101 Session 2007–2008. London: HMSO; 2007.

35 Jones MJ. Decision analysis using spreadsheets. *Eur J Oper Res.* 1986; **26**; 385–400.

36 Tan K, Dear PRF, Newell SJ. Clinical decision support systems for neonatal care. *Cochrane Database Syst Rev.* 2005; **2**: CD004211.

37 Ramnarayan P, Tomlinson A, Rao A, *et al.* ISABEL: a web-based differential diagnosis aid for paediatrics: results from an initial performance evaluation. *Arch Dis Child.* 2003; **88**: 408–13.

38 Graber ML, Mathew A. Performance of a web-based clinical diagnosis support system for internists. *J Gen Intern Med.* 2008; **23**(Suppl. 1): 37–40.

Index